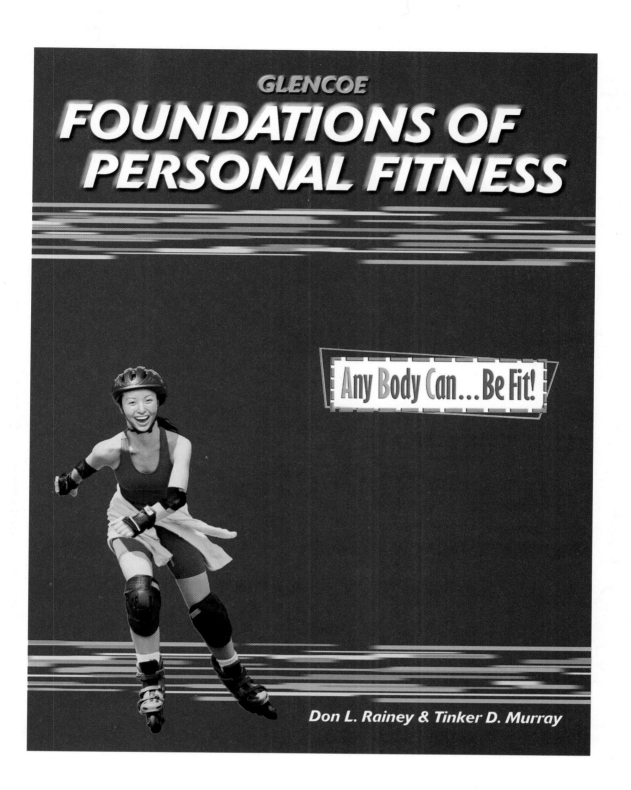

GLENCOE

FOUNDATIONS OF PERSONAL FITNESS

Any Body Can... Be Fit!

Don L. Rainey & Tinker D. Murray

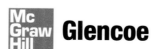 **Glencoe**

New York, New York   Columbus, Ohio   Chicago, Illinois   Peoria, Illinois   Woodland Hills, California

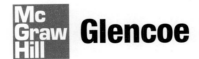

Glencoe

The *McGraw-Hill* Companies

Send all inquiries to:
Glencoe/McGraw-Hill
21600 Oxnard Street, Suite 500
Woodland Hills, California 91367

ISBN: 0-07-845127-2 (Student Edition)
ISBN: 0-07-845128-0 (Teacher Wraparound Edition)

Printed in the United States of America.

4 5 6 7 8 9 0   027   08 07 06 05

Don L. Rainey Don L. Rainey is a lecturer and director of the Physical Fitness and Wellness Program in the Health, Physical Education, and Recreation Department at Texas State University in San Marcos, Texas. He earned a Master of Science in Health and Physical Education at Lamar University. He was a founding member of the Texas Association for Health, Physical Education, Recreation and Dance (TAHPERD) Foundations of Personal Fitness Course Committee and taught the course at Marcus High School, where he coordinated health and physical education programs for 12 years. Don received the TAHPERD Honor Award in 1995. He has conducted over 100 workshops about the Foundations of Personal Fitness Course

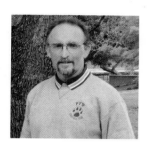

for educators. He was a subcommittee member for the Governor's Commission on Physical Fitness which developed the Fit Youth Today Program. He is also certified as a Strength and Conditioning Specialist by the National Strength and Conditioning Association (NSCA). Since 1989 he has worked with Tinker Murray to conduct and publish research in school physical education settings to promote physical activity in adolescents.

Tinker D. Murray Tinker D. Murray is a professor of Exercise and Sports Science in the Health, Physical Education, and Recreation Department at Texas State University. He earned his Ph.D. in Physical Education from Texas A&M University. He was a founding member of the Texas Association for Health, Physical Education, Recreation, and Dance (TAHPERD) Foundations of Personal Fitness Course Committee and has conducted over 60 workshops about the Foundations of Personal Fitness Course for educators. Tinker was given the TAHPERD Honor Award in 1995. He was a subcommittee member for the Governor's Commission on Physical Fitness, which developed the Fit Youth Today Program. He has been a

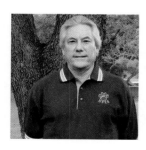

lecturer and examiner for the USA Track and Field Level II Coaching Certification Program since 1988. He is a fellow of the American College of Sports Medicine (ACSM) and certified as an ACSM program director. Since 1989, he has worked with Don Rainey to conduct and publish research in school physical education settings to promote physical activity in adolescents.

Physical Education Consultants

Kymm Ballard, M.S.
Physical Education Consultant
North Carolina Department of Public
    Instruction
Raleigh, North Carolina

Roberta L. Duyff, R.D., C.F.C.S.
Food and Nutrition Education Consultant
St. Louis, Missouri

D. Marian Franck, M.S., M.Ed.
Physical Education Teacher of the Year
National Association for Sport and
    Physical Education (NASPE)

Mark Giese, Ed.D.
Chair of the Health and Human
    Performance Department
Northeastern State University
Tahlequah, Oklahoma

Bonnie Mohnsen, M.A., Ph.D.
Physical Education Consultant
Cerritos, California

Scott Powers, Ph.D., Ed.D.
Professor and Director, Center for
    Exercise Science
University of Florida, Gainesville

Susannah Turney, M.S., C.A.P.E.
Adapted Physical Education Specialist
Irving Independent School District
Irving, Texas

Steven P. Van Camp, M.D.
Cardiologist, Alvarado Medical Group
Former President of American College of
    Sports Medicine
San Diego, California

Teacher Reviewers

Roy Alaniz, M.S.
Adjunct Professor, University of Texas
Curriculum Specialist
Brownsville Independent School District
Brownsville, Texas

Bill Bundy
Director of Athletics, Health, and Physical
    Education
Katy Independent School District
Katy, Texas

Nancy Duncan, M.A.
Physical Education Teacher
Fort Worth Independent School District
Fort Worth, Texas

Michael Rulon, M.A.
Health/Physical Education Teacher
Johnson Junior High School
Adjunct Faculty, Laramie County
    Community College
Cheyenne, Wyoming

Table of Contents

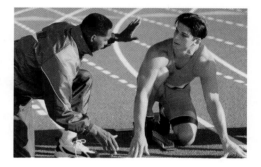

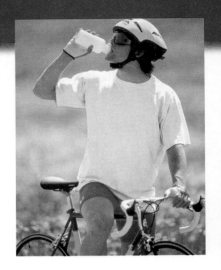
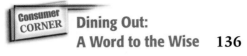

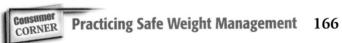

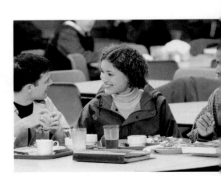

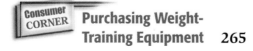

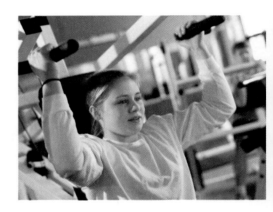

Fitness Check

Active Mind Active Body

Improving YOUR Personal Fitness
with your *Foundations of Personal Fitness* textbook

- Why should physical activity be part of your daily routine?
- How can you make the most of a personal fitness program?
- What are the benefits of having a high level of personal fitness?

Follow the guidelines and features below to make the most of your book.

What You Will Do ——————

Check the objectives to preview concepts covered in the lesson.

Terms to Know ——————

Find the terms listed at the beginning of each lesson.

Photos and Captions ——————

Study the photos and answer the caption questions as you learn more about each fitness topic.

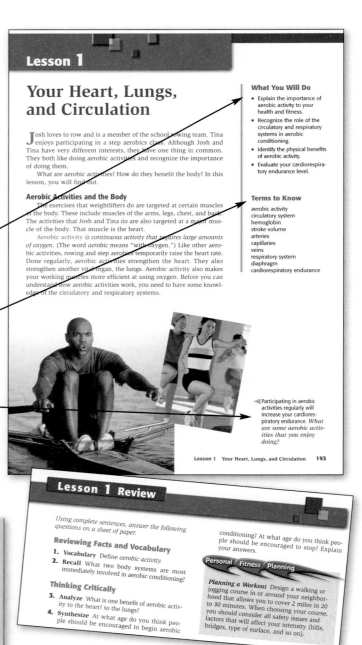

Lesson 1

Your Heart, Lungs, and Circulation

Josh loves to row and is a member of the school rowing team. Tina enjoys participating in a step aerobics class. Although Josh and Tina have very different interests, they have one thing in common. They both like doing aerobic activities and recognize the importance of doing them.

What are aerobic activities? How do they benefit the body? In this lesson, you will find out.

Aerobic Activities and the Body

The exercises that weightlifters do are targeted at certain muscles of the body. These include muscles of the arms, legs, chest, and back. The activities that Josh and Tina do are also targeted at a major muscle of the body. That muscle is the heart.

Aerobic activity *is continuous activity that requires large amounts of oxygen.* (The word *aerobic* means "with oxygen.") Like other aerobic activities, rowing and step aerobics temporarily raise the heart rate. Done regularly, aerobic activities strengthen the heart. They also strengthen another vital organ, the lungs. Aerobic activity also makes your working muscles more efficient at using oxygen. Before you can understand how aerobic activities work, you need to have some knowledge of the circulatory and respiratory systems.

What You Will Do

- Explain the importance of aerobic activity to your health and fitness.
- Recognize the role of the circulatory and respiratory systems in aerobic conditioning.
- Identify the physical benefits of aerobic activity.
- Evaluate your cardiorespiratory endurance level.

Terms to Know

aerobic activity
circulatory system
hemoglobin
stroke volume
arteries
capillaries
veins
respiratory system
diaphragm
cardiorespiratory endurance

◄ Participating in aerobic activities regularly will increase your cardiorespiratory endurance. *What are some aerobic activities that you enjoy doing?*

Lesson 1 Your Heart, Lungs, and Circulation **193**

Lesson 1 Review

Using complete sentences, answer the following questions on a sheet of paper.

Reviewing Facts and Vocabulary

1. **Vocabulary** Define *aerobic activity.*
2. **Recall** What two body systems are most immediately involved in aerobic conditioning?

Thinking Critically

3. **Analyze** What is one benefit of aerobic activity to the heart? to the lungs?
4. **Synthesize** At what age do you think people should be encouraged to begin aerobic

conditioning? At what age do you think people should be encouraged to stop? Explain your answers.

Personal Fitness Planning

Planning a Workout Design a walking or jogging course in or around your neighborhood that allows you to cover 2 miles in 20 to 30 minutes. When choosing your course, you should consider all safety issues and factors that will affect your intensity (hills, bridges, type of surface, and so on).

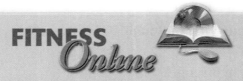

FITNESS *Online*

Stop...Think...Evaluate...Proceed...

Complete the **STEP Personal Inventory.** This will tell you more about your current level of personal fitness. Review what you have learned by completing **Online Vocabulary Activities** and by taking an **Online Quiz.** Design and implement your personal fitness program using the **Online Fitness Journal.**

Lesson Review

Complete the Lesson Review to check your understanding of the lesson concepts. Set your own fitness goals in the Personal Fitness Planning section of the review.

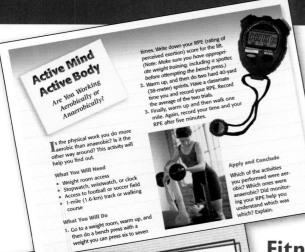

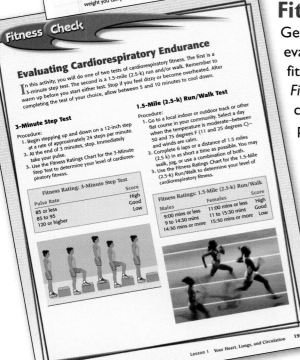

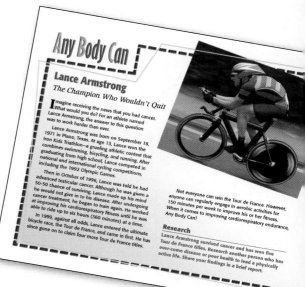

Active Mind—Active Body

Each *Active Mind—Active Body* feature provides an opportunity that lets you investigate an important concept for improving your fitness. Follow the steps under **What You Will Do** to get started, and summarize your experience in **Apply and Conclude.**

Fitness Check

Get up, get moving, and evaluate your physical fitness levels with the *Fitness Check* in each chapter. Follow the procedure for each activity and evaluate your performance by checking your Fitness Ratings.

Any Body Can

Watch for these special features, high-lighting well-known individuals whose accomplishments inspire others.

Consumer Corner

In these features, learn more about analyzing marketing claims and being a wise consumer.

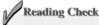

✓ Reading Check

Explain Explain in detail one of the benefits of maintaining a high level of cardiorespiratory fitness.

Reading Check

Stop and review what you have read by explaining key points.

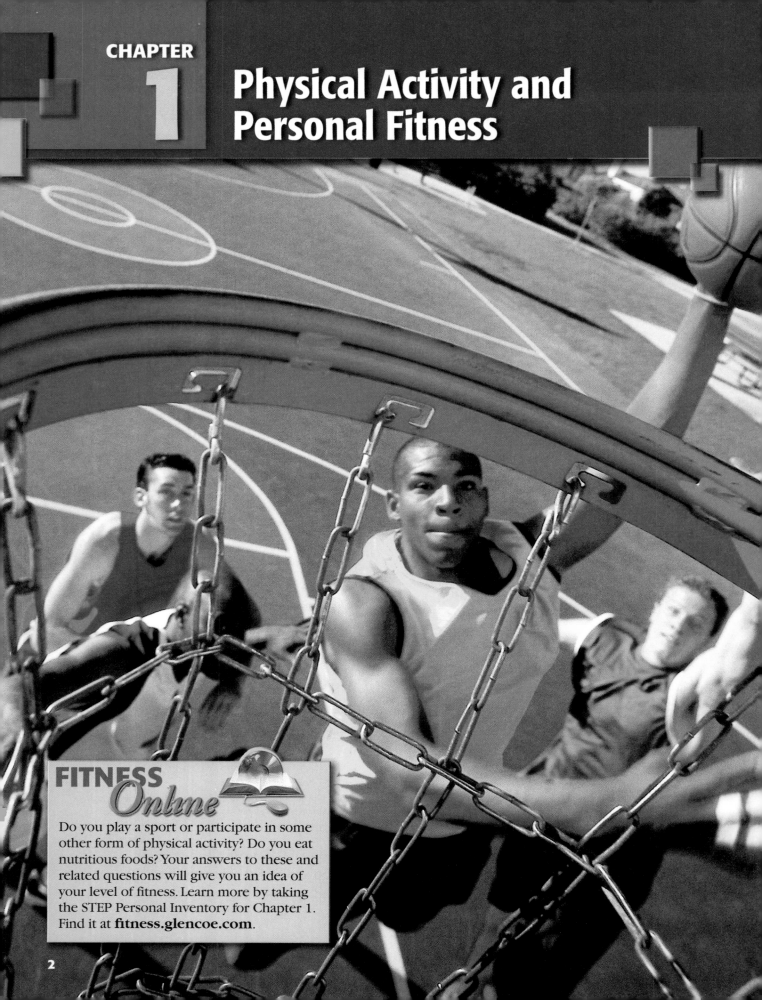

FITNESS
Online

Do you play a sport or participate in some other form of physical activity? Do you eat nutritious foods? Your answers to these and related questions will give you an idea of your level of fitness. Learn more by taking the STEP Personal Inventory for Chapter 1. Find it at **fitness.glencoe.com**.

Physical Activity, Exercise, and Health

Welcome to your course on the foundations of personal fitness! This course is different from other physical education courses you have taken. Previously, they may have consisted mainly of games and sports activities. In this course you will learn the **ABC**s of total, personal fitness: **A**ny **B**ody **C**an develop a plan to become and stay physically active for life.

Throughout this course, you will face a number of challenges concerning your personal fitness. These challenges include the following:

- Assessing your level of physical fitness and progress in the course
- Learning about changes in personal habits that you may need to make
- Taking responsibility for planning, developing, and maintaining a healthy and active lifestyle
- Designing a physical-activity and fitness program that can meet your individual needs throughout your life

As you can see, there is much work to do. Let's get started.

What You Will Do

- Define the importance of physical activity and personal fitness.
- Explain the relationship between health and fitness.
- Analyze the role of fitness in recognizing and resolving conflicts effectively.
- Describe methods of evaluating health-related fitness.
- Participate in activities to evaluate your health-related fitness.

Terms to Know

physical activity
exercise
physical fitness
personal fitness
health
wellness
functional health
sedentary
self-esteem
conflicts
functional fitness
skill-related fitness
health-related fitness

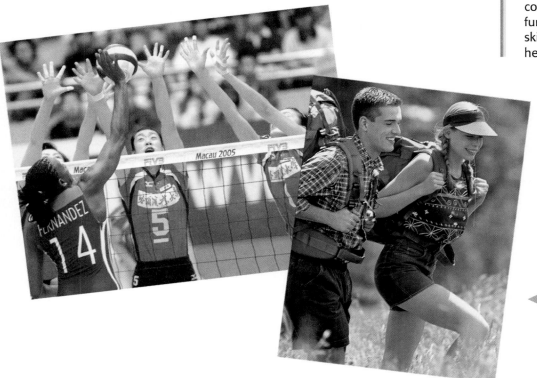

There is a variety of physical activities that can benefit your personal fitness. *What type of physical activities do you enjoy?*

What Is Physical Activity?

The human body is made up of many moving parts. Physical activity keeps those parts in working condition. **Physical activity** is *any movement that works the larger muscles of the body, such as arm, leg, and back muscles.* Physical activity can take several forms.

- It may be recreational, as in the case of sports, dancing, swimming, and other leisure-time activities.
- It may be incidental to some other activity, such as doing household chores, working at a part-time job, or volunteering for a neighborhood cleanup program.

Exercise is *physical activity that is planned, structured, and repetitive, and that results in improvements in fitness.* Throughout this book, you will learn about exercises that work different areas of the body, including internal organs such as the heart and lungs.

Physical activity and exercise are important to your health. Physically active people live longer, healthier lives. Physical activity and exercise add more than just years to your life; they add life to your years by making you look and feel better.

Why Are Physical Activity and Exercise Important?

Regular physical activity and exercise help keep your body physically fit. **Physical fitness** is *the body's ability to carry out daily tasks and still have enough reserve energy to respond to unexpected demands.*

Exercise is not the only way to improve physical fitness. Many forms of physical activity can provide fitness benefits. Participating in sports or action-oriented, leisure-time activities, such as dancing or ice-skating, are effective—and enjoyable—ways of staying fit. The diagram in **Figure 1.1** shows a variety of activities arranged in terms of energy level and time. Which of these activities do you enjoy doing?

Personal Fitness

Regular physical activity is central to physical fitness but, by itself, does not make a person totally fit. To achieve *total* or **personal fitness,** you should try to

- maintain acceptable levels of physical fitness.
- participate in regular physical activity.
- eat nutritious foods.
- sleep 8 to 9 hours each night.
- have regular medical checkups.
- maintain an appropriate weight.
- avoid harmful substances, such as tobacco, alcohol, and other drugs.

Physical fitness is not the same thing as personal fitness. It is only one component. Think about an all-around athlete who lives almost

FIGURE 1.1

PHYSICAL ACTIVITIES ARRANGED BY ENERGY LEVEL AND TIME

The activities at the top of the arrow take more time but are less vigorous. Those at the bottom take less time but are more vigorous. *Which type of activities could a person do daily? Which might be done weekly?*

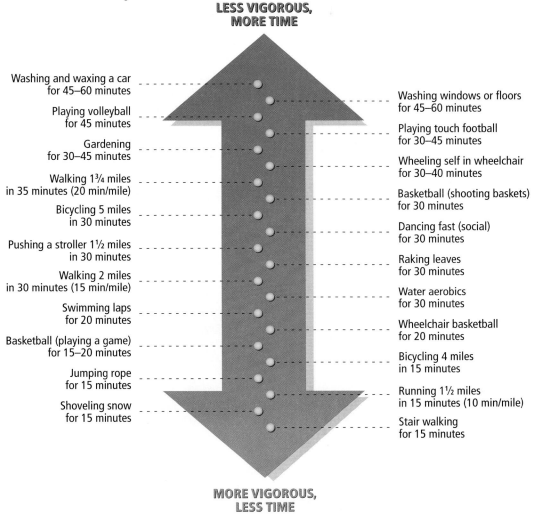

LESS VIGOROUS, MORE TIME

Washing and waxing a car for 45–60 minutes

Playing volleyball for 45 minutes

Gardening for 30–45 minutes

Walking 1¾ miles in 35 minutes (20 min/mile)

Bicycling 5 miles in 30 minutes

Pushing a stroller 1½ miles in 30 minutes

Walking 2 miles in 30 minutes (15 min/mile)

Swimming laps for 20 minutes

Basketball (playing a game) for 15–20 minutes

Jumping rope for 15 minutes

Shoveling snow for 15 minutes

Washing windows or floors for 45–60 minutes

Playing touch football for 30–45 minutes

Wheeling self in wheelchair for 30–40 minutes

Basketball (shooting baskets) for 30 minutes

Dancing fast (social) for 30 minutes

Raking leaves for 30 minutes

Water aerobics for 30 minutes

Wheelchair basketball for 20 minutes

Bicycling 4 miles in 15 minutes

Running 1½ miles in 15 minutes (10 min/mile)

Stair walking for 15 minutes

MORE VIGOROUS, LESS TIME

Source: U.S. Department of Health and Human Services, Centers for Disease Control and Prevention, 2003.[1]

entirely on high-fat food. Imagine a teen who loves aerobic dance but abuses harmful substances. Has either of these teens achieved total, personal fitness?

✔ Reading Check

Analyze Is it possible to be physically active without exercise? Explain.

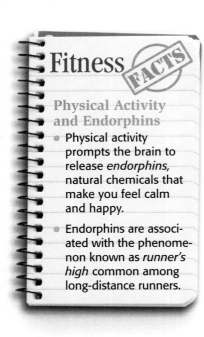
Fitness, Health, and Wellness

Fitness is an important part of maintaining your health—and health means much more than the absence of physical illness. Health is defined as *a combination of physical, mental/emotional, and social well-being.* The term wellness refers to *total health in all three areas.* Personal fitness is essential to maintaining your overall health.

Fitness and The Health Triangle

Health and wellness are sometimes represented by a triangle (see **Figure 1.2**). Personal fitness is essential to all three sides of the triangle. High levels of personal fitness promote *all* aspects of health.

Physical Health. People with high levels of personal fitness experience many benefits to their physical health. These physical benefits include

- a higher energy level.
- improved strength, flexibility, and muscle tone.

FIGURE 1.2

THE HEALTH TRIANGLE
Notice that all sides of the triangle are equal. *Is your health triangle well-balanced?*

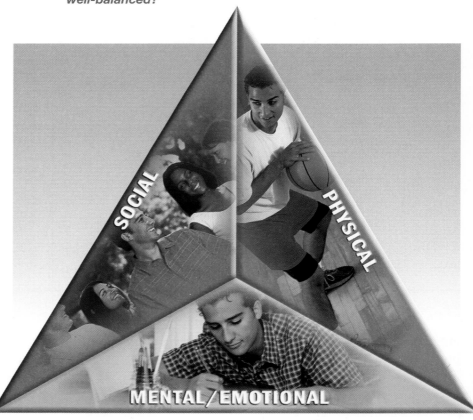

- better heart and lung function.
- stronger bones.
- healthier weight and reduced body fat.
- improved coordination.
- more restful sleep.

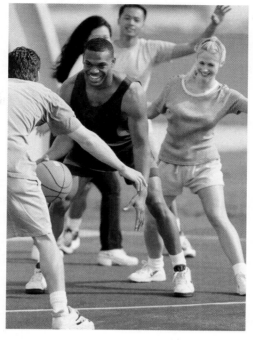

These teens are engaging in behaviors that benefit their health. *Which sides of the health triangle are they focusing on?*

Another aspect of physical health is functional health, *the ability to maintain high levels of health and wellness by reducing your risks of developing health problems.* Physical activity is one way to maintain your functional health. Physically active people have a lower risk for physical problems that are related to a sedentary (SED-uhn-tayr-ee), or *physically inactive,* lifestyle. These problems include

- **heart disease.**
- high blood pressure.
- stroke.
- diabetes.
- certain forms of cancer, including colon cancer.

Mental/Emotional Health. The benefits of personal fitness go beyond physical health. Fitness also improves mental/emotional health. People who are personally fit are typically able to

- think more clearly and concentrate on work or school.
- better handle the stress and challenges of everyday life.
- experience higher self-esteem, or *feelings of self-confidence and personal worth.*

Social Health. Achieving personal fitness, whether it is playing on a team or working out with a partner, will also benefit your social health. Personally fit individuals are better able to

- develop and maintain friendships.
- work well as part of a group.
- effectively recognize and resolve conflicts. Conflicts are *struggles or disagreements.* Playing a sport especially teaches individuals how to resolve disagreements without resorting to name-calling or fighting.

Reading Check

Summarize What is the relationship between health and fitness?

heart disease
For more on heart disease and its prevention through physical activity, see Chapter 7, page **200.**

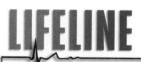

Dealing with Conflicts
Volleyball, basketball, and other competitive sports are a great way to stay in shape and improve social health at the same time. When you play a game as part of a team, you also get a chance to socialize and build social skills.

Just remember that it is a game. When tempers flare, everyone loses. Should this happen, keep your cool. Talk it out, take a break, or do both. Encourage others to do the same.

Methods for Evaluating Health-Related Fitness

In this activity, you will participate in a variety of activities that develop health-related fitness. You will learn more about health-related fitness in Chapter 3. Before you start, be sure to warm up.

Cardiovascular Fitness: Jumping Jacks

Procedure:
1. Begin with your feet together and arms spread as in **Figure 1.3a.**
2. Jump, spreading your arms and legs as in **Figure 1.3b.**
3. Bring your arms together, hands touching, directly over your head, as in **Figure 1.3c,** then return to the starting position.
4. Repeat these movements for a total of thirty seconds. Once you stop, rest for an additional thirty seconds.
5. Take your pulse, as instructed by your teacher.
6. Use the Fitness Ratings Chart for Jumping Jacks to assess your performance.

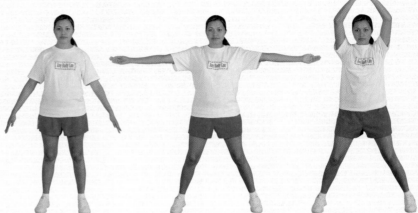

Figure 1.3a   **Figure 1.3b**   **Figure 1.3c**

Fitness Ratings: Jumping Jacks	
Beats per 30 seconds	**Rating**
Under 60 beats	Pass
Over 60 beats	Needs work

Body Composition: Finger Pinch Test

Procedure:
1. Sit in a chair and place both feet flat on the floor.
2. Place the end of your little finger on your kneecap.
3. Spread your fingers. Extend the thumb as far up your thigh as possible.

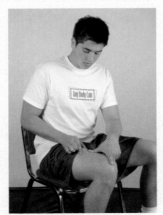

Figure 1.4

4. With your other hand, pinch a fold of skin at the end of your thumb as in **Figure 1.4.**
5. Use the Fitness Ratings Chart for the Finger Pinch Test to assess your current body composition. (NOTE: *Body composition* is the ratio of body fat to lean body tissues, such as muscle and bone.)

Fitness Ratings: Finger Pinch Test	
Skin Pinch Width	**Rating**
Narrower than thumb	Pass
Wider than thumb	Needs work

Flexibility: Zipper Stretch

Procedure:

1. Raise your right arm, bending your elbow. Reach down behind your back as far as possible.
2. At the same time, bend your left elbow and reach around your back as in **Figure 1.5.** Try to clasp your right hand. Your goal is to touch or overlap your right hand.
3. Switch arms and repeat the test. You may find that you do better on one side than the other. This is common because many individuals are more flexible on one side than the other.
4. Use the Fitness Ratings Chart for Zipper Stretch to assess your performance.

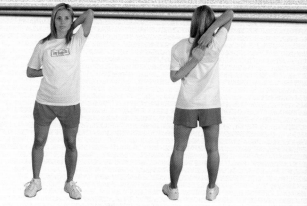

Figure 1.5

Fitness Ratings: Zipper Stretch

Ability to Touch	Rating
Touch or overlap	Pass
Inability to touch	Needs work

Muscular Strength: Push-ups

Procedure:

1. Extend your elbows and push your body up to a fully extended arm position, as in **Figure 1.6.** Keep your back straight at all times.

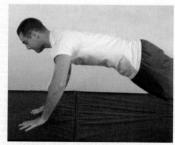

Figure 1.6

2. Gradually lower your body to the point where your chest just about touches the ground.
3. Repeat this motion as many times as you can.
4. Use the Fitness Ratings Chart for Push-ups to assess your performance.

Fitness Ratings: Push-ups

Number of Push-ups		Rating
Males:	5 or more	Pass
	Less than 5	Needs work
Females:	3 or more	Pass
	Less than 3	Needs work

Muscular Endurance: Wall Sit

Procedure:

1. Find a wall that you can lean back against comfortably and safely.
2. Stand 1 to 1½ feet from the wall. Place your feet shoulder width apart.
3. Lean back against the wall so that your back is straight and your shoulder blades touch the wall.

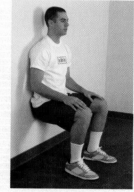

Figure 1.7

4. Squat down until your knees are at a 90-degree angle. (See **Figure 1.7.**) Try to hold this position for fifteen seconds.
5. Use the Fitness Ratings Chart for Wall Sit to assess your performance.

Fitness Ratings: Wall Sit

Time	Rating
15 seconds or more	Pass
Less than 15 seconds	Needs work

Functional Fitness

Maintaining high levels of health and fitness yields an additional benefit: functional fitness. This is *a person's physical ability to function independently in life, without assistance.* Functionally fit individuals maintain high levels of health and wellness and a reduced risk of chronic problems.

Like health itself, functional fitness may be thought of as a triangle. **Figure 1.8** shows the Physical Activity Pyramid. The base of the pyramid lists physical activities that should be done daily. The second level lists goals for physical activities and exercises that should be done three to five times a week. The third level lists activities and exercises that should be done two to three times per week. The top level of the triangle highlights physical inactivity, which should occur infrequently.

FIGURE 1.8

THE PHYSICAL ACTIVITY PYRAMID

This pyramid provides guidelines for how to divide your time when doing various types of physical activity. *What physical activities do you do daily?*

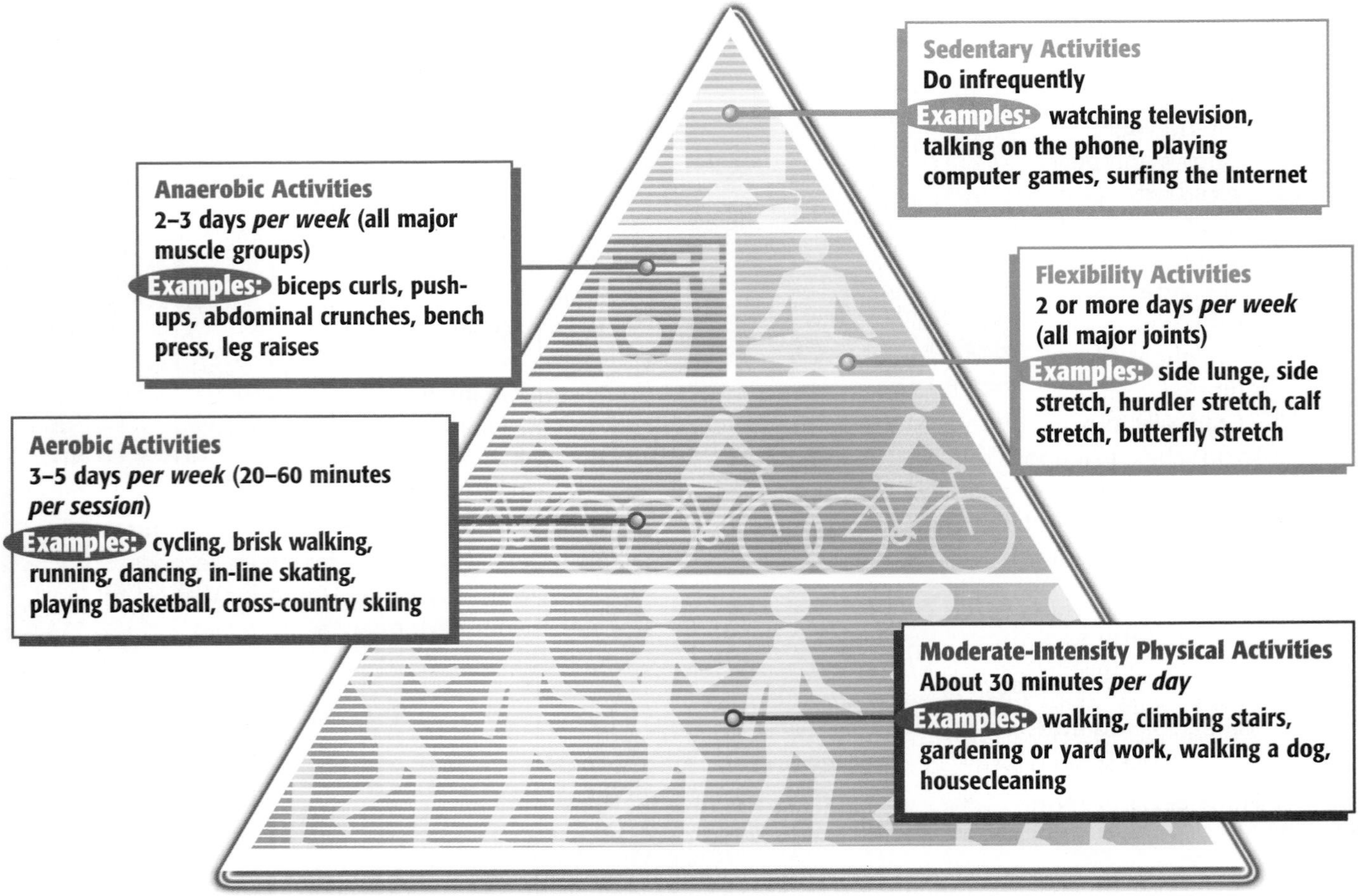

Sedentary Activities
Do infrequently
Examples: watching television, talking on the phone, playing computer games, surfing the Internet

Anaerobic Activities
2–3 days *per week* (all major muscle groups)
Examples: biceps curls, push-ups, abdominal crunches, bench press, leg raises

Flexibility Activities
2 or more days *per week* (all major joints)
Examples: side lunge, side stretch, hurdler stretch, calf stretch, butterfly stretch

Aerobic Activities
3–5 days *per week* (20–60 minutes *per session*)
Examples: cycling, brisk walking, running, dancing, in-line skating, playing basketball, cross-country skiing

Moderate-Intensity Physical Activities
About 30 minutes *per day*
Examples: walking, climbing stairs, gardening or yard work, walking a dog, housecleaning

Healthy People 2010 and Fitness

The United States government has launched *Healthy People 2010*, an initiative designed to encourage all Americans to make health and fitness a top priority. The goal, to be achieved by the year 2010, is for all Americans to reach and sustain high levels of fitness in one or both of the following:

- **Skill-related fitness.** This is *your ability to perform successfully in various games and sports.* It is also known as *performance fitness.* There are six components, or measures, of **skill-related fitness:** *agility, balance, power, speed, coordination, and reaction time.*
- **Health-related fitness.** This is *your ability to become and stay physically healthy.* There are five components of **health-related fitness:** *cardiovascular fitness, body composition, muscular strength, muscular endurance, and flexibility.*

Improving your health-related fitness will be the focus of many of the remaining chapters of this book. Each chapter will contain a "Fitness Check" that will allow you to assess your fitness level.

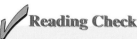 **Reading Check**

List What are the components of skill-related fitness? of health related-fitness?

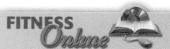
Go to **fitness.glencoe.com** for information about the President's Challenge for Physical fitness.

Activity Using the information provided at this site, create a plan for your school to become an Active Lifestyle Model School.

For more on **skill-** and **health-related fitness,** see Chapter 3, pages **72–76.**

Lesson 1 Review

Using complete sentences, answer the following questions on a sheet of paper.

Reviewing Facts and Vocabulary

1. **Vocabulary** What is *physical activity?* What is *physical fitness?*

2. **Recall** What is the relationship between *physical fitness* and *health?*

Thinking Critically

3. **Analyze** Explain how participating in physical activity with others can help you develop skills to recognize and resolve conflicts.

4. **Synthesize** Explain why it might be possible to say that someone who does not exercise could still be physically active. Explain why it might be possible for someone to be physically active without having personal fitness.

5. **Describe** Carlos is preparing to start a fitness program. Before he begins, he is eager to evaluate how he rates in all areas of his health-related fitness. Briefly describe methods he can use to evaluate his health-related fitness in all five areas.

Personal Fitness Planning

Evaluating Physical-activity Level Make a log and record the physical activities and exercises you do for one week. Based on your log, determine whether you are currently very active, moderately active, or inactive. Write down ways you could adjust your weekly schedule to become more active than you currently are.

What You Will Do

- Identify changeable risk factors that affect your levels of health and personal fitness.
- Describe lifestyle choices that can improve overall levels of fitness and offset negative factors.
- Define *stress* and describe activities that you can use for stress reduction.
- Identify risk factors for developing heart disease.

Terms to Know

risk factors
heredity
stress

Risk Factors and Your Behavior

The average life expectancy in the United States is about seventy-seven years. More and more people, however, are living into their hundreds. Your life expectancy and the quality of those years will be influenced by how well you maintain your functional health and fitness.

Personal Fitness and Risk Factors

Achieving and maintaining a high level of functional health and fitness is often made more difficult by risk factors, or *conditions and behaviors that represent a potential threat to an individual's well-being.* Where personal fitness is concerned, these are factors that put you at risk for certain diseases, including heart disease, lung disease, and bone disease. **Figure 1.9** shows several of these diseases and lists the risk factors for each.

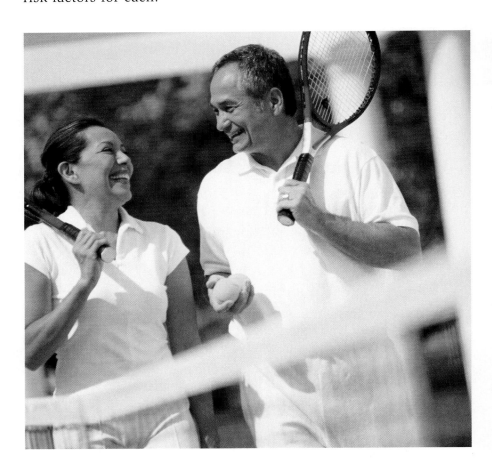

▶ Physical activity and exercise are ways to lower your risk of developing health problems as you age. *What other measures can you take?*

FIGURE 1.9

DISEASES AND RISK FACTORS

Heredity and a sedentary lifestyle, in combination with other risk factors, increase the risk for developing all of these diseases. *Which risk factors are changeable?*

Disease	Contributing Risk Factors	Disease	Contributing Risk Factors
High Blood Pressure	• Heredity • Overweight • Sedentary lifestyle • Unhealthful eating plan	Heart Disease	• Diabetes • Heredity • High blood pressure • Overweight • Sedentary lifestyle • Smoking • Stress • Unhealthful eating plan
Colon Cancer	• Heredity • Sedentary lifestyle • Unhealthful eating plan		
Diabetes	• Heredity • Overweight • Sedentary lifestyle • Unhealthful eating plan	Stroke	• Heredity • High blood pressure • Overweight • Sedentary lifestyle • Unhealthful eating plan
Osteoporosis	• Heredity • Sedentary lifestyle • Unhealthful eating plan		

Risk Factors You Can't Modify

Some risk factors are largely beyond your control. However, it is important to be aware of how they affect you and how you can counteract their influence on your health and fitness.

Age

As we age, our chances of developing diseases such as heart disease, high blood pressure, and cancer increases. Although you cannot change your age, learning about and developing healthful habits now can make a positive difference in your levels of personal fitness throughout your life.

Heredity

To a degree, your personal fitness potential was determined before you were born. You are a product of heredity—*the sum of the physical and mental traits that you inherit from your parents.* Included are such features as eye color, hair color, and height.

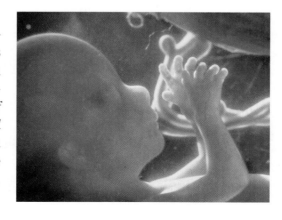

Traits such as speed and power are determined before you are born. *What other traits are predetermined by heredity?*

Active Mind Active Body

Identifying Risk Factors for Heart Disease

A first step toward reversing the effects of harmful risk factors in your life is identifying them. In this activity, you will assess the factors in your life that put you at risk for developing heart disease.

What You Will Need

- Pen or pencil
- Paper

What You Will Do

Copy the chart that follows onto a separate sheet of paper. Review each of the risk factors. Place a check mark in the *Yes* column of those that apply to you personally. (For some factors, you may need to consult an adult family member.) If you check *yes,* mark whether this is a risk factor you can modify.

Apply and Conclude

In which of these areas did you find potential risk factors in your life? What are some of the specific risks facing you? Which of these can you change for the better? In your private fitness journal, write an explanation about how you can go about making necessary changes.

	Yes	Can Modify	Cannot Modify
1. Heredity			
2. Gender			
3. Sedentary lifestyle			
4. Smoking			
5. Food choices			
6. Excessive stress			
7. Obesity			
8. Diabetes			

hotlink

heredity
For more on heredity and its role in fitness, see Chapter 7, page **208.**

As a risk factor, **heredity** determines your likelihood of developing certain diseases and disorders. These include high blood pressure, heart disease, diabetes, and certain types of cancers. Like your age, your genetic makeup cannot be changed, but the risks it may pose can be reduced by maintaining a healthy lifestyle.

Gender. One aspect of heredity that can have far-reaching implications to personal fitness is gender. Natural differences between males and females exist. For example, females possess about 38 percent of the upper-body strength and 45 percent of the lower-body strength of males. It is also a fact that males are at higher risk for heart disease than are women.

 Reading Check

Explain What is the relationship between heredity and your health?

Changeable Risk Factors

Although you cannot control risk factors such as heredity or age, you *can* lessen their impact on your health and fitness. You can reduce or eliminate some of your risks, because they stem from something you can control—your behavior.

Becoming Physically Active

One changeable risk factor for developing health problems is physical inactivity. Research has shown that adults who are sedentary develop chronic diseases at a much higher rate than do more active individuals. Choosing a physically active lifestyle is one way to reduce your risks of developing disease and to live a longer, healthier life. It is essential to maintaining your future functional health and fitness.

Practicing Healthful Eating Habits

How much food you eat—and the types of food—are considerations that greatly impact your health and fitness. For example, limiting the amount of fat intake, sodium intake, and cholesterol intake in the foods you eat can reduce your risk of developing certain diseases, including heart disease. Maintaining a healthy body weight and making nutritious, balanced food choices will also reduce your risk of becoming overweight or obese. **Obesity** is a major risk factor for developing **type 2 diabetes.** You will learn more about the connections between nutrition, body composition, and disease in later chapters.

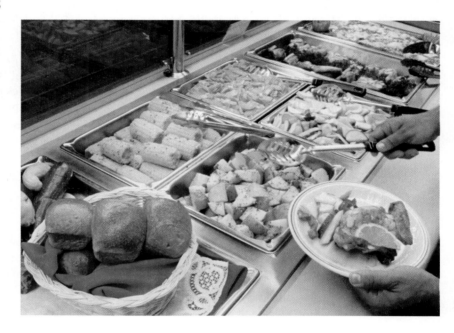

▼ Knowing what to eat can make a difference in your health and fitness. *Do you know which foods to eat in moderation?*

Avoiding Smoking and the Use of Tobacco Products

One of the most important steps you can take to promote your health is to make a decision not to smoke or use tobacco products. Studies have shown that people who smoke for ten years or more are at far greater risk of heart and lung disease than are nonsmokers. People using smokeless tobacco, such as chewing tobacco and other products, face similar risks. These include cancer of the throat. You will learn more about harmful substances and how to avoid them in Chapter 2.

Reading Check

Explain Identify two diseases that are affected by your eating plan.

hot link

obesity
For more on obesity, see Chapter 5, page **150.**

type 2 diabetes
For more on type 2 diabetes, see Chapter 6, page **173.**

Any Body Can

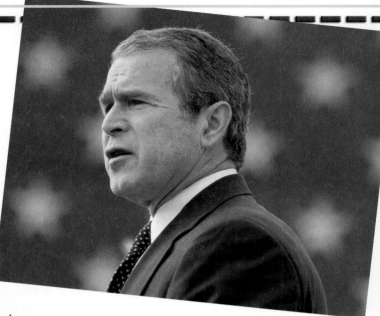

George W. Bush
The Fitness Challenge

The presidency of the United States is a job with tremendous responsibilities. You would think that with all a president has to do, the last thing on the commander in chief's mind would be personal fitness. However, George W. Bush, the forty-third president of the United States, makes time in his demanding schedule to keep fit.

George W. Bush was born on July 6, 1946, in New Haven, Connecticut. He graduated from Yale in 1968 and earned a business degree from Harvard in 1972. Bush was elected governor of Texas in 1994 and again in 1998. His leadership of this huge state paved the way for his presidency.

President Bush's life has been a model for a physically active lifestyle. In addition to participating in sports, he regularly jogs several miles and lifts weights two to three times per week. On June 20, 2002, he challenged all Americans to get healthier by becoming more physically active; by getting preventive health screenings; by choosing nutritious foods; and by avoiding alcohol, tobacco, and other drugs.

On June 22, 2002, President Bush, at age 55, set an example for all Americans by participating in a fitness challenge at Ft. McNair in Washington, D.C., where he ran 3.1 miles in under 21 minutes. That is less than 7 minutes per mile.

Not everyone can be the president. However, Any Body Can try to follow President Bush's physical activity goals.

Presentation

Working in groups, create a television commercial that promotes the four challenges George Bush has given to the American people to become healthier. Your commercial should be designed especially for a teen audience and should include visual aids and/or demonstrations, if possible.

Managing Stress in Your Life

You are probably all too aware of stress in your daily life. Stress is *the mind and body's response to the demands and threats of everyday life.* Stress is perfectly normal. Everyone experiences stressful moments. You may not be aware, however, that too much stress can take a toll on your health. It can lead to sleeplessness, depression, and other health problems.

Fortunately, there are strategies for coping positively with stress. These include the following recommendations:

- **Adjust your eating habits.** In particular, limit your intake of caffeine. This is a stimulant drug found in chocolate, soft drinks, some sports drinks, and coffee.

- **Spend some time alone.** Taking a break and allowing yourself time to unwind can improve your mood and reduce your feelings of worry or stress. Spend time reading a favorite magazine or listening to soothing music. Writing about the concerns in your life can also be an effective way of managing stress.
- **Maintain a high level of physical activity.** Physical activity, whether it's playing a sport or working out alone is a positive outlet for stress. It allows you a way to redirect your energies and escape from stressful thoughts. Any type of exercise or physical activity can be an outlet for stress, including: weight lifting, jogging, dancing, and household chores, such as washing the car or cleaning your room.

Dealing with stress in a positive way is a challenge that will arise periodically throughout your life. It is important to redirect your energy, keep a positive outlook, and seek out support, if necessary. To help you understand and handle stress, the chapters to come will present coping strategies geared to the specific chapter topic. You will find these under the heading "Stress Break" in the margins.

 Reading Check

Identify What are the negative effects of stress?

Lesson 2 Review

Using complete sentences, answer the following questions on a sheet of paper.

Reviewing Facts and Vocabulary

1. **Vocabulary** What are *risk factors*?
2. **Vocabulary** What is *stress*?
3. **Recall** Name three changeable risk factors that can impact your functional health.

Thinking Critically

4. **Analyze** Todd has a family history of heart disease on both sides of his family. Because he is male, his risk of developing heart disease is higher than if he were female. Todd believes there is no point in worrying about this as a teen because, as he ages, he will develop heart disease, no matter what. What advice would you give Todd?

5. **Extend** Many people have their own ways of coping with stress, such as listening to music, speaking with a close friend, or doing something physically active. List physical activities that you have used in the past or could use in the future to reduce stress in your life. Share your list with your classmates.

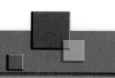

Personal Fitness Planning

Researching Risks Visit **fitness.glencoe.com** to learn more about the specific health risk factors for developing type 2 diabetes. Evaluate the health risk factors of a close relative of yours and determine if that person is at low, medium, or high risk for type 2 diabetes.

Developing a Positive Fitness Attitude

What You Will Do

- Investigate positive and negative attitudes toward personal fitness.
- Evaluate the role of peer influence in the decisions you make.
- Evaluate consumer issues, including marketing claims in the media, in your attitude toward fitness.
- Identify the benefits of adhering to a commitment to personal fitness.

Terms to Know

attitude
peers
media
commitment
adherence
self-concept

The secretary of the U.S. Department of Health and Human Services has called physical activity "a passport to good health for all Americans." Similar endorsements have been made for other lifestyle behaviors that promote wellness. However, current government statistics reveal that about a third of all teens nationwide are sedentary. Not surprisingly, the same percentage of American youth is overweight.

Your Attitudes

Although people might be aware of the importance of personal fitness, some find it difficult to develop and maintain a personally fit lifestyle for themselves.

One reason for this is attitude. Attitude is *your mindset or outlook toward a given topic or subject.* Your attitudes, especially during adolescence, play a major role in the decisions you make.

Your personal beliefs shape your attitudes about physical activity. Your beliefs about physical activity will change as you age and your

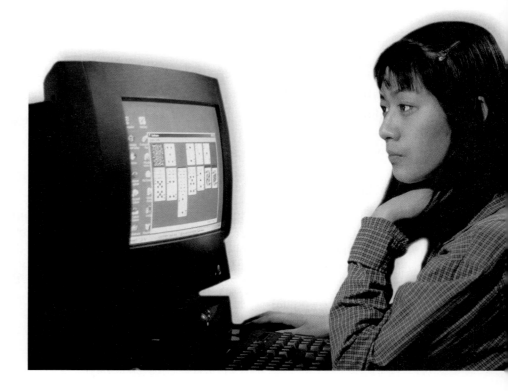

▶ Your attitudes and choices about how you spend your free time will affect your health and fitness levels. *Do you make physical activity and exercise part of your daily routine?*

knowledge about physical activity increases. The following are some common attitudes toward the subject of personal fitness. How many of these are familiar to you? How many have you expressed yourself?

- Exercise is boring.
- I'll start watching what I eat when I get to be an adult.
- I'm too busy for sports right now.
- I don't have time for breakfast in the morning.
- Exercise doesn't work.
- Sleep is for babies.
- I don't want to hurt myself.
- Physical activity is strictly for "athletes."
- I'm too tired to exercise today; I'll start tomorrow.
- I only need about 4 hours of sleep a night to function fully the next day.
- There has to be an easier way to get in shape!

In the "Active Mind—Active Body" activity on page **21**, you'll explore other attitudes that affect personal fitness.

Peer Influence

Where do negative attitudes like these come from? One source may be your peers. Peers are *people the same age who share a common range of interests and beliefs.* As a teen, your peers include your friends, classmates, and other students you see at school and around the community. Peer influence is the effect these individuals' words and actions have on your attitudes and behaviors. As shown in **Figure 1.10,** this influence can be either direct or indirect, positive or negative.

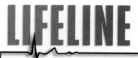

Positive Peer Influence

You may know other teens that have a negative attitude about behaviors and habits that promote good health. They might even encourage you to engage in behaviors that harm your health.

Remember, just as your peers influence you, you also influence them.

Think about the kind of friend you are and your attitudes. Know that a positive outlook will not only benefit you, but it has the power to positively influence others.

FIGURE 1.10

EXAMPLES OF PEER INFLUENCE

Peer influence can be positive or negative. *Can you think of another example of each type of peer influence?*

	Positive	Negative
Direct	Volunteering time at a nursing home based on encouragement from a friend who thinks you would be great at it	Accepting a dare to do something physically dangerous
Indirect	Developing good study habits because you see your friends studying hard	Adopting an unhealthful habit, such as smoking, because other people are doing it

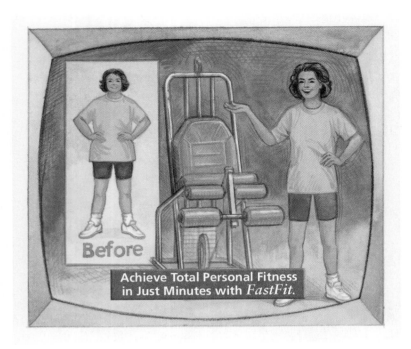

Achieve Total Personal Fitness in Just Minutes with *FastFit*.
Before

▶ Ads for some products suggest that achieving fitness should be fast and easy. *How can such messages contribute to a negative attitude about fitness?*

The Media

Another source that may promote negative attitudes about physical activity is the media. The term **media** is used to denote *the collective forms of mass communication found within society at any given time.* The media today include TV, radio, the movies, books, newspapers, magazines, music, and the Internet. Advertisements found on these sources are also examples of media.

Although these media can provide positive messages, many foster negative attitudes and inaccurate information. Take for example an advertisement for a belt that claims to tone the abdominal muscles without any kind of workout, or another for a pill that promises to burn fat. Ads like these reinforce the attitudes that exercise is too difficult and that there must be an easy shortcut to fitness.

✓ **Reading Check**

Explain How can an advertisement that is selling a fitness product lead to a negative attitude about fitness?

A Commitment to Change

As a teen, you may not feel the necessity of developing your personal fitness. The health risks of sedentary living may seem years away. You may be telling yourself that there will be plenty of time to "turn things around."

The truth, however, is that your adult years are just around the corner. There is no time like the present to make a commitment to personal fitness. A **commitment** is *a pledge or promise.* By making a commitment to fitness, you are making a promise to develop and maintain positive fitness behaviors.

Begin by examining your attitudes toward each of the lifestyle factors that promote fitness. The self-inventory in the "Active Mind—Active Body" activity on page **21** will help you explore some of your attitudes. Be honest with yourself and take your answers seriously. If your attitudes are negative, make the commitment to work at changing them. If your attitudes are positive, you have already taken a step in the right direction.

In the next lesson, you will learn how to put your positive thoughts and attitudes into action. You will learn how to launch and maintain a program that will keep you fit for life.

Adherence

Adherence refers to *the ability to stick to a plan of action.* If you adhere to a fitness program, you will succeed. Sometimes, people who start personal fitness programs fail to adhere to them. Many of the reasons for this were explained earlier in this lesson. By developing an awareness of negative attitudes, you can increase your chances for succeeding in a fitness program. Remember, to be a healthy individual, it is your responsibility to develop your personal fitness.

 Reading Check

Compare What is the difference between commitment and adherence?

Active Mind Active Body

Investigating Attitudes about Personal Fitness

Evaluating your attitudes is the first step toward changing those that are negative. This activity will help you do that.

What You Will Need

- Pen or pencil
- Paper

What You Will Do

The 20 statements that follow are designed to evaluate your current attitudes about fitness-related lifestyle factors. Copy the statements onto a separate sheet of paper. After each statement, write a number from 1 through 5, where 5 means "strongly agree" and 1 means "strongly disagree." Be as truthful as you can. There will be no grade assigned to this activity.

Apply and Conclude

Did you respond honestly to every statement? Which positive attitudes do you currently have toward your fitness? What areas, if any, do you need to improve?

1. I don't have time to exercise.
2. I eat breakfast every day.
3. I am not very athletic.
4. I seldom weigh myself.
5. I have always enjoyed participating in physical activities and exercise.
6. I enjoy physical education classes.
7. I have a moderate-to-high level of health and physical fitness.
8. I get 8 to 9 hours of sleep every night.
9. I take the stairs instead of the elevator or escalator whenever possible.
10. I like team games and sports.
11. I like to lift weights.
12. I enjoy eating healthful snacks.
13. I like to engage in physical activities with friends.
14. Exercising twice a week is all I need to do to stay in shape.
15. I prefer to ride rather than walk, even to go short distances.
16. Learning about personal fitness will be valuable to me later in life.
17. I find physical education classes boring.
18. I eat three balanced meals every day.
19. I have trouble sleeping.
20. I spend more than 25 hours a week watching TV.

Fitness and Your Social Health

Remember that physical fitness is essential to all sides of the health triangle. When you are personally healthy and fit, you have a positive self-image that allows you to work well with others. Describe one example when a person who has a high level of personal health can be helpful in recognizing a conflict in a team sport before it develops into a major conflict.

Benefits of Personal Fitness

During your teen years, you will experience periods of growth and many physical changes. As discussed in Lesson 1, regular physical activity or exercise, combined with a sound nutrition plan, will provide many benefits to your physical health as you grow and change. In the remaining sections of this lesson, you will take a closer look at some other benefits related to mental/emotional health, as well as your overall functional fitness throughout life.

Enhancement of Self-Esteem

Most people agree that self-esteem is a powerful force within each individual. It enables people to cope better with the basic challenges of life. Healthy, fit people are more likely to experience feelings of happiness and higher self-esteem. They also have a more positive **self-concept.** This is *the view you have of yourself.* Simply put, people who are fit, healthy, and feel good about their health and physical appearance are more likely to live an enjoyable, productive life. **Figure 1.11** shows some of the more important factors affecting your self-esteem and your physical self-concept.

FIGURE 1.11

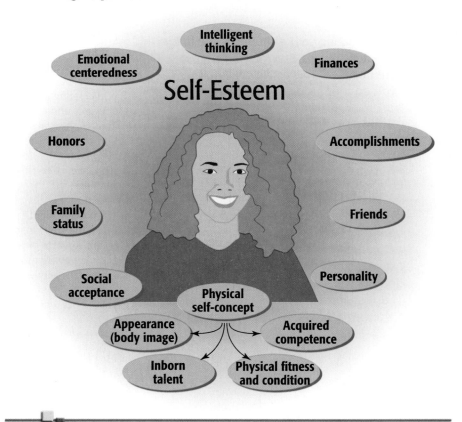

FACTORS INFLUENCING SELF-ESTEEM
Put yourself in the circle at the center of this diagram. *How do you regard yourself in each of these areas?*

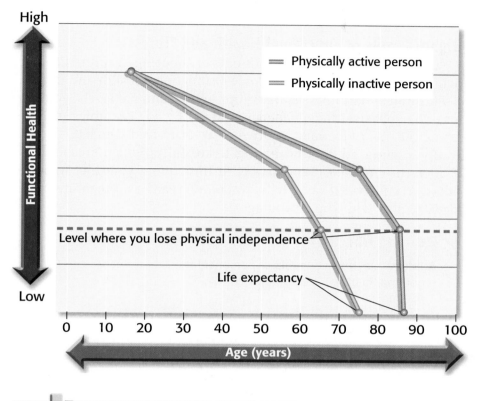

FIGURE 1.12

THE INFLUENCE OF PHYSICAL ACTIVITY ON FUNCTIONAL HEALTH AND FITNESS

Physical activity improves functional fitness. *Where does your current level of activity fall on this graph? What changes, if any, do you need to make?*

High

Functional Health

— Physically active person
— Physically inactive person

Level where you lose physical independence

Life expectancy

Low

0   10   20   30   40   50   60   70   80   90   100

Age (years)

STRESS BREAK

Types of Stress

Not all stress is negative. Technically speaking, there is *good stress* and *bad stress*. Bad stress, also known as "distress," can increase your risk for chronic disease.

By contrast, positive stress—or "eustress" is enjoyable. It is the kind of stress that accompanies scoring high on a difficult exam, winning an important game, or being elected class president.

You can increase the amount of eustress, simultaneously decreasing the amount of distress, by making physical activity a lifelong habit.

Stress Reduction

As noted earlier in this chapter, managing stress is part of maintaining a healthy lifestyle. One of the benefits of personal fitness is stress reduction. Regular physical activity or exercise is an effective stress reducer. For example, regular physical activity lowers blood pressure and can reduce hormone levels that cause stress.

Improvements in Academic and Physical Performance

Regular participation in physical activity, exercise, or both has been shown to enhance performance in school. Teens who are physically active often have enhanced concentration spans, have higher energy levels, and miss fewer days of school.

Increased Life Expectancy

Physical activity and exercise increase muscular strength and endurance. Researchers have discovered that an active lifestyle also improves blood **cholesterol** and **triglyceride** levels. As you will see in

hot link

For more on **cholesterol** and **triglycerides,** see Chapter 4, pages **119–120.**

Chapter 4, these are substances in the blood that increase a person's risk of cardiovascular disease.

Physically active people are also less likely to smoke or begin smoking. Thus, physical activity and exercise decrease disease risks and increase life expectancy. **Figure 1.12** compares the aging process of a physically active person with a physically inactive person. The physically inactive person has a shorter life expectancy than the physically active person.

Higher Levels of Functional Health and Fitness

One of the most important benefits of choosing healthful lifestyle habits is that it increases your level of functional health and fitness. If your functional-fitness status drops below minimal levels, you can lose your physical independence in daily living. Examples include losing the ability to walk, to drive a car, or to feed yourself.

By staying active and eating healthfully, you increase your chances of remaining functionally fit throughout your life. In addition, the positive lifestyle habits that you learn as a teen are more likely to stay with you as you age.

 Reading Check

Analyze List three benefits of personal fitness to mental/emotional health.

Lesson 3 Review

Using complete sentences, answer the following questions on a sheet of paper.

Reviewing Facts and Vocabulary

1. Recall Explain how your attitudes affect your level of fitness.

2. Vocabulary What are *peers?* What is *peer influence?*

3. Recall What is a *commitment?*

Thinking Critically

4. Evaluate Sean is a straight-A student. He does not participate in any type of physical activity regularly. Between the academic demands of school and the stress he feels meeting those demands, he says he has no time for exercise. What advice would you give him about the relationship among physical activity, stress, and academic performance?

5. Analyze Kevin believes that physical activity is the only lifestyle behavior anyone needs to follow. He tells his friends, "If you work out, you can eat anything you want." Assess Kevin's attitude toward total personal fitness.

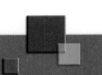

Personal Fitness Planning

Evaluating Claims For the next week, take note of any advertisements you see for fitness products. Evaluate which of these consumer issues fosters a negative attitude toward physical activity and which emphasizes a positive attitude toward physical fitness. Be prepared to share your findings with your class.

Guidelines for Getting Started

What You Will Do

- Design a personal fitness program by using specific guidelines.
- Define different levels of physical activity.
- Evaluate your current level of physical activity.

Terms to Know

behavioral-change stairway
regular physical activity
   or exercise
moderate physical activity
   or exercise
vigorous physical activity
   or exercise

Don't put off 'til tomorrow what you can do today. Have you heard this saying? It makes a good motto for someone who has made a commitment to become and stay personally fit. Is that someone you? If so, it is time to get started.

In this lesson, you will take your first steps toward developing an effective program of fitness. The chapters ahead will provide details you will need to put your plan into action.

Setting Fitness Goals

As discussed in Lesson 3, sticking to your fitness plan is essential to becoming personally fit. The following guidelines will help you design a plan that enables you to stick with your commitment.

- Make a contract with yourself to show your commitment to improving your personal fitness.
- Make a list of goals that are both reasonable and specific.
- Make a schedule of your fitness activities that fits in with your other obligations and responsibilities.
- Be patient: begin slowly and progress gradually.
- Enjoy it. Make it a social experience by participating with others in a variety of activities that you like doing.

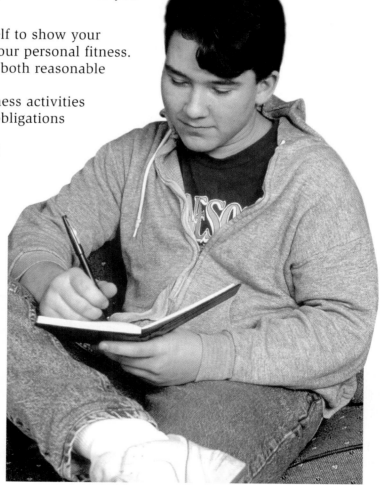

▶ Designing a fitness plan involves careful planning. *Why do you think it is important to write down your goals?*

Choosing Your Physical Activities

When designing your fitness program, choose activities that will be both effective and safe. As you begin your program, the activities you choose should be of moderate intensity. While you want to challenge yourself, it is important that you do not take on more than you can physically handle. Activities should be low-impact and lower weight-bearing, such as walking or lap swimming. Choose a variety of activities and consider safety. Avoid activities that can cause injury or personal harm.

 Reading Check

Explain What written steps should you take when planning your fitness program?

The Behavioral-Change Stairway

One approach that has helped many people achieve and maintain lasting overall fitness is the behavioral-change stairway. This is *a step-by-step approach for helping people achieve their fitness goals.* The steps in this approach are shown in **Figure 1.13.** By taking fitness one step at a time, anyone—including you—can reach your fitness objectives.

Beginning to Climb. It may surprise you to learn that one of the hardest legs of the upward journey is the first. Moving from Step 1 (not thinking about fitness) to Step 2 (beginning to think about fitness) requires conscious effort. This is why making a contract with yourself can be very helpful.

FIGURE 1.13

BEHAVIORAL-CHANGE STAIRWAY
Improving fitness happens one step at a time. *What step on the behavioral-change stairway are you currently at in regard to personal fitness?*

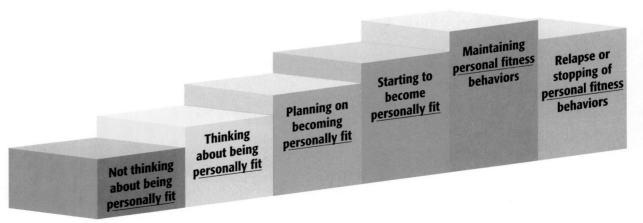

Source: U.S. Department of Health and Human Services, Centers for Disease Control and Prevention, 1999.[2]

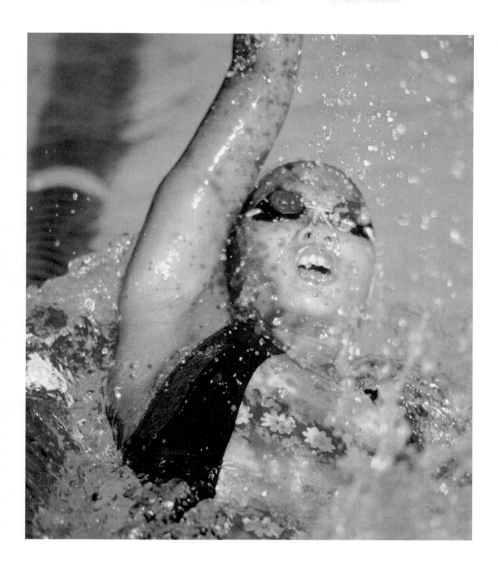

◀ Achieving goals involves making a realistic plan. *How can this teen achieve her goal of swimming one mile nonstop? Why is having a plan of action helpful?*

Once you have reached Step 2, you need to think "actively." Assess your current behaviors, taking note of which need the most work. Be on the lookout at this stage for any negative attitudes that may still be holding you back.

Planning Your Journey. At Step 3, you develop your game plan, including setting goals and a realistic schedule. Begin by asking yourself, "What is my goal?" Then devise a regular schedule of activity to follow. Allow a reasonable time for achieving your goal. Consider Martha's goal: to be able to swim one mile nonstop. To achieve this goal, she will need to start slowly, maybe doing five minutes at first, then adding a few minutes more in each following session. By exercising patience as well as her muscles, Martha will eventually reach her fitness objective.

Staying on Track. Step 4 of the journey is the point where some people begin to slide back. Once you have developed a plan for your program, make up your mind to stick with it. You may have "off" days; everyone does. However, if you can stick with your routine until it becomes habit, you will be well on your way to success.

Staying at the Top. Once you have reached Step 5, your goal should be to stay there. This might involve trying new activities and including a friend or family member. Make physical activity or exercise a social experience as well as a physical one.

Don't worry if you have an occasional relapse. That's normal. If you do, just be sure to get back into a regular routine as soon as possible. Most important of all, engage in physical activities and exercises that you like to do. Vary your routine by doing different activities on different days. Be creative.

 Reading Check

Identify Briefly summarize what happens at Step 4 and Step 5 of the behavioral-change stairway.

Physical Activity and Exercise Guidelines

As you will discover in this program, a relationship exists between the amount of energy you burn in performing an exercise or activity and the benefits you receive. **Figure 1.14** shows the relationship between the level of physical activity and the amount of benefits to your health and fitness. In general, the harder you work, the greater the rewards to your health and fitness.

In order to compare activities and exercises in terms of the energy they require, fitness experts have devised three ratings. These are *regular, moderate,* and *vigorous.* You will come across these terms frequently throughout this program.

Note that the definition of the terms depends on two factors: **frequency** (how often an activity or exercise is done) and **intensity** (how much energy is expended). As a teen, you should strive to do a minimum of 225 minutes of activity or exercise per week. Adults should do a minimum of 150 minutes per week.

Regular Physical Activity or Exercise

Regular physical activity or exercise is *any activity or exercise performed most days of the week, preferably daily.* Such activity may also be done

- 5 or more days of the week if moderately intense activities are done.
- 3 or more days per week if vigorous activities are done.

Moderate Physical Activity or Exercise

Moderate physical activity or exercise is *any activity or exercise that ranges in intensity from light-to-borderline-heavy exertion.* Examples of such activities and exercises are walking briskly, mowing the lawn, dancing, swimming, and cycling on level terrain. To achieve moderate intensity, any of these activities or exercises must:

hot link

frequency and intensity
For more on frequency and intensity, see Chapter 3, pages **84–87.**

FIGURE 1.14

BENEFITS OF PHYSICAL ACTIVITY AND EXERCISE

This graph shows the effect that physical activity and exercise have on health and fitness. *What is the relationship between physical fitness and health as explained in this graph?*

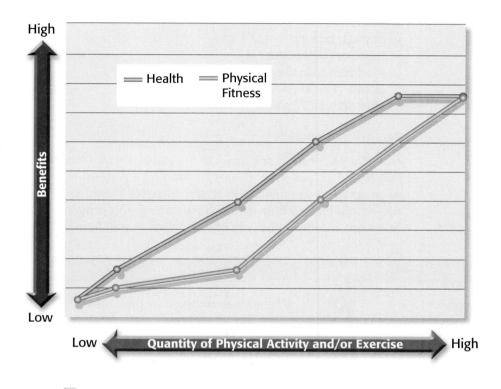

- Reach a rating of perceived exertion of 11 through 14. As you will see in Chapter 3, **rating of perceived exertion (RPE)** is a measure of how hard you *feel* you are working during physical activity or exercise.
- Burn 3.5 to 7 calories per minute. You will learn more about the relationship between calories and activities in Chapter 5.

Vigorous Physical Activity or Exercise

Vigorous physical activity or exercise is *any activity or exercise that ranges in intensity from heavy-to-maximum exertion.* Examples of such activities and exercises are jogging, shoveling snow, high-impact aerobic dance, swimming continuous laps, and cycling uphill. In a later chapter you will learn other strategies for determining the intensity level of an exercise or activity. To achieve vigorous intensity, any of these activities or exercises must

- reach a rating of perceived exertion of 15 or higher.
- burn more than 7 calories per minute.

hot link

rating of perceived exertion (RPE)
For more on the RPE scale, see Chapter 7, page **209.**

Active Mind Active Body
How Physically Active Are You Now?

This activity will help you determine your current activity level.

What You Will Need
- Pen or pencil
- Paper

What You Will Do

Respond to the statements that follow. For each "yes" response, write the point value shown. When you have finished, add your points to determine your current level of physical activity:

Inactive (0–5 points)
Moderately active (6–11 points)
Active (12–20 points)
Very active (21 points or higher)

Apply and Conclude

How did you score? Look again at the statements for which you recorded "yes" responses. Can you find a pattern? In what areas do you need to improve? Take this inventory again from time to time as you work through this program. See what improvements you make to your overall fitness.

Points	Statement
1	1. I usually walk to and from school and work.
1	2. I usually take the stairs rather than use elevators or escalators.
	3. My typical daily physical activity is best described as:
0	a. Light (such as walking to class, sitting in class, or sitting at home).
4	b. Moderate (such as fast walking).
9	c. Vigorous (such as playing football, volleyball, basketball, or working out in the gym).
1	4. I spend a few hours each week in light leisure activity (such as walking or slow cycling).
1	5. I hike or bicycle at a moderate pace once a week or more on the average.
1	6. At least once a week, I participate for an hour or more in vigorous dancing, such as aerobic or folk dancing.
2	7. I play racquetball or tennis at least once a week.
1	8. I often walk for exercise or recreation.

Points	Statement
1	9. When I feel bothered by pressures at school, work, or home, I use exercise as a way to relax.
3	10. Two or more times a week I perform calisthenic exercises (sit-ups, push-ups, and so on) for at least 10 minutes per session.
2	11. I regularly participate in yoga or perform stretching exercises.
4	12. Twice a week or more, I engage in weight training for at least 30 minutes.
	13. I participate in active recreational sports such as volleyball, baseball, or softball:
2	a. about once a week.
4	b. about twice a week.
7	c. three times a week or more.
	14. I participate in vigorous fitness activities like jogging or swimming for a minimum of 20 minutes per session:
3	a. about once a week.
5	b. about twice a week.
10	c. three times a week or more.

Source: **Health: Making Life Choices, 2nd Edition,** *2000. Activity adapted from Russell Pate (University of South Carolina, Department of Exercise Science).*[3]

Jump Starting Your Personal Fitness Program

In this course you will participate in a conditioning program that will allow you to experience the benefits of physical activity and regular exercise in a positive way. The conditioning program will focus on health-related fitness components, including a cardiovascular component (such as walking, jogging, cycling, or aerobic dance), a muscular strength and endurance component (such as weight lifting or calisthenics), and a flexibility component (for example, stretching or range-of-motion activities). You will learn more about each of these components of fitness as you read this text.

It is important for you to get started *now* on your personal-conditioning program. That way you can begin to assess your fitness levels accurately and safely in the "Fitness Check" activities in each chapter. It is also important that you follow the personal-conditioning program for several weeks prior to your physical evaluations. Doing so will help you improve your levels of physical fitness.

Begin your conditioning program at a low-to-moderate level. Gradually increase this level over a period of several weeks to reduce injury risk. When you first start your program, it will be difficult to include all the fitness components at one time. It is best to start with the cardiovascular and flexibility components. Add the muscular-strength and endurance components later. Remember to be patient when you first start your program. This will help you move successfully through the behavioral-change stairway to a lifetime of personal fitness.

Lesson 4 Review

Using complete sentences, answer the following questions on a sheet of paper.

Reviewing Facts and Vocabulary

1. **Vocabulary** What is the *behavioral-change stairway?*

2. **Recall** Between which two steps does the behavioral-change stairway descend? Explain.

3. **Recall** How often should teens perform regular physical activity?

Thinking Critically

4. **Extend** Two friends, Wanda and Kay, are both 15. Wanda is just beginning the behavioral-change stairway. Kay is at Step 5. What can Kay do to motivate her friend to maintain a commitment to physical activity and exercise?

5. **Evaluate** Using the recommended days per week and recommended intensity levels for a person beginning a fitness program, how many days per week should a beginner participate in physical activity or exercise?

Personal Fitness Planning

Designing and Implementing a Program
Using the guidelines listed at the beginning of this lesson, write out a plan for your personal fitness program. Include a contract, a list of goals, and a schedule. You should also make a list of ways to motivate yourself to move toward the maintenance stage of the behavioral-change stairway and a list of the reasons why you might fall into the relapse stage.

TRUE/FALSE

On a sheet of paper, write the numbers 1–10. Write True *or* False *for each statement below.*

1. The only way to develop fitness is to become an athlete.
2. Personal fitness is another name for physical fitness.
3. The fitness behaviors that you develop as a young adult will have little effect on you and your health as an adult.
4. Heredity is one risk factor that can threaten your health.
5. You can lessen the impact risk factors have on your health and fitness through the behaviors you choose.
6. The foods you eat have little to do with the possibility of developing heart disease.
7. Your peers can have a positive or negative influence on your attitudes.
8. Making a commitment to keep fit is lying to yourself.
9. Adherence is another word for commitment.
10. The *Healthy People 2010* objectives are designed to encourage all Americans to develop and maintain healthy, active lifestyles.

MULTIPLE CHOICE

On a sheet of paper, write the letter of the word or phrase that best completes each statement.

11. Physical fitness affects
    a. physical health.
    b. social health.
    c. mental and emotional health.
    d. all of the above.
12. People who are personally fit do all of the following EXCEPT
    a. lose at least 20 pounds.
    b. eat healthfully.
    c. get adequate rest.
    d. avoid tobacco.
13. People who lead sedentary lifestyles
    a. live longer.
    b. are inactive.
    c. experience less stress.
    d. make great athletes.
14. Which of the following is a changeable risk factor?
    a. Age
    b. Gender
    c. Genetics
    d. Stress
15. A major risk factor for developing diabetes is
    a. smoking.
    b. obesity.
    c. gender.
    d. stress.
16. The average life expectancy for adults in the United States today is about ___ years.
    a. seventy-five
    b. seventy
    c. seventy-seven
    d. eighty-seven
17. The media includes all of the following EXCEPT
    a. the Internet.
    b. movies.
    c. peers and classmates.
    d. music.
18. Peer influence in your life can be all of the following EXCEPT
    a. direct.
    b. negative.
    c. from a teacher.
    d. from a classmate.
19. When starting a fitness program, your best advice is to
    a. take it slow at first.
    b. stop if you don't see results.
    c. look for shortcuts.
    d. do without food.
20. *Healthy People 2010* seeks to get all Americans to do each of the following EXCEPT
    a. become physically active.
    b. take turns exercising.
    c. get regular health screenings.
    d. avoid tobacco.

DISCUSSION

Using complete sentences, answer the following questions on a sheet of paper.

21. **Evaluate** Explain how two 75-year-old adults could both have their functional health but at the same time differ in terms of their functional-fitness levels. Give examples.
22. **Analyze** Explain how a person can adjust his or her lifestyle and behaviors to reduce his or her risk for early death due to heredity.
23. **Discuss** What is the relationship between personal fitness and health?

VOCABULARY

On a sheet of paper, write the letter of the term in Column B that best fits the definition in Column A.

Column A

24. Conditions and behaviors that represent a potential threat to an individual's well-being.
25. The mind and body's response to the demands and threats of daily life.
26. The body's ability to carry out daily tasks and still have enough reserve energy to respond to unexpected demands.
27. Total health.
28. Pledge or promise.
29. Inactive.
30. The collective forms of mass communication found within society at any given time.

Column B

a. wellness
b. physical fitness
c. risk factors
d. sedentary
e. commitment
f. media
g. stress

CRITICAL THINKING

Using complete sentences, answer the following questions on a sheet of paper.

31. **Extend** How can developing your personal fitness benefit your social health?
32. **Compare and Contrast** What advantages does a physically fit person have over a person with a low level of physical fitness on a day-to-day basis? Explain your answer.
33. **Evaluate** A friend who doubts that a physically active lifestyle can improve your academic performance points to a player on the school football team, who is an average student. Explain the flaw in your friend's reasoning.

CASE STUDY

RAUL CUTS CLASS

Raul is a junior who avoids physical education classes. Since his first days in middle school, he has managed to develop a bag of tricks that allows him to sit out more days than he participates. His problems with physical education are that:

- He dislikes other students making fun of his inability to pass fitness tests.
- He is overweight and finds it embarrassing to be seen in gym shorts and a T-shirt.
- There is a history of heart trouble in his family. Raul thinks he heard somewhere that there is a connection between heart attacks and working out.

HERE IS YOUR ASSIGNMENT:

Assume that you are Raul's friend. Write a letter to Raul trying to convince him not only to attend physical education class this semester but also to work hard during this class to get himself into shape. Use information from this chapter to support your case.

KEYS TO HELP YOU

- Consider Raul's lifestyle and behaviors.
- Consider Raul's attitudes and beliefs.
- Consider Raul's self-esteem.
- Consider Raul's health risks.
- Consider the potential benefits of physical activity for Raul's overall health.

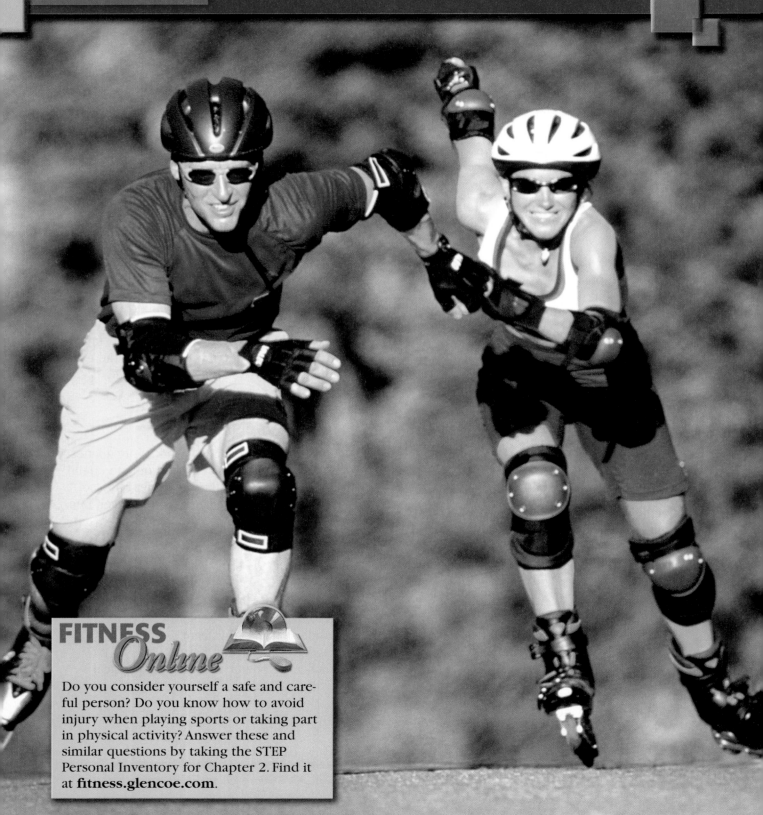

FITNESS
Online

Do you consider yourself a safe and careful person? Do you know how to avoid injury when playing sports or taking part in physical activity? Answer these and similar questions by taking the STEP Personal Inventory for Chapter 2. Find it at **fitness.glencoe.com**.

Personal Fitness Screening

What You Will Do

- Define medical screenings and identify who needs them.
- Identify the types of information gathered during a medical screening.
- Describe the role your medical history plays in your overall levels of fitness.

Terms to Know

medical screening
obesity
chronic disease
asthma
hernia
medical history

After being sedentary for years, April decided to take up tennis. Some of her friends already played tennis, so she asked them for advice on getting started. One suggestion, which came as a surprise, was to have a medical screening. "What's a medical screening?" April asked. "What does it have to do with tennis?"

Do you know the answer to April's questions? After reading this lesson, you will.

Medical Screening

A **medical screening** is *a basic assessment of a person's overall health and personal fitness.* It includes a physical examination and may be performed by a doctor, nurse, or other health care professional.

A medical screening measures, among other things, the individual's physical readiness to take part in strenuous activity. It also tests for previously undetected medical problems that may be aggravated by vigorous activity.

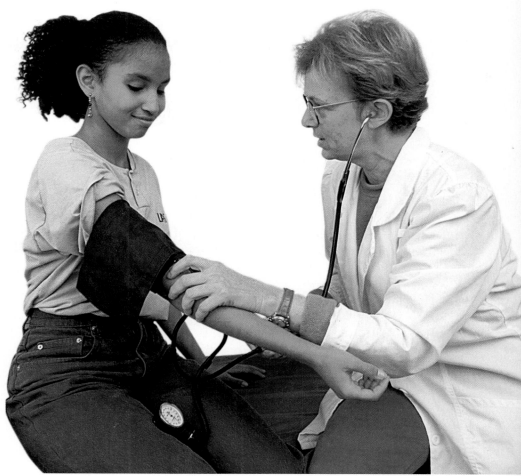

► A medical screening is an important step in personal fitness planning. *Why do you think it is important to have a medical screening before beginning a new sport or fitness program?*

Who Should Have a Medical Screening?

In general, everyone should have a medical screening before starting a program of vigorous physical activity. Such an examination is especially important for people who fit one or more of the following descriptions:

- **People with poor lifestyle habits.** This includes people who have been physically inactive.
- **People over 40.** Middle-aged and older adults need to be particularly mindful of the importance of medical screenings.
- **People who are overweight or suffer from obesity.** Obesity is *a medical condition in which a person's ratio of body fat to lean muscle mass is excessively high.* Obesity and overweight are major health problems in the United States today.
- **People with a known chronic disease.** A chronic disease is a disease *that is ongoing.* One such disease that affects a person's ability to perform physically demanding activities is asthma (AZ-muh). This is *a disease in which the small airways of the lungs become narrowed, making it difficult to breathe.* Two other chronic illnesses are **heart disease** and **diabetes.**

In addition to an initial medical screening, everyone is advised to have a periodic follow-up evaluation. There are no absolute guidelines for how often this needs to occur. The chart in **Figure 2.1** gives some basic recommendations, based on age.

Reading Check

Identify Who should have a medical screening?

hot link

heart disease
For more on heart disease, see Chapter 7, page 200.

diabetes
For more on diabetes, see Chapter 6, page 173.

Fitness FACTS

Obesity
- 60 percent of American adults are overweight or obese.
- Over 80 percent of people with diabetes are overweight or obese.
- High blood pressure is twice as common in obese adults than in those who are at a healthy weight.

Source: The Surgeon General's Call to Action to Prevent and Decrease Overweight and Obesity, 2001.[1]

FIGURE 2.1

MEDICAL SCREEN TIMETABLE
The necessity of a medical screening varies with age. *What trend do you notice in the frequency of visits as a person gets older?*

Age	Frequency of Screening
6 to 15	Every 3 years
16 to 34	Every 2 years
35 to 59	Once a year
60 and up	Twice a year

Active Mind Active Body

What Is Your PAR-Q?

Preparation for any program of physical activity should include the use of a Physical Activity Readiness Questionnaire, or PAR-Q. Answering these questions correctly will help you understand your own readiness for beginning a program of physical activity. In this activity you may want to answer these questions along with your parents or guardian to ensure correct answers.

What You Will Need

- Pen or pencil
- Paper
- PAR-Questionnaire (page **38**)

What You Will Do

1. On a separate sheet of paper, answer as many of the seven PAR-Q questions as you can. Leave a blank for any questions you are unable to answer.
2. Discuss the questions you were unable to answer with a parent or other adult in the home. Complete the questionnaire.
3. Discuss the PAR-Q answers with your physical education teacher.
4. Design a modified program of exercise or physical activity with the guidance of your physician and physical education instructor.

Apply and Conclude

Based on the answers of the PAR-Q, how ready are you to begin a physical-activity program? What modifications, if any, should you consider for your physical-activity program? Will you need special equipment?

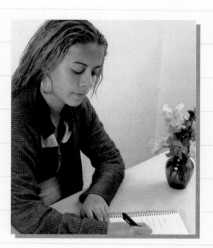

What Happens During a Medical Screening?

A medical screening may consist of just a few tests or a full medical examination. The following are some of the tests and measurements that might be performed:

- A complete blood count, or CBC. This is a test in which a sample of blood is drawn. The sample is then sent to a laboratory where it is tested for possible indicators of diseases and disorders.
- Your height and weight.
- An examination of your eyes, ears, nose, and throat.
- Your **blood pressure.** Blood pressure is the force of the blood in the blood vessels of the body.
- An examination of your lungs to make sure they are clear.
- An examination of your heart to make sure the heartbeat is regular and normal.
- For males, a test for hernia, *a condition that occurs when muscle fibers from the intestine protrude through the wall of the abdomen.* Hernias are painful and often require surgery. People with hernias are advised not to lift weights or participate in other activities that may aggravate the condition.

blood pressure For more on blood pressure, see Chapter 7, page **206.**

PAR - Q & YOU
(Physical Activity Readiness—Questionnaire)

(A Questionnaire for People Aged 15 to 69)

Regular physical activity is fun and healthy, and increasingly more people are starting to become more active every day. Being more active is very safe for most people. However, some people should check with their doctor before they start becoming much more physically active.

If you are planning to become much more physically active than you are now, start by answering the seven questions in the box below. If you are between the ages of 15 and 69, the PAR-Q will tell you if you should check with your doctor before you start.

Common sense is your best guide when you answer these questions. Please read the questions carefully and answer each one honestly: check YES or NO.

YES	NO	
☐	☐	1. Has your doctor ever said that you have a heart condition and that you should only do physical activity recommended by a doctor?
☐	☐	2. Do you feel pain in your chest when you do physical activity?
☐	☐	3. In the past month, have you had chest pain when you were not doing physical activity?
☐	☐	4. Do you lose your balance because of dizziness or do you ever lose consciousness?
☐	☐	5. Do you have a bone or joint problem that could be made worse by a change in your physical activity?
☐	☐	6. Is your doctor currently prescribing drugs (for example, water pills) for your blood pressure or heart condition?
☐	☐	7. Do you know of any other reason why you should not do physical activity?

NOTE: If the PAR-Q is being given to a person before he or she participates in a physical activity program or a fitness appraisal, this section may be used for legal or administrative purposes.

I have read, understood, and completed this questionnaire. Any questions I had were answered to my full satisfaction.

NAME _____ DATE _____

DATE _____ WITNESS _____

SIGNATURE _____

WITNESS _____

SIGNATURE OF PAR...

If you answered

YES to one or more questions

Talk with your doctor by phone or in person BEFORE you start becoming much more physically active or BEFORE you have a fitness appraisal. Tell your doctor about the PAR-Q and which questions you answered YES to.

- You may be able to do any activity you want—as long as you start slowly and build up gradually. Or, you may need to restrict your activities to those which are safe for you. Talk with your doctor about the kinds of activities you wish to participate in and follow his/her advice.
- Find out which community programs are safe and helpful for you.

NO to all questions

If you answered NO honestly to all PAR-Q questions, you can be reasonably sure that you can

- start becoming much more physically active—begin slowly and build up gradually. This is the safest and easiest way to go.
- take part in a fitness appraisal—this is an excellent way to determine your basic fitness so that you can plan the best way for you to live actively.

DELAY BECOMING MUCH MORE ACTIVE:

- if you are not feeling well because of a temporary illness such as a cold or a fever— wait until you feel better; or
- if you have other medical conditions, talk to your doctor

Please note: If your health changes so that you then answer YES to any of the above questions, tell your fitness or health professional. Ask whether you should change your physical activity plan.

▲ The PAR-Q helps you assess your readiness for beginning a program of physical activity.

Source: Canada's Physical Activity Guide to Healthy Active Living, 2002.[2]

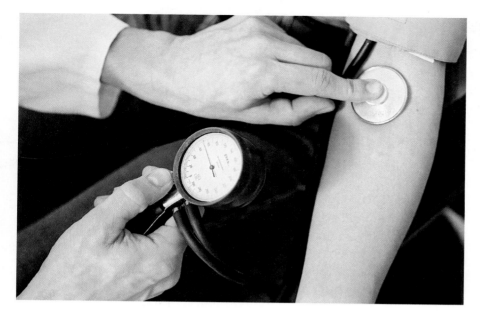

During a medical screening, your health care provider will check your blood pressure. *What other tests might he or she perform?*

Your Medical History. A medical screening carried out by a physician usually includes an update of your medical history, *a record of past health problems and illnesses.* The doctor will ask about any medications you may be taking. He or she will also ask about the health of other members of your family. This will help determine whether you are at risk of diseases relating to **heredity.**

 Reading Check

Summarize Name five tests that might be done during a medical screening.

h t link

heredity For more on heredity, see Chapter 1, page 13.

Lesson 1 Review

Using complete sentences, answer the following questions on a sheet of paper.

Reviewing Facts and Vocabulary

1. **Vocabulary** Define *medical screening.*
2. **Recall** What are some diseases that make a complete medical screening necessary before beginning a fitness program?

Thinking Critically

3. **Recall** How is your medical history a factor in your overall levels of fitness?
4. **Extend** Seth has never had a medical screening before, and feels a little nervous. How would you explain to Seth what is involved, to put his mind at ease?

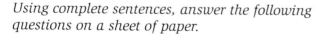 **Personal Fitness Planning**

Evaluating Health Review your results for the PAR-Q, then take the survey home to help your family or friends to determine their readiness for physical activity. What differences did you notice among the responses? If the answers to the questions were *Yes* on the questionnaire, how should these individuals prepare for physical activity?

What You Will Do

- Explain how environmental conditions can influence the safety of your fitness program.
- Describe the relationship among fluid balance, physical activity, and loss of water and salt.
- Plan a program of physical activity to reduce environmental risks.

Terms to Know

fluid balance
dehydration
heat cramps
heat exhaustion
heatstroke
acclimatization
rehydrate
heat-stress index
hypothermia
frostbite
wind-chill factor

Environmental Concerns

It is early Saturday morning on the day of the big race. Tony has been planning and training for months now. Today's weather forecast calls for high temperatures and humidity. Most of Tony's training has been in cooler temperatures with low humidity. What precautions should Tony consider before, during, and after the race? What are some of the dangers of being physically active in very hot or very cold weather? In this lesson, you will find out.

Environmental Conditions and Physical Activity

Climate is a potential risk factor in personal health and fitness. This is especially true for people who are physically active or play sports on days when the temperature reaches extreme highs or lows. Does this mean you should avoid physical activity on such days? Not necessarily. As long as you use common sense and follow a few simple rules, most activities can be carried out safely.

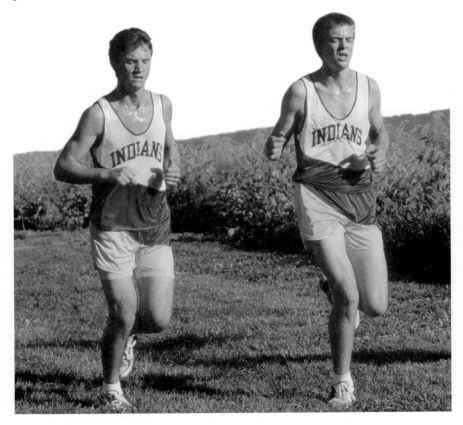

▶ Physical activity in hot weather can lead to dehydration and heat-related injury. *What precautions should you take when exercising on a hot day?*

Extreme Heat and Fluid Balance

During physical activity, your body produces heat. This causes your body temperature to rise above normal. To prevent overheating, your body perspires. The sweat you produce evaporates on your skin. This, in turn, cools your body.

Hot and humid weather can cause you to perspire too much and affect your fluid balance. This is *the body's ability to balance the amounts of fluid taken in with the amounts lost through perspiration or excretion.* In extreme heat, you perspire so heavily that your body loses too much water and important body chemicals such as salt. This is called dehydration, or *body fluid loss,* and it can put you at risk of several heat-related injuries.

Heat Cramps. Heat cramps are *muscle spasms resulting from the loss of large amounts of salt and water through perspiration.* These contractions are due, at least in part, to the loss of sodium caused by dehydration. Heat cramps are the mildest form of heat injury. They can be minimized by drinking plenty of fluids before and during physical activity. This will help you to maintain a normal body fluid balance.

Heat Exhaustion. Heat exhaustion is *an overheating of the body resulting in cold, clammy skin and symptoms of shock.* Other symptoms of heat exhaustion include weakness, headache, rapid pulse, stomach discomfort, dizziness, and heavy sweating. Body weight may drop due to loss of water. Individuals who display these symptoms should stop physical activity immediately and get to a cool, dry place and drink plenty of fluids. They should not resume physical activity for a day or two, or until they have returned to their normal body weight.

Heatstroke. The most serious of the heat-related injuries is heatstroke, *a condition in which the body can no longer rid itself of heat through perspiration.* Its symptoms include a very high body temperature, rapid pulse, and loss of consciousness. The skin becomes hot and dry to the touch. Heatstroke requires immediate medical attention. If you suspect someone is suffering from heatstroke, call 911. Move the person to a cool place and sponge him or her with cold water until help arrives.

hot link

fluid balance For more on your body's fluid balance and how to maintain it, see Chapter 4, page 125.

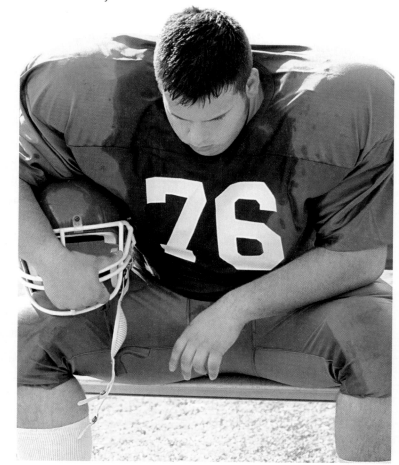

▼ Learning to recognize the symptoms of heat-related injury during physical activity and exercise is important. *What are the symptoms of heat cramps? Heat exhaustion? Heatstroke?*

✔ Reading Check

List Name some common symptoms of the three heat-related illnesses described.

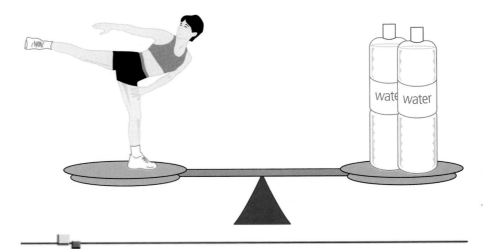

FIGURE 2.2

MAINTAINING WATER BALANCE

Think about how much water there is in a 1.5 liter bottle of water. In an hour-long workout, your body can sweat the equivalent of 2 bottles this size. *How can you avoid dehydration?*

How to Avoid Heat-Related Injury

Although heat-related injury is a serious concern, you can avoid such injury and still enjoy physical activity on hot days. When exercising in the heat, gradually increase the intensity of your activity. The following are some other strategies for preventing heat-related injuries.

Acclimatization. Acclimatization is *the process of allowing your body to adapt slowly to weather conditions.* You can become acclimatized to working out in the heat after five to ten days. The first few physical-activity or exercise sessions should be light. They should also be brief, lasting no more than twenty minutes.

Fluid Intake. During physical activity in hot weather, your body can lose up to 3 liters of water per hour through perspiration. (See **Figure 2.2.**) To prevent dehydration, you need to rehydrate—*restore lost water*—by drinking plenty of fluids before, during, and after physical activity. Here are some guidelines:

- **Before.** Consume between $1^{1}/_{2}$ and $2^{1}/_{2}$ cups of cool water or sports drink 10 to 20 minutes *before* exercising in the heat. (1 cup = 8 ounces.)
- **During.** During physical activity in the heat, attempt to match fluid loss with fluid intake, approximately $1^{1}/_{2}$ cups to $3^{1}/_{4}$ cups (12 to 36 ounces) of water every hour.
- **After.** Drink 2 cups of water or sports drink for every pound lost. It may take up to 12 hours to achieve complete fluid replacement after strenuous exercise in the heat.

For most situations, water works as well as any beverage in preventing dehydration. You can also choose one of the many sports drinks on the market. Avoid beverages that are carbonated and/or

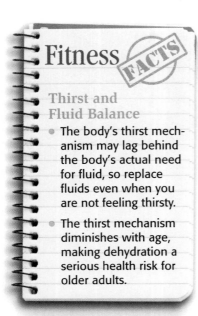

Fitness FACTS

Thirst and Fluid Balance

- The body's thirst mechanism may lag behind the body's actual need for fluid, so replace fluids even when you are not feeling thirsty.

- The thirst mechanism diminishes with age, making dehydration a serious health risk for older adults.

that contain caffeine. Such beverages are absorbed at a much slower rate than plain water. Caffeine, in addition, may slow rehydration.

Clothing. When choosing clothing for sports or activities in the heat, choose lightweight material. Cotton fabrics are best, since they absorb moisture rapidly and promote evaporation and cooling. Garments should be loose-fitting and light in color. Tight clothes do not allow air to circulate between the skin and the clothing. Dark clothing absorbs heat. Wearing a brimmed hat or cap can provide protection from the sun. Sunscreen should be used on all areas of exposed skin.

Setting Limits. One of the most important safeguards against heat-related injury is learning to use the heat-stress index. This is *a scientific measure of the combined effects of heat and humidity on the body.* Take a moment to examine the chart in **Figure 2.3.** Observe that a reading of 105 degrees or higher places you at high risk of injury. You can reduce this risk by limiting strenuous outdoor activity or exercise when the heat-stress index is in the red zone. In general, try to exercise during the cooler parts of the day, such as early morning or evening.

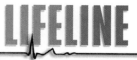

FIGURE 2.3

HEAT-STRESS INDEX

Using the heat-stress index chart can help you avoid heat-related injury. *What would the heat-stress index be if it were 90 degrees and the humidity were 70 percent?*

Relative Humidity	Air Temperature (°F)										
	70°	75°	80°	85°	90°	95°	100°	105°	110°	115°	120°
0%	64	69	73	78	83	87	91	95	99	103	107
10%	65	70	75	80	85	90	95	100	105	111	116
20%	66	72	77	82	87	93	99	105	112	120	130
30%	67	73	78	84	90	96	104	113	123	135	148
40%	68	74	79	86	93	101	110	123	137	151	
50%	69	75	81	88	96	107	120	135	150		
60%	70	76	82	90	100	114	132	149			
70%	70	77	85	93	106	124	144				
80%	71	78	86	97	113	136					
90%	72	80	91	108							

Low Risk 90 or Less	Medium Risk 91 to 105	Higher Risk 106 to 130	Probable Injury 131 or More

RISK OF HEAT INJURY

Physical Activity in Extreme Cold

When you are physically active or exercise in cold weather, you are at risk of hypothermia, *a condition in which your body temperature drops below normal.* Hypothermia can also result from long exposure in windy or rainy weather. When hypothermia occurs, body temperature becomes dangerously low. The brain cannot function at a low temperature, and body systems may cease to function properly. Hypothermia can lead to death. A person with hypothermia may act disoriented and lose motor control. Seek medical help as soon as possible.

In extremely cold conditions you also significantly increase your risk of frostbite, *tissue damage from freezing.* It occurs most often on the head, face, feet and hands. If you notice a lack of feeling in your toes, fingers, nose, or ears while exercising in cold weather, go indoors to warm up.

When you plan to exercise or be physically active in cold weather, pay attention to weather forecasts. Note in particular the wind-chill factor. This is *the combined influence of wind and temperature on the body* (see **Figure 2.4**). Avoid spending extended periods outdoors when the wind-chill factor is below –22 degrees. When you do go

---

FIGURE 2.4

WIND-CHILL INDEX

The wind-chill index will help you determine if it is unsafe to exercise outdoors. *If it were 15 degrees Fahrenheit and the wind were blowing at 30 mph, what would the wind-chill factor be?*

Wind Speed (mph)	Air Temperature (°F)														
Calm	40°	35°	30°	25°	20°	15°	10°	5°	0°	–5°	–10°	–15°	–20°	–25°	–30°
5	37	33	27	21	16	12	6	1	–5	–11	–15	–20	–26	–31	–35
10	28	21	16	9	4	–2	–9	–15	–21	–27	–33	–38	–46	–52	–58
15	22	16	11	1	–5	–11	–18	–25	–36	–40	–45	–51	–58	–65	–70
20	18	12	3	–4	–10	–17	–25	–32	–39	–46	–53	–60	–67	–76	–81
25	16	7	0	–7	–15	–22	–29	–37	–44	–52	–59	–67	–74	–83	–89
30	13	5	–2	–11	–18	–26	–33	–41	–48	–56	–63	–70	–79	–87	–94
35	11	3	–4	–13	–20	–27	–35	–43	–49	–60	–67	–72	–82	–90	–96
40	10	1	–6	–15	–21	–29	–37	–45	–53	–62	–69	–76	–85	–94	–101

Low Risk Warmer than –21	Increasing Risk –22 to –67	High Risk Colder than –67

RISK OF FROSTBITE

out, wear warm, loose-fitting clothing in layers. These layers will help trap warm air as it leaves the body. Protect your extremities—your hands, feet, head, and ears—from extreme cold. These are the places where much of your body heat is lost.

 Reading Check

Compare In what ways are the risks of exercising in extreme heat similar to those of exercising in extreme cold?

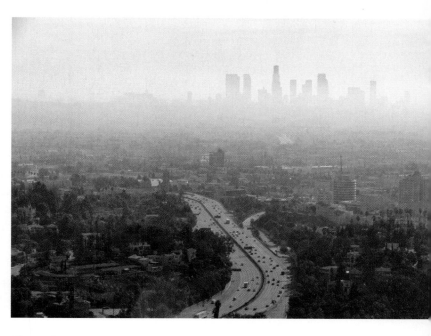

<figure>▼ Air pollution can make physical activity and exercise hazardous. *What steps can you take to reduce your risks from air pollution?*</figure>

Other Outdoor Environmental Concerns

Weather-related concerns are important when participating in outdoor sports and activities. However, other potential environmental factors can also pose a risk.

Air Pollution

Air quality is an important factor to consider when participating in outdoor physical activity. Gases and particles emitted from factories, motor vehicles, and other sources can worsen air quality. Exercising outdoors when air quality is poor increases the amount of pollutants that enter the body, increasing the risk of **lung diseases.** Carbon monoxide is a particularly harmful gas because it absorbs into the blood more readily than does oxygen.

However, there are several steps you can take to reduce the health risks associated with air pollution. First, pay attention to daily media reports of the air quality index, which reports local air quality. During periods of poor air quality, limit or avoid outdoor exercise. In addition, identify the areas and times of day that have less motor vehicle traffic. Finally, find suitable indoor physical activity and exercise opportunities as an alternative to outdoor activities on days when air quality is poor.

Altitude

Do you live in a mountainous or other high-altitude region? High altitudes begin at about 5,000 feet above sea level. The air at higher altitudes is thinner than at lower altitudes. Less oxygen is available to the heart and lungs. This can reduce your ability to exercise or perform strenuous work. It can also cause you to tire more quickly than you would at sea level.

If you move from a low altitude to a high altitude, gradually increase the amount you exercise over a period of days. If possible, change altitude slowly over several hours. Drink plenty of water, because dehydration is more likely to occur at high altitudes.

lung diseases For more on respiratory problems and their causes, see Chapter 7, page 203.

Personal Safety

It is important to protect your personal safety when participating in physical activities. You can reduce the risk of becoming a victim of crime by developing an awareness of risk factors. Here are some guidelines to keep in mind.

- Take time to examine and plan your outdoor routes.
- Exercise in well-lit areas.
- Exercise with friends, especially at night.
- Wear reflective clothing.
- Avoid exercising in high-crime neighborhoods.
- Avoid isolated trails or paths.
- Always let someone know where you are going. Make sure to say when you expect to return as well.

Unleashed Dogs

As you exercise outdoors, be alert for dogs not on leashes. If you encounter a dog, do not unnecessarily frighten or threaten it. If confronted by a dog that appears vicious, it may be best to face it and yell, "Bad dog! Stop!" Then walk slowly away—never run.

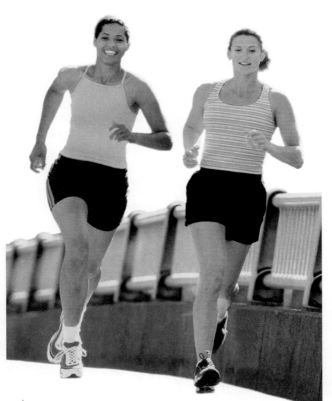

▲ Jogging with a partner is one way of maintaining safety while exercising. *What other actions can you take?*

Reading Check

List What are the environmental factors that can put your physical and personal safety at risk?

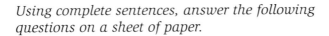

Lesson 2 Review

Using complete sentences, answer the following questions on a sheet of paper.

Reviewing Facts and Vocabulary

1. **Vocabulary** Define *frostbite.*
2. **Recall** How can you prevent dehydration?

Thinking Critically

3. **Explain** How can environmental conditions affect your body's fluid balance? Explain what causes loss of water and salt during exercise.
4. **Synthesize** Before exercising, what precautions should you take to reduce risks in each of the following areas: *hot weather, cold weather, pollution, crime?*

Personal Fitness Planning

Analyzing Risks Make a list of all the places you were physically active or exercised during the past thirty days. Identify any of the environmental concerns discussed in this lesson that were factors in the success of your workout or game. Tell how you will avoid these in the future. Identify other activities you could do that might be safer.

Safety Gear and Clothing

It was the first day of school. At the end of fourth-period physical education class, students were given a checklist of items they would need to buy. "Two pairs of cotton socks—why cotton?" Elias asked his friend. "Socks are socks."

Contrary to what Elias believes, when it comes to physical activity, not all clothing choices are equal. Neither is all safety equipment, such as protective headgear. In this lesson, you will learn how to make informed purchases in both areas.

Clothing

Clothing does not need to be expensive to be effective for physical activity and exercise. It does, however, need to be suited to the particular activity or exercise. If you will be doing a lot of stretching or bending, such as aerobic dance, you will want material that is not too tight and that allows you to move comfortably. If you will be doing a rugged activity such as rock climbing, you will want fabrics with durability.

For outdoor activities, choose a fabric that breathes, while absorbing perspiration. Cotton does both. New state-of-the-art fabrics are lightweight, highly breathable, and can provide warmth for a variety of temperatures. You may also want to consider fabrics that are wind and water-resistant.

Another prime consideration in choosing any sportswear or active wear is comfort. Select clothing that fits well but that stretches so you can move freely.

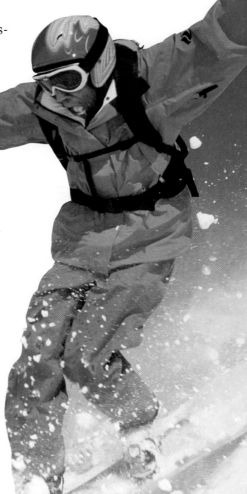

▶ Choosing appropriate clothing for physical activities can ensure comfort and reduce the risk of injury. *What type of clothing is appropriate for outdoor activities?*

What You Will Do

- Identify appropriate clothing for your personal fitness program.
- Demonstrate the basics of choosing appropriate, nonskid footwear.
- Explain how to reduce your risk of activity-related injury.

Terms to Know

pronation
supination
toe box

Footwear

The starting point for most fitness activities is footwear. No matter what type of training you're interested in, you should always choose nonskid footwear. A nonskid shoe can significantly reduce your risk for injuries.

When shopping for footwear, think about the activities you will be doing. For example, if you are going to play basketball, select a shoe specifically designed for that sport. To give ankle support, you should consider getting a high-top shoe. If you will be doing a variety of activities, consider all-purpose cross-training shoes. **Figure 2.5** shows the features you should look for in an exercise shoe.

FIGURE 2.5

FEATURES OF AN EXERCISE SHOE
Learning the parts of a shoe can help you make a more informed choice.

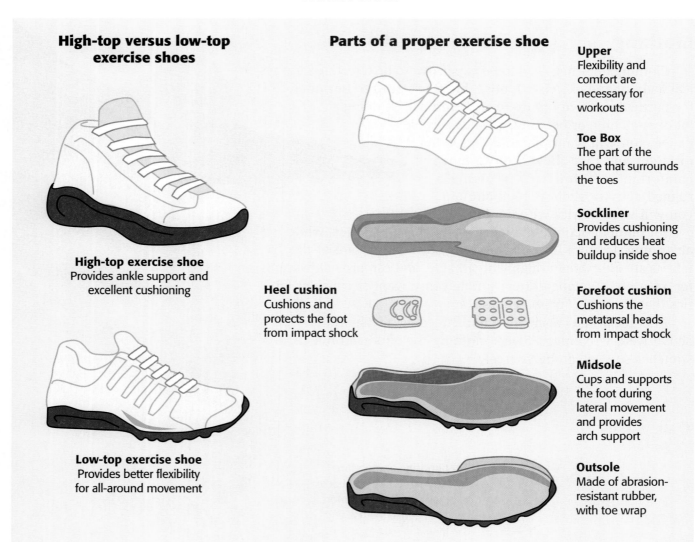

High-top versus low-top exercise shoes

High-top exercise shoe
Provides ankle support and excellent cushioning

Low-top exercise shoe
Provides better flexibility for all-around movement

Parts of a proper exercise shoe

Upper
Flexibility and comfort are necessary for workouts

Toe Box
The part of the shoe that surrounds the toes

Sockliner
Provides cushioning and reduces heat buildup inside shoe

Heel cushion
Cushions and protects the foot from impact shock

Forefoot cushion
Cushions the metatarsal heads from impact shock

Midsole
Cups and supports the foot during lateral movement and provides arch support

Outsole
Made of abrasion-resistant rubber, with toe wrap

FIGURE 2.6

TYPES OF FEET AND ARCHES

Not everyone has the same shape of foot or type of arch. *Which foot most resembles yours? Which tread is more like your own?*

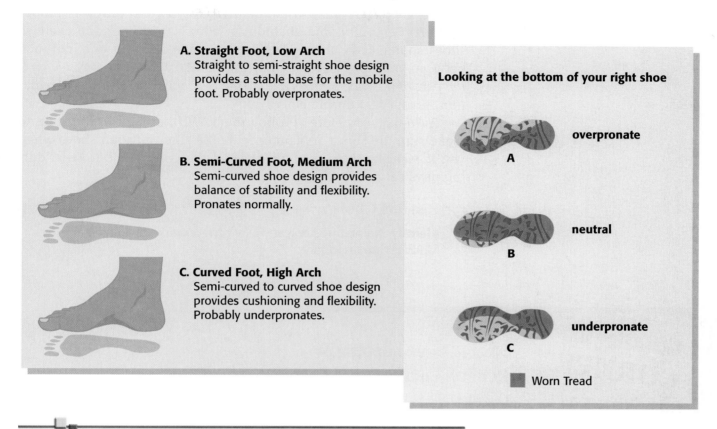

A. Straight Foot, Low Arch
Straight to semi-straight shoe design provides a stable base for the mobile foot. Probably overpronates.

B. Semi-Curved Foot, Medium Arch
Semi-curved shoe design provides balance of stability and flexibility. Pronates normally.

C. Curved Foot, High Arch
Semi-curved to curved shoe design provides cushioning and flexibility. Probably underpronates.

Looking at the bottom of your right shoe

A — overpronate

B — neutral

C — underpronate

■ Worn Tread

Stride Irregularities

One factor you need to consider when shopping for shoes is stride irregularities, such as overpronation and underpronation. **Pronation** is *the normal motion of the foot as you walk or run, from the outside of the heel striking the ground through the normal inward roll of the foot.* In normal pronation, the body's weight is distributed evenly over the surface of the foot. In overpronation, the motion of the foot rolls inward too far. This may cause pain to the inside of the knees or legs.

Supination is *the normal outward roll of the foot as it hits the ground.* Too much supination, or underpronation, causes the weight to shift to the outside of the foot. This can cause soreness and injury to the outside of your knees and thighs.

Figure 2.6 shows the profiles of a foot that pronates normally, along with those that over- and underpronate. It also shows the amount of shoe wear that occurs in each situation.

If you stride normally, an average shoe without special features should work for you. If you tend to overpronate, you may need a shoe that provides greater stability. If you underpronate, you may need a shoe that has greater cushioning and flexibility.

Buying Shoes

Before you buy shoes for physical activity or exercise, it's wise to visit a local sporting goods store. Seek the advice of a knowledgeable salesperson. You might also ask your physical education instructor for advice.

The best shoe for you is one that fits you and provides proper support, flexibility, and cushioning. Physical-activity and exercise shoes should have a snug heel and a space of about one half-inch between your longest toe and the end of the shoe. A roomy **toe box,** *the part of the shoe that surrounds the toes,* will allow proper circulation in your feet during activity.

Try on shoes before you buy them. Walk around in the store to make sure the shoes are comfortable. Be sure to try on shoes when you're wearing the same type of socks that you intend to wear during physical activity.

 Reading Check

Identify Name three reasons why correct workout clothing and footwear are important.

Consumer CORNER

Smart Shoe Shopping: Quality, Comfort, and Cost

You can spend anywhere from $25 to $150 for a pair of exercise shoes. If you plan to be physically active—and hopefully you do—you need to purchase a pair of quality shoes. Here are some tips for making a smart purchase:

- **Look for quality.** When it comes to shoes, be sure not to compromise on comfort and fit. A quality pair of shoes will last longer than an inexpensive brand.
- **Choose nonskid footwear.** The soles of your shoes should be nonskid, especially for activities such as skateboarding, weight lifting, and basketball.
- **Choose comfortable shoes over shoes that look good.** If you feel you must have the latest shoe from companies with well-known names, don't settle for a poor fit because of its look.
- **Know when to replace shoes.** Knowing when to replace your shoes is as important

as any other shopping consideration. Once an exercise shoe starts to lose its sole and support, it should no longer be used for fitness activities. Such a shoe could cause injuries to your feet and joints.

- **Have a spare pair.** If possible, you may want to have a second pair of exercise shoes and alternate their use. This will give one pair time to dry out and regain its cushioning effect. This strategy will provide you with the support you need and can extend the life of your shoes significantly.

Comparison Shopping

Compare prices for a single brand and style of exercise shoe online or in print resources. Which stores or Web sites appear to have the best prices?

Active Mind Active Body

Wet Foot Test

Choosing the right shoe for the right activity begins with knowing the shape of your foot, specifically your arch. Does your foot have a low arch, semi-curved arch, or curved arch? Finding out is easy. In this activity you examine the shape of your arch and become better able to choose the footwear you need.

What You Will Need

- Bucket or pan of water
- Paper (colored preferred) and pencil

What You Will Do

1. Place the bottom of either foot into the water.
2. Lightly press your wet foot on the colored paper.
3. Trace the outline of the water impression on the paper.
4. Examine the shape to determine your arch category.

Apply and Conclude

Refer back to **Figure 2.6** on page **49** to compare your arch impression. What type of arch do you have?

- Straight feet (Type A) leave an imprint that is oval shaped.
- Semi-curved feet (Type B) show the forefoot and the heel connected by a band about 2 inches wide or more.
- Curved feet (Type C) have a narrow band connecting the forefoot and heel.

Have you been using the correct type of footwear? How will knowing the shape of your arch influence you the next time you purchase a pair of exercise shoes?

Safety Equipment

If you participate in an activity such as bicycling, skateboarding, downhill skiing, snowboarding, or in-line skating, you should always wear protective equipment. The most important piece of equipment you can buy is a safety helmet. Statistics show that the likelihood of head injury is reduced 85 percent when a helmet is worn. When skateboarding or in-line skating, wear helmets, light gloves, elbow pads, knee pads, and wrist guards.

Helmet Specifics

A protective helmet should have a foam liner inside to absorb impact to the head in case of a fall. Choose a helmet that meets the standards set by either the American National Standards Institute (ANSI) or the Snell Memorial Foundation. Make sure the helmet has a snug but comfortable fit. Finally, the helmet should have a chin strap and buckle, so it will stay securely fastened. Other safety precautions might include the following.

Mind OVER Matter

Etiquette and Safety

There are many ways you can use your understanding of fitness principles to avoid injury to yourself or others. Give four examples where you can apply etiquette during physical activity. Explain how thinking of the other person can help you prevent injuries at the gym or during certain sports and games.

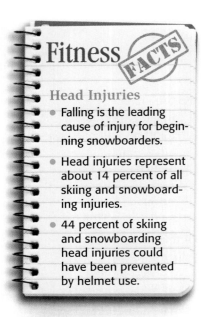
- Take extra care around pedestrians and vehicles.
- Always control your speed.
- Pay close attention to the pavement for holes or obstructions.
- If you do fall, prepare your body for the blow by curling up into a ball and rolling as you hit the ground. This will help reduce the chance of serious injury.
- Replace your helmet if it has any damage.

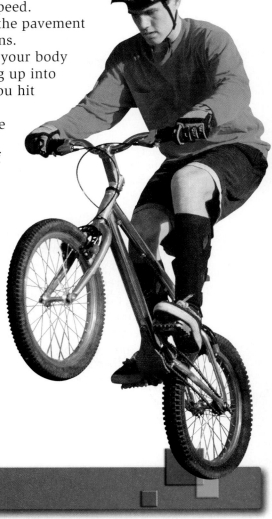

▶ Most head injuries could be avoided if riders wore proper head gear. *What features should you look for when choosing a helmet?*

Lesson 3 Review

Using complete sentences, answer the following questions on a sheet of paper.

Reviewing Facts and Vocabulary

1. **Vocabulary** Define *pronation* and *supination.*

2. **Recall** Give two reasons for wearing a safety helmet while skateboarding, cycling, and snowboarding.

Thinking Critically

3. **Extend** Name a sport that might require a clothing fabric that easily stretches. What sport would demand durability in a fabric?

4. **Analyze** Why is nonskid footwear important for safe physical activity?

5. **Synthesize** Alex and Calvin play one-on-one basketball on a regular basis. Alex has been complaining about the discomfort of his shoes for some time. Calvin has recently read about pronation and other concerns associated with purchasing shoes. What advice could Calvin give to Alex about purchasing new shoes?

Personal Fitness Planning

Evaluating Equipment Take time to evaluate all of your workout clothing and equipment. Are the soles of your shoes wearing out? Has the cushion support of your shoes diminished? Are there any cracks in your helmet or tears in the chin strap? Make a note of any problems. If possible, make arrangements to replace damaged shoes or other equipment.

Preventing Fitness Injuries

Charlie has been jogging regularly now for three months. He has not experienced any soreness since the early weeks of his fitness program. However, recently he has been experiencing a slight pain in his lower back. He is curious about the cause of this injury. He is concerned about whether continued exercise will cause serious back problems.

Do you know the potential causes of minor back pain? Do you know what treatments Charlie might consider? After reading this lesson, you will learn how to avoid common fitness-related injuries.

What You Will Do

- Apply the biomechanical principle of force to walking and jogging.
- Describe examples of unsafe walking/jogging technique.
- Identify common fitness-related injuries.
- Explain how to treat and prevent common fitness injuries.

Terms to Know

biomechanics
tendons
ligaments
cartilage
shinsplint
strain
sprain
RICE
stress fracture

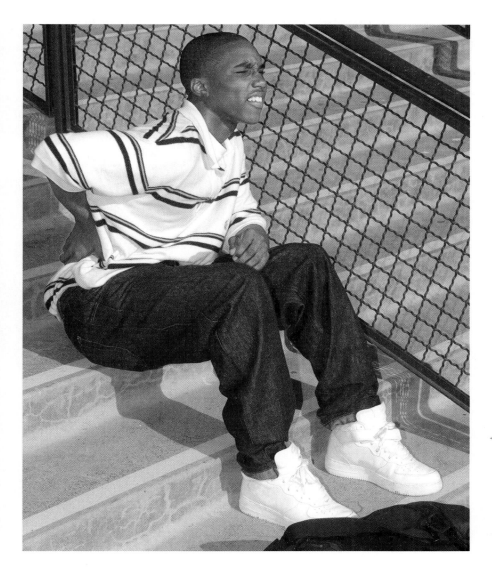

◄ Understanding biomechanics can help you avoid fitness-related injury or soreness. *Have you ever experienced soreness after a workout? What action did you take to relieve the discomfort?*

Biomechanics

Charlie's back pain relates to biomechanics. Biomechanics is both *the study and the application of principles of physics to human motion.*

The laws of biomechanics dictate that when you jog slowly, your foot strikes the ground with a force that is three to five times your body weight. This activity places tremendous force and stress on the feet, lower legs, knees, upper legs, hips, and back. By understanding and reacting to these principles, you can minimize this stress and the injuries that can result. This holds true not only for jogging but also for in-line skating, tennis, and many other recreational sports.

The following suggestions will help you walk and jog safely and efficiently from a biomechanical standpoint.

- Start slowly. Follow the recommendations for efficient, gentle walking and jogging shown in **Figure 2.7.**
- Breathe deeply through your nose and mouth, rather than through your nose only.
- Relax your fingers, hands, arms, shoulders, neck, and jaw.
- Bend your arms at the elbows at an angle of about 90 degrees.
- Swing your arms straight forward and back instead of across your body.
- Stand upright.
- Hold your head up, and minimize your head motion.
- Develop a smooth, even stride that feels natural and comfortable to you.
- When your foot strikes the ground, it should land on the heel.
- Try to point your toes straight ahead as your heel strikes the ground. Push off on the ball of your foot.
- Do not pound noisily as you walk or jog.
- Avoid slapping your feet and excessive bouncing.
- Try to walk or jog on a soft surface, such as a dirt road, track, or grassy area, as compared to a concrete or asphalt surface.
- Avoid hilly surfaces, because they can place unusual stress on your muscles and joints.

Use the "Fitness Check" activity on page **56** to evaluate your walking and jogging form. This information will help you prevent injuries and may improve your form. Correct biomechanical form is important for all physical activities that place stress on the body. In Chapter 11, you will learn more about biomechanics and how to apply biomechanically correct form to daily activities such as lifting.

 Reading Check

Explain Describe the biomechanically correct way your foot should strike the ground when jogging.

FIGURE 2.7

CORRECT AND INCORRECT JOGGING FORM

For effective, gentle jogging, start slowly and follow the mechanics illustrated by the top runner. *How could the bottom runner correct his form?*

Correct Form

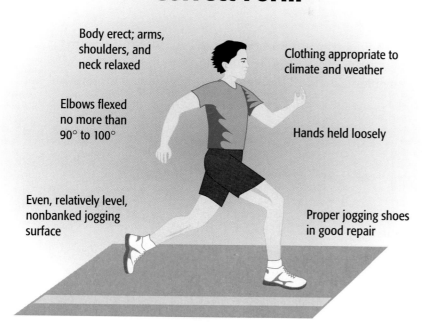

Body erect; arms, shoulders, and neck relaxed

Clothing appropriate to climate and weather

Elbows flexed no more than 90° to 100°

Hands held loosely

Even, relatively level, nonbanked jogging surface

Proper jogging shoes in good repair

Incorrect Form

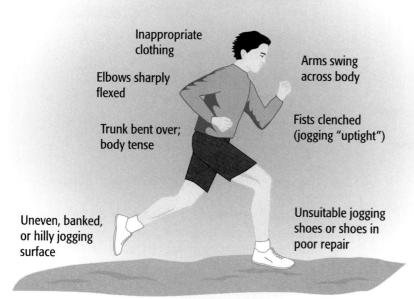

Inappropriate clothing

Arms swing across body

Elbows sharply flexed

Trunk bent over; body tense

Fists clenched (jogging "uptight")

Uneven, banked, or hilly jogging surface

Unsuitable jogging shoes or shoes in poor repair

Applying Biomechanics: Correct Walking and Jogging Checklist

Practicing correct biomechanical technique is an important part of your fitness program. Often you may not be aware that you are using incorrect technique. In this activity, you will work with a partner to identify any biomechanical problems that may affect your jogging or participation in other activities.

Biomechanic Walk/Jog Test

Procedure:

1. Select a smooth surface at least 20 yards in length.
2. Before beginning to jog, arrange with your partner to observe your jogging technique from three different perspectives and check for any biomechanical technique problems. Your partner should refer to **Figure 2.7** on page **55** in assessing your technique.
3. With your back to your partner, jog for 15 to 20 yards.
4. Turn and jog the same distance back toward your partner.
5. Finally, jog left to right to allow your partner to observe you from the side.
6. Have your partner use the Biomechanical Checklist to assess your performance. You should receive a point for each item in the list that you are doing correctly.
7. Repeat the activity while attempting to correct any needed improvement.
8. Use the Fitness Ratings Chart for Biomechanical Form to assess your performance.
9. Reverse roles with your partner and repeat steps 1 through 8.

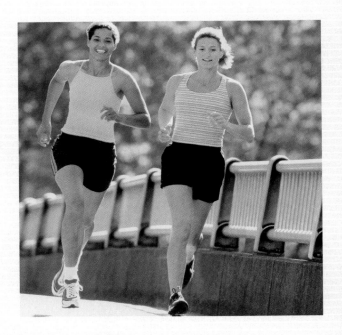

Biomechanical Checklist

✔ Breathing is relaxed and rhythmical.
✔ Hands, arms, shoulders, neck, and jaw are relaxed.
✔ Elbows are at about 90 degrees with arms swinging straight forward and back, not across the body.
✔ The upper body is erect, with minimal head motion.
✔ The stride is comfortable—the steps do not appear to be too long or too short.
✔ The foot stride is from heel to toe, with toes pointed straight ahead.
✔ There is no excessive bouncing or slapping of the feet, while applying the proper force.

Fitness Ratings for Biomechanical Form	
Points	**Rating**
6 or 7	Excellent
4 or 5	Fair
3 or less	Needs work

Common Fitness Injuries and Treatment

When people are active and in motion, injuries can happen. Luckily, most of the injuries you encounter in keeping fit will probably be minor. However, you should always pay close attention to any injury. Seek medical attention if the injury interferes with your ability to perform daily tasks or take part in your fitness program for more than a few days. The most common types of fitness injuries are to the skin, muscles, connective tissue, and bones.

Skin Injuries

Common skin injuries include cuts, scrapes, bruises, and blisters. Minor cuts and scrapes usually heal in a few days if you keep them clean. Apply antiseptic medicine to the injured area, and cover the injury with a bandage. Most minor bruises will not need treatment and will disappear in a week.

Blisters are usually caused by excessive friction between the skin and another surface. Foot blisters are common when you first start physical conditioning. They can be prevented by gradually breaking in your shoes and wearing socks that fit well. If you get a blister, treat it as you would a cut or scrape, and do not let it dry out.

Muscle Injuries

One of the most common muscle injuries is a muscle cramp. These are painful spasms that can occur during physical activity or exercise. Muscle cramps may be associated with dehydration or an imbalance of **minerals** in the body. A cramp in the side or sides of your abdomen is often referred to as a side stitch. These are commonly experienced during vigorous activities that involve running.

You can avoid most muscle cramps by making sure you follow a proper warm-up and cooldown routine, and stay hydrated. If you experience a muscle cramp, it is best to stretch the muscle and firmly massage the area. You may also want to apply moist heat to the affected area. If the cramp does not go away, you should see a doctor or health care provider.

Connective Tissue Injuries

Other common fitness-related injuries involve connective tissue. Connective tissue is the soft material that helps hold bones and joints of the body in place. There are three types of connective tissues, as shown in **Figure 2.8** on page **59**. **Tendons** are *bands of connective tissue that connect muscles to bones.* **Ligaments** are *bands of tissue that connect bone to bone and limit the movement of joints.* **Cartilage** is *tissue that surrounds the ends of bones at a joint to prevent the bones from rubbing against each other.*

Inflammation of a tendon or muscle in the leg is known as a **shin-splint.** A shinsplint is often the result of overuse. Improper footwear, running or jogging on hard surfaces, or incorrect jogging form can also cause shinsplints.

Mind OVER Matter

Exercise for Life

Physical activity, as you have seen, can improve your appearance and make you feel better. You should try, therefore, to fit workouts into your daily routine.

If you have a busy schedule, don't worry. Deal with your priorities and, as soon as possible, get back to your workout routine.

Taking time off from your routine may be good. You may find that after a break you are more relaxed and enjoy your workout even more.

hot link

minerals
For more about minerals and their role in physical activity, see Chapter 4, page **125**.

FITNESS
Online

Be prepared for emergencies. Go to **fitness. glencoe.com** for injury prevention information from the American Heart Association.

Activity Based on what you learned at this site, discuss ways to recognize sports injuries and how to respond in emergency situations.

A pull or rip in a muscle or tendon is a **strain.** Strains may result from insufficient warm-up, lack of flexibility, or overuse. Strains are painful and often result in bruising and swelling of the injured area. Never immediately apply heat to a strain. Doing so can cause additional swelling and slow the recovery process.

A tear of a ligament is called a **sprain.** They result from a sudden twisting force to a joint, such as the wrist or ankle. Like strains, they result in pain and swelling, and may be minor or severe. However, sprains are a more serious injury and should be evaluated by a health care professional for proper care.

Treatment for Connective Tissue Injuries

If you are uncertain about any pain or injury you experience during or after physical activity or exercise, it is always best to seek medical attention as soon as possible. In the event of a strain or sprain, you should immediately use the **RICE** formula. This is *a first-aid procedure for strains and sprains that become swollen.* The letters in RICE correspond to each step of the formula.

- **R**est the injured area.
- **I**ce the area to reduce swelling. (Do not apply ice directly to the skin. Use an ice pack or ice wrapped in a towel.)
- **C**ompress the area by wrapping it in an elastic bandage.
- **E**levate, or raise, the body part.

▶ The RICE formula is used to relieve muscle strains. *What is the proper treatment for muscle cramps?*

FIGURE 2.8

A JOINT AND ITS CONNECTIVE TISSUE

Connective tissue can be injured by overuse. *What types of injuries can occur to these tissues? What should you do for each type of injury?*

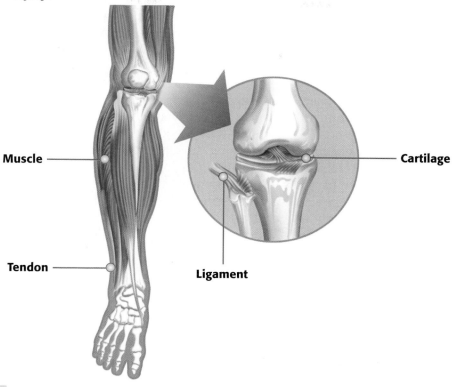

Muscle

Tendon

Ligament

Cartilage

Injuries to Bones

Injuries to bones are serious and require medical care. A **stress fracture,** one such injury, is *a break in the bone caused by overuse.* Your doctor may not be able to diagnose a stress fracture until several weeks after it occurs. Stress fractures start as a small crack in a bone. There is usually pain above and below the crack in the bone, and it is very tender to touch. Over time (four to six weeks), the stress fracture will worsen. At that time it can often be detected through X-ray examination.

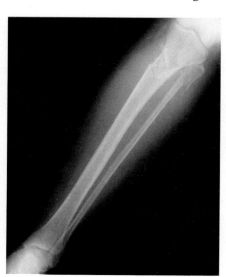

◀ An X ray might be necessary in order to detect a stress fracture. *What causes a stress fracture?*

hot link

warm-up For more on warm-up, see Chapter 3, page 102.

cooldown For more on cooldown, see Chapter 3, page 108.

FITT For more on FITT, see Chapter 3, page 83.

Preventing Injuries

While it is important for you to become physically active, it is equally important to take proper caution and avoid injury. To prevent or safely treat common injuries, follow these guidelines.

- Pay attention to your body. If you feel unusually sore or fatigued, postpone activity or exercise until you feel better.
- Include a proper **warm-up** and **cooldown** in your personal fitness program. You'll learn about warm-ups and cooldowns in the next chapter.
- Monitor the frequency, intensity, time, and type (**FITT**) of your exercise closely. Progress slowly but steadily.
- If you run or walk along busy streets, always face oncoming traffic.
- Wear reflective clothing during night physical activities or exercise, such as walking or jogging.
- Use proper safety equipment for activities with a higher injury risk, such as skateboarding, snowboarding, in-line skating, and cycling.
- Always seek out proper medical advice when you have an injury.

✓ Reading Check

Explain Tell how RICE can be used to treat muscles, connective tissue, and bone injuries.

Lesson 4 Review

Using complete sentences, answer the following questions on a sheet of paper.

Reviewing Facts and Vocabulary

1. **Vocabulary** Define *biomechanics*.
2. **Vocabulary** What do the letters in *RICE* stand for?
3. **Recall** What are the three types of connective tissue? What are two common connective tissue injuries?

Thinking Critically

4. **Summarize** Describe examples of unsafe walking/jogging techniques.

5. **Extend** During his morning run, Ian got a muscle cramp. What are two steps he can take to minimize the risk of this happening again?

Personal Fitness Planning

Investigating Fitness Plan a visit to your school's or a local athletic training facility. Interview any of the trainers about the variety of athletic injuries and treatments they administer regularly. Discuss with them the equipment used to treat injuries. Make note of the treatments used on the most common injuries.

Avoiding Harmful Substances

Each year, more people die in the United States from smoking cigarettes than from motor vehicle crashes, murders, and fires combined. Smoking diminishes a person's lung capacity, making it harder for the person to take part in physical activity. Over the long run, smoking severely compromises a person's functional health and fitness.

Why then do people choose to smoke? In this lesson, you will find some answers to that question. You will also find some compelling reasons to avoid using tobacco, alcohol, and other illegal drugs.

Why Some People Use Harmful Substances

Smoking can have serious health consequences. The consequences of using alcohol and illegal drugs, as you will see, are similarly grave. Considering these facts, why do you think so many people take such extreme risks?

What You Will Do

- Explain common myths about substance abuse.
- Identify the effects of substance abuse such as alcohol, tobacco, and other drugs on physical performance.

Terms to Know

substance abuse
addiction
smokeless tobacco
anabolic steroids

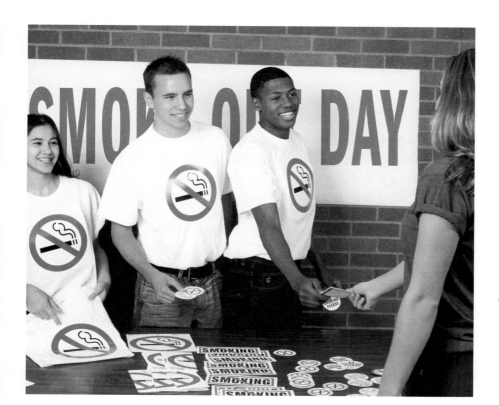

◀ While some people may find reasons to abuse harmful substances, many more find reasons to avoid them. *How many reasons can you think of to avoid harmful substances?*

Active Mind Active Body

Myths About Substance Abuse

It is important that you have a clear understanding about the myths associated with harmful substance abuse. Review the following myths. See if you already understand why they are myths. Then complete the follow-up activity provided.

What You Will Need

- Pen or pencil
- Paper

What You Will Do

- Review each of the three myths shown.

- List the reasons(s) why you believe each is a myth.
- Discuss your answers with your physical education teacher.
- Complete the follow-up activity provided.

Myth #1: Smoking is glamorous.
Reality: Smoking can speed up the aging process, making a person look older than he or she is. It also decreases your physical working ability.

Myth #2: If an alcoholic really wanted to control his or her drinking, he or she could.
Reality: Alcohol is an addictive drug. If used habitually, it can lead to the disease of alcoholism, which may require professional intervention.

Myth #3: Steroid use is an easy, painless way to become stronger.
Reality: Steroids alone will not make a person stronger. A person must also work out in order to make strength gains. In addition, there are many dangerous side effects that can accompany steroid use. These include a tendency to become violent ("roid rage"), to lose hair, and to gain unwanted hair.

Apply and Conclude

Conduct a survey to see how many people believe one or more of the myths presented here. Present the results to your class.

hotlink

peer influence For more on peer influence during the teen years, see Chapter 1, page 19.

One reason commonly cited by people is **peer influence.** Peer influence is the effect people your own age have on your thoughts and actions. Many teens claim to use these substances because they *believe* others their age are doing so. In many cases, this assumption is incorrect.

Another reason given is that smoking and drinking are viewed as cool. However, there is nothing cool about taking risks with your health and future.

Athletes who choose to take performance-enhancing drugs such as anabolic steroids claim they do so to excel at sports. As you will see, steroid use is very dangerous. This is why it is banned from professional sports.

As you may realize, a number of myths surround the use of these substances. How many of these myths are you aware of? Find out by completing the "Active Mind—Active Body" activity on this page.

Substance Abuse and Its Effects

Substance abuse is *any unnecessary or improper use of chemical substances for nonmedical purposes.* This includes alcohol, nicotine, illegal drugs, and over-the-counter medications. Alcohol, which is classified as a drug, is an abusable substance. Since it is illegal for teens to drink, consuming any amount of alcohol also constitutes a crime. It is also illegal in most localities for teens to buy cigarettes, which contain *nicotine,* a powerful stimulant drug. Any time a person uses a chemical substance or drug for recreation or any other purpose than the one intended, he or she is guilty of substance abuse.

When a person abuses harmful substances, he or she risks the possibility of damaging or ruining his or her functional health and fitness. The habitual use of many drugs and other harmful substances can lead to addiction—*physical and mental dependence.* This causes the body and mind to crave more and more of the substance.

In the remaining sections of this chapter, you will take a closer look at the health risks associated with the use of tobacco, alcohol, and steroids.

Tobacco

Cigarettes contain over 40 poisonous chemicals. Among these are the poisons arsenic and cyanide, and the gas carbon monoxide. It should be noted that smoking cigarettes is harmful not only to the smoker but to others who breathe in the smoke. Some of the health problems caused by this secondhand smoke are the same as those associated with inhaling directly.

Smoking interferes with the normal working of the lungs. Habitual smokers are three times more likely than nonsmokers to experience shortness of breath during exercise or physical activity. Smokers are also more prone to coughs and lung infections, which can hamper daily routine, including work or school.

Tobacco contains a stimulant drug, nicotine. This causes the hearts of smokers and other tobacco users to beat faster. Nicotine is also powerfully addictive, making it difficult for smokers to quit when they want to. The graphic in **Figure 2.9** on page **64** shows some other effects of smoking on the body.

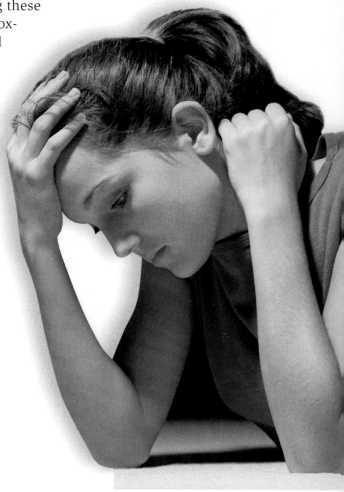

▶ Substance abuse can take a toll on the emotional and physical health of the user as well as the user's family and friends. *What are some other dangers of substance abuse?*

FIGURE 2.9

EFFECTS OF TOBACCO USE

Tobacco use seriously damages the respiratory system. *What other body systems are negatively affected by tobacco use?*

Nervous System
Short-term Effects:
Changes take place in brain chemistry. Withdrawal symptoms (nervousness, shakes, headaches) may occur as soon as 30 minutes after the last cigarette. The heart rate and blood pressure increase.

Long-term Effects: There is an increased risk of stroke due to decreased flow of oxygen to the brain.

Respiratory System
Short-term Effects: User has bad breath, shortness of breath, reduced energy, coughing, and more phlegm (mucus). Colds and flu are more frequent. Allergies and asthma problems increase. Bronchitis and other serious respiratory illnesses increase.

Long-term Effects: Risk of lung cancer, emphysema, and other lung diseases increases.

Circulatory System
Short-term Effects:
Heart rate is increased. Energy is reduced because less oxygen gets to body tissues.

Long-term Effects: Blood vessels are weakened and narrowed. Cholesterol levels increase. Blood vessels are clogged due to fatty buildup. Oxygen flow to heart is reduced. Risk of heart disease and stroke is greater.

Digestive System
Short-term Effects: User has upset stomach, bad breath, stained teeth, dulled taste buds, and tooth decay.

Long-term Effects: Risk of cancer of the mouth and throat, gum and tooth disease, stomach ulcers, and bladder cancer increases.

Smokeless Tobacco. One form of tobacco that has been popular among some athletes, and especially baseball players, is smokeless tobacco. This is *tobacco that is sniffed through the nose or chewed.* Although the use of this product has declined among athletes, who have become aware of its dangers, its teen users still number in the millions. The following are some of the facts about smokeless tobacco.

- It releases 10 times the amount of cancer-causing substances into the bloodstream than cigarettes do.
- Long-term use of smokeless tobacco can lead to an elevated heart rate and high blood pressure.
- It causes cancer of the mouth, lips, and gums.

Alcohol

Alcohol is a depressant drug. This means that it slows down the central nervous system, impairing vision, reaction time, and coordination. It also affects the function of internal organs, such as the stomach and kidneys. This may result in nausea, vomiting, and dehydration.

One of the most serious short-term dangers of using alcohol is impaired judgment, often increasing risk-taking behaviors. Combined with slowed reaction time, this factor makes drinking and any physical activity a dangerous combination.

Long-term drinking increases the risk for high blood pressure, heart rhythm disorders, heart muscle disorders, and stroke. It is also associated with the development of many cancers and liver disease. In teens, alcohol use can interfere with growth and development. The graphic in **Figure 2.10** shows some other effects of alcohol on the body.

FIGURE 2.10

EFFECTS OF ALCOHOL USE ON THE BODY

Alcohol has both short- and long-term effects on the body.
What organs are damaged by long-term alcohol use?

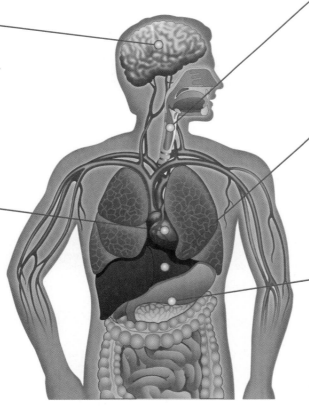

Brain and Nervous System
Short-term Effects: Speech is slurred and vision is blurred. Drinker has difficulty walking.

Long-term Effects: Brain cells, many of which cannot be replaced, are destroyed. Damage occurs to nerves through the body, resulting in numbness in the hands and feet.

Heart and Blood Vessels
Short-term Effects: Perspiration increases and skin becomes flushed.

Long-term Effects: High blood pressure and damage to the heart muscle is common. Blood vessels harden and become less flexible.

Mouth and Esophagus
Short-term Effects: Tongue, gums, and throat are affected. Breath smells of alcohol.

Long-term Effects: Damage occurs to tissues of the esophagus, resulting in possible bleeding.

Liver
Short-term Effects: Liver changes alcohol into water and carbon dioxide.

Long-term Effects: Liver is damaged, possibly resulting in **cirrhosis** (suh-ROH-sis), scarring and destruction of the liver.

Stomach and Pancreas
Short-term Effects: Stomach acids increase, which often results in nausea and vomiting.

Long-term Effects: Irritation occurs in the stomach lining, causing open sores called ulcers. Pancreas becomes inflamed.

Anabolic Steroids

Anabolic steroids are *chemicals similar in structure to the male hormone testosterone.* Steroids are used as a medicine to treat specific chronic diseases. All other uses of steroids are illegal and dangerous. Anabolic steroids are taken as pills or by injection, using syringes and needles. If needles are shared or contaminated, anabolic steroid users run a serious risk of exposure to disease-causing bacteria and viruses, including the HIV virus that causes AIDS. The federal Anabolic Steroids Act of 1990 made illegal manufacture, distribution, possession, and use of anabolic steroids a crime in all states. There is no valid medical reason for a healthy person to use steroids. This is why nonmedical use of anabolic steroids is a crime, punishable by law.

Effects of Steroid Use. Athletes sometimes use steroids in an attempt to increase weight, strength, and muscle mass. Others might use them to boost confidence and aggressiveness. However, steroid use has harmful effects on a person's physical, mental, and social health.

FIGURE 2.11

EFFECTS OF ANABOLIC STEROIDS

Anabolic steroids have serious effects for both males and females. *Which of the effects listed are the most threatening to your physical health?*

Males	Females
• Lower sperm count	• Infertility (inability to have children)
• Smaller testicles	• Deeper voice
• Increased risk of testicle or prostate cancer	• More facial hair
• Larger breasts	• Smaller breasts

Both Males and Females	
• Hair loss or baldness	• Acne
• Sleeping problems	• Upset stomach
• Rapid weight gain	• Difficulty urinating

Although steroids might increase muscle size, the tendons and ligaments that attach those muscles to the bones are not made stronger by steroid use. This imbalance between muscles and their connective tissues can result in serious injury that can take a long time to heal and can end an athlete's career. Steroids also have serious physical effects on other body systems. These are shown in **Figure 2.11.**

People who are on anabolic steroids can have wide mood swings. Happy one minute, users can suddenly feel angry and bad-tempered. Some users become impulsive and try dangerous stunts. Others get depressed and may contemplate—or commit—suicide. Both males and females can become much more aggressive on anabolic steroids. Bursts of anger called "roid rage" can result in violence; users risk harming themselves and others and may face arrest and jail time. Athletes who test positive for steroids can face exclusion from an event, expulsion from the team, monetary fines, and possibly jail time. All steroid use other than that prescribed by a doctor or physician has serious consequences to a person's health and fitness.

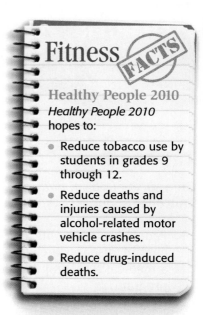

Fitness FACTS

Healthy People 2010

Healthy People 2010 hopes to:

- Reduce tobacco use by students in grades 9 through 12.
- Reduce deaths and injuries caused by alcohol-related motor vehicle crashes.
- Reduce drug-induced deaths.

Source: Modified from the National Healthy People 2010 Objectives as measured by the National Youth Risk Behavior Survey, 2001.[5]

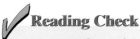 **Reading Check**

Summarize What is one physical risk associated with using anabolic steroids?

Lesson 5 Review

Using complete sentences, answer the following questions on a sheet of paper.

Reviewing Facts and Vocabulary

1. **Vocabulary** What is *addiction*?
2. **Recall** How can addiction to a substance negatively affect your functional health and fitness?
3. **Recall** Name three harmful effects of smokeless tobacco.

Thinking Critically

4. **Evaluate** Choose one substance detailed in the lesson and identify how it is harmful to physical performance.

5. **Extend** Johnny and Harrell are both age 15. They have both heard that by taking anabolic steroids and lifting weights they can increase their muscle mass more quickly than by just using weights. What advice can you give them about using anabolic steroids?

Personal Fitness Planning

Understanding Risks Research the negative effects of alcohol, tobacco, or a particular drug. Explain how the substance affects overall health, including physical performance, emotional health, and social relationships. Share your report with the class.

True or False

On a sheet of paper, write the numbers 1–8. Write True or False for each statement below.

1. People with poor lifestyle habits or known chronic diseases are strongly advised to have a medical screening before starting an exercise program.
2. In cold weather, exercise clothing should be made of a heavy material and be tight fitting to help prevent heat loss.
3. Carbon monoxide, a dangerous pollutant, is more readily absorbed by the bloodstream than oxygen.
4. It is always a good idea to try on exercise shoes with socks before you purchase them.
5. RICE stands for rest, ice, compression, and elevation.
6. Shinsplints are a type of safety equipment that should be worn to protect injury to the knees and ankles.
7. The regular use of many drugs and other harmful substances can lead to physical and mental dependence.
8. Smokeless tobacco is a less harmful tobacco product than cigarettes.

Multiple Choice

On a sheet of paper, write the letter of the word or phrase that best completes each statement.

9. Of the following, the one that is NOT an example of a chronic disease is
   a. heart disease.
   b. asthma.
   c. diabetes.
   d. common cold.
10. Of the following, all are questions that might be asked during a medical history EXCEPT
    a. what medications you may be taking.
    b. what health problems and illnesses you have had.
    c. what health problems and illnesses members of your family have had.
    d. how fast you are able to run.

11. The biological reason for perspiration during physical activity in hot weather is
    a. it cools down the body.
    b. it removes harmful chemicals that build up in the body during intense activity.
    c. it enables you to play better.
    d. none of the above.
12. Anyone exercising in extreme cold conditions is exposed to all of the following health risks EXCEPT
    a. frostbite.
    b. hypothermia.
    c. wind-chill factor.
    d. none of the above.
13. Of the following, the one that is NOT a guideline for exercising in high altitudes is
    a. drink plenty of fluids.
    b. gradually change altitude.
    c. eat meals more often to prevent altitude sickness.
    d. gradually increase exercise over a period of time.
14. An important consideration when purchasing a new pair of athletic shoes is
    a. the shape of your foot.
    b. proper support.
    c. nonskid sole.
    d. all of the above.
15. All of the following are things to look for when selecting a protective helmet EXCEPT
    a. a foam liner inside to absorb blows to the head in case of a fall.
    b. a racing stripe that shows other bikers or skaters that you mean business.
    c. a snug but comfortable fit.
    d. a chin strap and buckle so that the helmet will stay securely fastened.
16. All of the following are aspects of good biomechanical technique EXCEPT
    a. breathing deeply through your nose and mouth.
    b. keeping your arms straight down at your sides.
    c. standing nearly erect, with your head up.
    d. choosing a soft surface, such as a dirt road or grassy area as opposed to concrete or asphalt.
17. Of the following, the one that is NOT a connective body tissue is
    a. shinsplint.
    b. cartilage.
    c. ligament.
    d. tendon.

DISCUSSION

Using complete sentences, answer the following questions on a sheet of paper.

18. **Explain** Tell why it is important to know the air temperature and the amount of humidity in the air when exercising or taking part in a vigorous physical activity.
19. **Identify** List two possible non-weather-related dangers of your exercise environment. Give two safety recommendations for each.
20. **Summarize** Tell what you should consider and do before you buy a pair of physical-activity or athletic shoes.

VOCABULARY

On a sheet of paper, write the letter of the term in Column B that best fits the definition in Column A.

Column A

21. The normal motion of the foot as you walk or run.
22. A tear of a ligament.
23. Ongoing, as in a disease that continues for an extended time.
24. The study of the principles of physics applied to human motion.
25. A drop in body temperature to below normal.
26. A physical or mental dependence.

Column B

a. chronic disease
b. hypothermia
c. sprain
d. pronation
e. addiction
f. biomechanics

CRITICAL THINKING

Using complete sentences, answer the following questions on a sheet of paper.

27. **Analyze** What are the steps involved in administering the RICE treatment to injuries?
28. **Synthesize** Most serious fitness injuries can be prevented by the use of safety equipment. Give reasons why people, especially teens, may be reluctant to use safety equipment.

29. **Explain** Detail the importance of using replacement fluids during and after vigorous exercise in the heat. Tell which fluids to use and which to avoid, giving reasons in each case.

CASE STUDY

CASE STUDY—DAVID'S FITNESS PROGRAM

David is an unfit, overweight fifteen-year-old who has lived all his life in Minnesota. His family recently moved to central Texas. David has never been very athletic or physically active, and he has not paid much attention to his health or personal fitness.

Now that he has moved to a warmer climate, he would like to make some changes in his fitness habits. His goals are to lose 20 pounds and to become more physically fit overall.

David has no experience with personal fitness programs and knows little about them. He does realize that he needs the help of someone knowledgeable in designing and implementing his fitness program. He needs someone like you!

HERE IS YOUR ASSIGNMENT:

Assume that you are David's neighbor and that he has asked you to help him plan his new physically active lifestyle. Organize a list of things David should consider and do before beginning a moderate to vigorous fitness program.

KEYS TO HELP YOU

- Consider David's current medical status.
- List the concerns David must deal with as he changes from his previous environment to his new environment.
- Consider David's needs and desires.

Designing a Personal Fitness Program

FITNESS Online

What is the first thing you should do before exercising or taking part in a sport? What is the last thing you should do? How do you set your fitness goals? To find out the answers to these questions, take the STEP Personal Inventory for Chapter 3. Find it at **fitness.glencoe.com**.

Health-Related and Skill-Related Fitness

Jack is on the school track team. His dream is to become an Olympic sprinter. The team coach believes Jack has real potential. "You just have to be willing to work hard," the coach has told him.

Jack is not sure what the coach means. How, he wonders, can a person work at becoming a better runner? Is it possible to increase your speed? After reading this lesson, you will know the answers to Jack's questions.

Health-Related Fitness vs. Skill-Related Fitness

As you learned in Chapter 1, total physical fitness includes both of the following:

- **Health-related fitness.** This is your ability to become and stay physically healthy.
- **Skill-related fitness.** This is your ability to maintain high levels of performance on the playing field.

While your level of skill-related fitness is reflected in how well you perform a physical activity, your level of health-related fitness provides a measure of your physical health. Improving in one area may lead to improvements in the other.

What You Will Do

- Identify the specific components of health-related and skill-related fitness.
- Compare and contrast health-related and skill-related fitness.
- Analyze factors that influence your health-related and skill-related fitness.
- Demonstrate the skill-related components of fitness.

Terms to Know

energy cost
agility
balance
coordination
speed
power
reaction time

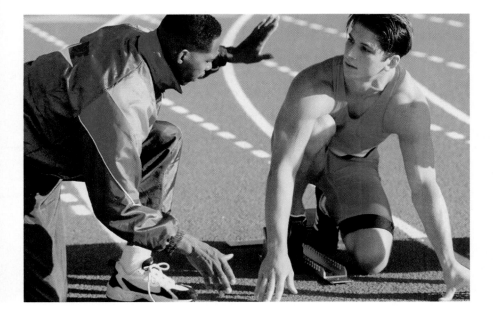

It is possible to improve both your health-related and skill-related fitness. *How do you think participating in a sport, such as track, can help you develop both health- and skill-related fitness?*

Health-Related Fitness

There are five components, or measures, of health-related fitness. These are:

- **Body composition.** This is the relative percentage of body fat to lean body tissue, including water, bone, muscle, and connective tissue.
- **Cardiovascular fitness.** This is the ability of your body to work continuously for extended periods of time. Because this involves your lungs as well as your heart and vessels, cardiovascular fitness is sometimes called **cardiorespiratory endurance.**
- **Muscular strength.** This refers to the maximum amount of force a muscle or muscle group can exert against an opposing force.
- **Muscular endurance.** This refers to the ability of the same muscle or muscle group to contract for an extended period of time without undue fatigue.
- **Flexibility.** This is the ability to move a body part through a full range of motion.

Levels of **health-related fitness** for any given component vary from person to person. These differences are due partly to heredity and partly to other, external factors. Some people, for example, are born with greater muscular strength, others with greater flexibility. As you will see, however, it is possible to improve in all of these areas.

 Reading Check

List Name the five components of health-related fitness.

Body Composition. For most people, the most critical factor in **body composition** is body fat. While some body fat is important, too much can impair your functional health and increase your risks for chronic disease. By the same token, too little body fat—being too lean—can also be problematic.

By adopting a physically active lifestyle, you can help control your percentage of body fat. When you engage in physical activities or exercise, you burn or expend energy. The source of this energy is found in calories from the foods you eat. Calories that are not expended are stored by the body as fat.

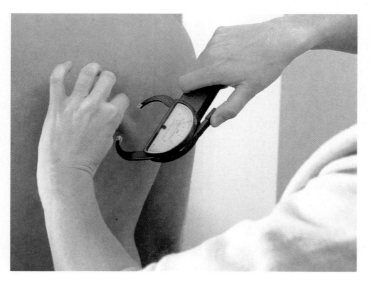

◀ One method for determining body composition is to measure a skin fold with a tool called a caliper. Males should carry 7 to 19 percent body fat, females 12 to 24 percent.

hot link

cardiorespiratory endurance
For more on cardiorespiratory endurance, see Chapter 7, page **198.**

body composition
For more on measuring body composition, see Chapter 5, page **162.**

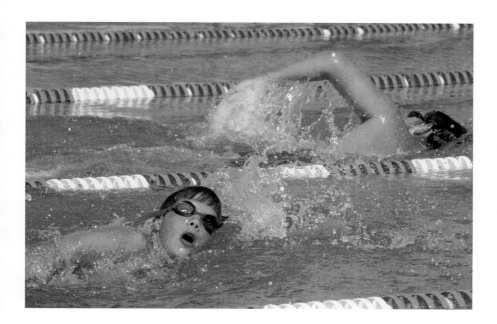

 Swimming laps is an excellent activity for increasing your muscular endurance. *What other component of health-related fitness does swimming improve?*

Cardiovascular Fitness. Cardiovascular fitness, or cardiorespiratory endurance, is a function of how well your heart and lungs do their job. Moderate to high levels of cardiovascular fitness have been shown to increase life expectancy, reduce the risk of cardiovascular disease, and improve functional health.

A number of activities and exercises promote cardiovascular fitness. These include brisk walking, hiking, jogging, dancing, skipping rope, rowing, swimming, and skating.

Muscular Strength. Muscular strength is partly determined by factors beyond your control. These include age, gender, and heredity. Individual levels of muscular strength can be increased, however, through weight training, **calisthenics,** or similar exercises. Work that requires heavy lifting will also lead to gains in muscular strength.

A moderate to high level of muscular strength improves functional health and fitness. It also helps reduce your risk for muscle, bone, and joint injuries. In addition, muscular strength contributes to more efficient movement and reduces your energy cost. Energy cost is *the amount of energy needed to perform different physical activities or exercises.*

Muscular Endurance. Like muscular strength, **muscular endurance** helps you move more efficiently. The higher your level of muscular endurance, the lower your energy cost. You are thus able to do more physical work without tiring.

Exercises such as sit-ups and push-ups can increase muscular endurance. So can work that requires repetitive heavy lifting. You will learn more about muscular endurance in Chapters 9 and 10.

✓ Reading Check

Compare Explain the difference between muscular strength and muscular endurance.

hot link

calisthenics
For more on calisthenics, see Chapter 9, page **266.**

muscular endurance
For more on measuring muscular endurance, see Chapter 9, page **267.**

▶ Flexibility enhances your performance in sports as well as helps you maintain a high level of functional fitness. *In addition to gymnastics, what other sports require a high level of flexibility?*

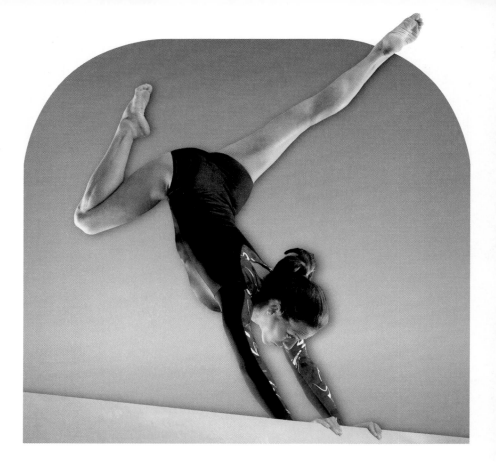

flexibility
For more on flexibility and exercises that can improve it, see Chapter 11, page **334**.

Stress and Stretching

It is not uncommon for people who sit most of the day to have headaches and neck aches. Do you suffer from either of these problems? They are caused by muscle stress. Messages from your body include clenched teeth and rigid shoulders.

Through basic stretching exercises, you can avoid muscle stress. Moving your shoulders in a circular motion will stretch the muscles, easing the tension.

Flexibility. A moderate to high level of **flexibility** is central to efficient physical movement. It can also

- help reduce your risk for muscle and bone injuries.
- improve performance fitness.
- reduce some types of muscle soreness following physical activity or exercise.
- improve functional health and fitness.

You can achieve moderate to high levels of flexibility through stretching activities, some of which are provided in Chapter 11.

Skill-Related Fitness

Why are some individuals capable of outstanding physical performance? How can a track star high jump seven feet? What enables the Olympic weight lifter to lift massive amounts of weight? Why aren't all people capable of such physical feats? The answer to these questions can be summed up in one term: *skill-related fitness.*

As noted in Chapter 1, another name for skill-related fitness is *performance fitness.* Skill-related fitness has six components, or measures. These are *agility, balance, coordination, speed, power,* and *reaction time.* Highly skilled athletes generally excel in most, and sometimes all six, areas.

Like health-related fitness, skill-related fitness can enhance your ability to complete daily chores and other physical tasks unrelated to exercise. Unlike health-related fitness, skill-related fitness will not necessarily reduce lifestyle-related health risks.

Agility. What do skilled football running backs have in common with successful soccer players? The answer is agility. This is *the ability to change and control the direction and position of the body while maintaining a constant, rapid motion.* Other skill-related components of fitness, such as speed and coordination, may influence your level of agility. Sports that require a high level of agility include football, soccer, basketball, baseball, and softball.

Balance. This is *the ability to control or stabilize the body while standing or moving.* A simple act such as walking requires a great deal of balance. The gymnast, golfer, and ice skater all need high degrees of balance. Balance helps you maintain control while coordinating your movements.

Balance in sports depends in large measure on biomechanics. As explained in Chapter 2, biomechanics is the application of principles of physics to human motion. Often, redistributing body weight will result in improved balance and, hence, performance in a sport. For example, many golfers are able to improve their swing by shifting their body weight so that the weight is evenly distributed. Basketball players can improve their defensive plays by widening their stance. This provides a wider base of support and lowers the center of gravity to improve balance and overall performance.

Coordination. This is *the ability to use the senses to determine and direct the movement of your limbs and head.* Gymnastics, cheerleading, and juggling demand a high level of coordination.

Coordination requires using a combination of different muscle groups at once. This ability can be sharpened with practice. Other components of skill-related fitness, such as speed, reaction time, and agility, may influence your level of coordination. Like balance, coordination can be improved by widening the base of support and lowering your center of gravity.

Agility is the component of skill-related fitness that accounts for this running back's "quick feet." *What other sports can you name that require a high degree of agility?*

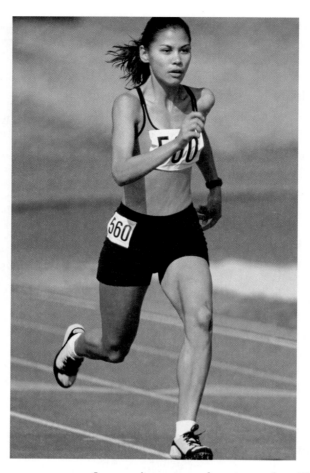

► This athlete possesses extraordinary levels of speed and power.

Speed. This is *the ability to move your body, or parts of it, swiftly.* Foot speed is usually measured over a short and straight distance, usually less than 200 meters. Other speed evaluations might include hand or arm speed. The baseball pitcher, boxer, sprinter, and volleyball spiker all require specific kinds of speed.

Although speed is largely determined by heredity, speed can be increased. Building muscular strength, for example, can lead to speed gains.

Power. This is *the ability to move the body parts swiftly while simultaneously applying the maximum force of your muscles.* Power is thus a function of both speed and muscular strength. The long jump, power lifting, and swimming all require high levels of power.

Increasing muscular strength will lead to improvements in power. Proper biomechanics can also enhance power by improving your balance, coordination, and speed.

Reaction Time. This is *the ability to react or respond quickly to what you hear, see, or feel.* The quicker your response, the better your reaction time.

Good reaction time is important to sprinters and swimmers, who must react to starts. The tennis player, boxer, and hockey goalie all require quick reaction times as well. Factors such as decreased motivation and increased fatigue can slow your reaction time. Finding ways to stay motivated and practicing regularly will improve your reaction time.

Some activities and sports mainly benefit skill-related fitness, while others might be more beneficial to health-related fitness. Some, like volleyball and cross-country skiing, benefit both areas of fitness. **Figure 3.1** lists several activities, each followed by an *S* if its benefits are mainly skill-related, an *H* if its benefits are health-related, or a *B* if it is beneficial for both. The chart also ranks each activity according to the individual components of skill- and health-related fitness.

✔ **Reading Check**

Extend Name a sport or activity that requires at least three components of skill-related fitness.

FIGURE 3.1

BENEFITS OF PHYSICAL ACTIVITIES

Which of these sports or activities are you currently involved in?
How do they compare in each of the 11 areas of skill- and health-related fitness?

Activity or Sport	Skill-Related Fitness						Health-Related Fitness				
	A	**B**	**R**	**P**	**S**	**C**	**CF**	**F**	**MS**	**ME**	**BC**
Archery *S*	1	3	1	1	3	4	1	2	3	1	1
Backpacking *H*	2	2	1	2	2	2	3	3	2	4	3
Ballet *B*	4	4	2	3	2	4	3	4	4	3	3
Baseball *S*	3	3	4	4	3	4	1	3	3	1	1
Basketball *B*	4	3	4	4	3	4	3	3	3	3	3
Bicycling *H*	1	4	2	1	2	2	4	2	2	4	3
Canoeing *B*	1	3	2	3	3	3	2	2	3	3	2
Circuit training *H*	2	2	1	3	3	2	2	3	3	4	3
Dance, aerobic *H*	3	2	2	1	1	4	4	3	2	3	4
Dance, social *H*	3	2	2	1	2	3	2	2	2	2	2
Fitness calisthenics *H*	3	2	1	2	2	2	1	4	2	3	2
Football *S*	4	3	4	4	4	3	2	2	4	2	2
Golf (walking) *B*	2	2	1	3	1	4	2	4	2	1	4
Gymnastics *B*	4	4	3	4	2	4	2	4	4	4	4
Handball *H*	4	2	3	3	3	4	4	3	2	3	3
Hiking *H*	2	2	1	2	1	2	3	2	2	4	3
Interval training *H*	2	2	1	1	2	2	4	1	3	3	4
Jogging *H*	1	2	1	1	1	2	4	1	2	3	4
Judo *S*	4	3	4	4	4	4	1	4	2	2	3
Karate *S*	4	3	4	4	4	4	1	4	4	2	3
Racquetball *B*	4	2	3	2	3	4	4	2	2	3	3
Rope jumping *H*	3	2	2	2	2	3	3	2	2	3	3
Rowing *H*	3	2	1	4	2	4	4	2	2	4	4
Skating, ice *B*	3	4	2	2	3	4	3	2	2	3	4
Skating, in-line *B*	3	4	1	2	3	4	3	2	1	3	4
Skiing, cross-country *B*	3	2	1	4	2	4	4	3	2	3	4
Skiing, downhill *B*	4	4	3	3	3	4	2	3	3	2	3
Soccer *B*	4	2	3	3	3	4	4	2	2	3	4
Softball (fast pitch) *S*	3	2	4	3	3	4	3	2	3	1	1
Softball (slow pitch) *S*	2	2	3	3	3	4	2	1	3	1	1
Surfing *B*	4	4	3	3	2	4	2	3	2	3	4
Swimming *H*	3	2	1	2	2	4	4	3	2	3	4
Tennis *B*	3	2	3	3	3	4	4	2	3	3	3
Volleyball *B*	3	2	3	2	3	4	3	2	3	2	3
Walking *H*	1	2	1	1	1	2	3	1	1	2	3
Weight training *H*	2	3	1	2	1	3	1	3	4	3	4

Legend

S = Skill-Related Fitness	2 = Fair	**P** = Power	**MS** = Muscular Strength
H = Health-Related Fitness	1 = Low	**S** = Strength	**ME** = Muscular Endurance
B = Both of the Above	**A** = Agility	**C** = Coordination	**BC** = Body Composition
4 = Excellent	**B** = Balance	**CF** = Cardiovascular Fitness	
3 = Good	**R** = Reaction Time	**F** = Flexibility	

Demonstrating Skill-Related Fitness

In this activity, you will do six tests, one for each of the six skill-related fitness components. As you progress through later chapters, you may want to retake one or more of these tests to assess your progress.

Demonstrating Agility: Picking Up Lines

Procedure:
1. Mark off two parallel lines 5 feet apart.
2. Start at one line. Run to the other line and bend over to touch the line with your hand, as in **Figure 3.2**.
3. Reverse your direction and return to the start, again bending over to touch the line.
4. Repeat steps 2 and 3. Do not stop running until you have completed two full circuits.
5. Use the Fitness Ratings Chart for Picking Up Lines to assess your performance.

Fitness Ratings: Picking Up Lines	
Time	Rating
Under 5 seconds	Pass
Over 5 seconds	Needs work

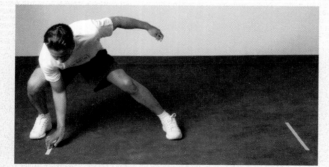

Figure 3.2

Demonstrating Balance: Blind One-Leg Stand

Procedure:
1. Stand on one foot.
2. Gently pull your other leg up and back. Do not pull back in a way that puts stress on your knee. Do not wobble or hop. Close your eyes (see **Figure 3.3**).
3. Try to hold this position for ten seconds.
4. Use the Fitness Ratings Chart for the Blind One-Leg Stand to assess your performance.

Fitness Ratings: Blind One-Leg Stand	
Time	Rating
10 seconds or more	Pass
Under 10 seconds	Needs work

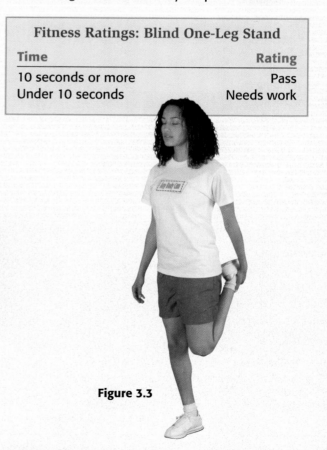

Figure 3.3

Demonstrating Coordination: Foot-and-Ball Volley

Procedure:
1. For this activity you will need a ball at least the size of a tennis ball or bigger.
2. Drop the ball over your dominant foot, as shown in see **Figure 3.4.** (Your dominant foot is the one you usually kick with.)
3. Try to bounce the ball off your foot three consecutive times.
4. Now try it with your other foot.
5. Use the Fitness Ratings Chart for Foot-and-Ball Volley to assess your performance.

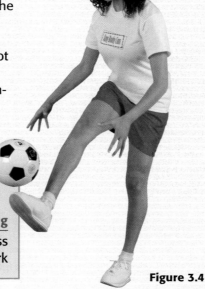

Fitness Ratings: Foot-and-Ball Volley

Number of Bounces	Rating
3 bounces or more	Pass
Under 3 bounces	Needs work

Figure 3.4

Demonstrating Power: Standing Long Jump

Procedure:
1. Lie on the floor.
2. Have a partner mark off two lines, one at the top of your head and one at your feet.
3. Stand up. Starting at either line, jump as far as you can toward the other line. (See **Figure 3.5.**)
4. Use the Fitness Ratings Chart for the Standing Long Jump to assess your performance.

Fitness Ratings: Standing Long Jump

Jump Height	Rating
Jump your height or greater	Pass
Jump less than your height	Needs work

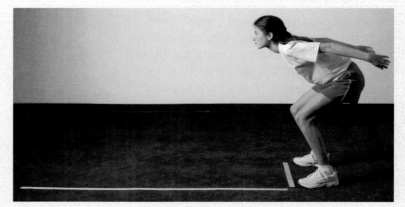

Figure 3.5

continued on next page

Demonstrating Speed: Push and Clap

Procedure:

1. Lie face down on the floor in a push-up position.
2. Place your hands on the floor so that they line up alongside your chest.
3. Push your body up in the air. Try to clap your hands twice before returning to the floor, as in **Figure 3.6.** Use a mat if one is available.
4. Use the Fitness Ratings Chart for Push and Clap to assess your performance.

Fitness Ratings: Push and Clap	
Number of Completions	**Rating**
1 completion	Pass
No completions	Needs work

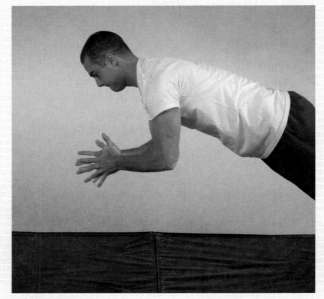

Figure 3.6

Demonstrating Reaction Time: Hand Slap

Procedure:

1. Stand facing a partner.
2. Have your partner place his or her hands palms up. Place your hands palms down over your partner's hands. Allow 4 inches of space between your hands and your partner's.
3. Your partner will quickly attempt to touch the top of your hands as in **Figure 3.7.** Try to remove your hands before they are touched.
4. Use the Fitness Ratings Chart for Hand Slap to assess your performance.

Fitness Ratings: Hand Slap	
Result	**Rating**
Do not touch	Pass
Touch	Needs work

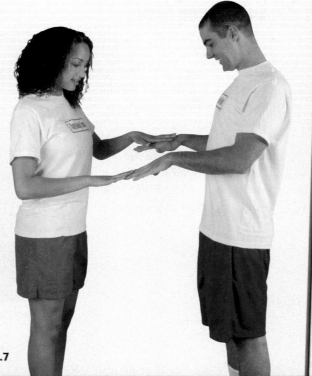

Figure 3.7

Health-Related Fitness, Skill-Related Fitness, and You

According to some estimates, heredity may account for as much as 70 percent of your skill-related fitness and 40 percent of your health-related fitness. Does this mean that only people born with the gift of speed or strength can achieve high levels of fitness in these areas? Not necessarily. Low levels of fitness do not have to be permanent. Any of these 11 components can be nurtured and developed. One key is practice.

Practice is important for anyone who wants to improve his or her skills and performance in a specific game or sport. Agility, coordination, and power, in particular, are skill-related components that can be improved through practice. Often, one skill-related ability requires the use of other skill-related components. For this reason, working to improve one skill may lead to benefits in other areas.

Health-related fitness can be improved by participating in many physical activities that are not necessarily related to sports or games. In fact, some of the most popular physical activities, such as swimming, bicycling, hiking, and jogging, are not sports- or game-related.

In the lessons and chapters to come, you will learn exercises and activities that will lead to improvements in your health-related and skill-related fitness. Whether you make these behaviors a part of your lifestyle is up to you. The next step is yours.

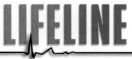

Hidden Benefits

Among the benefits of developing your health-related and skill-related fitness is your improved ability to demonstrate positive self-management and social skills needed to work with others. Think of an example when you have had an opportunity to recognize a potential conflict during a game, sport, or physical activity. Explain how you were able to apply positive behaviors and find a way to resolve the conflict so that you and your teammates could continue playing or participating in an activity.

Lesson 1 Review

Using complete sentences, answer the following questions on a sheet of paper.

Reviewing Facts and Vocabulary

1. **Recall** What physical activities require a high level of balance, coordination, and speed? Why?

2. **Vocabulary** List and define each of the five health-related fitness components.

Thinking Critically

3. **Compare and Contrast** What is the difference between health-related and skill-related fitness?

4. **Evaluation** Clint and Ellen are both 15. Clint is interested in developing his skill-related fitness, particularly his speed and agility. Ellen is interested in developing her health-related fitness, particularly her muscular endurance. Make a list of hints and tips you can give Clint and Ellen to help them meet their initial goals.

Personal Fitness Planning

Assessing Progress Make a chart of your Fitness Ratings on the "Fitness Check" activities in Chapters 1 and 3. In which health-related and skill-related activities do you perform well? Which are your weaker areas? Make a list and plan to improve in as many of those areas as possible.

What You Will Do

- List the components of exercise prescription.
- Describe the overload principle and how it applies to a fitness program.
- Apply the physiological principles of frequency, intensity, time, and type to a fitness program.
- Describe methods of evaluating levels of intensity in a workout.

Terms to Know

exercise prescription
overload principle
frequency
cardiovascular conditioning
intensity
heart rate
perceived exertion
talk test
time
type

▶ Exercise prescription is the "dose" of exercise you need to maintain a high level of fitness. *Why is it important to make sure your exercise prescription is the right "dose"?*

FITT and the Principle of Overload

Has a doctor ever prescribed a medication for you? Such medications come with a recommended dose on the label. A dose is the amount a person needs to receive the medication's benefit.

Did you know that physical activity and exercise are also dose-related? Unlike medications, these fitness behaviors never require a doctor's prescription. *You* control the dose. In so doing, you also control the benefits.

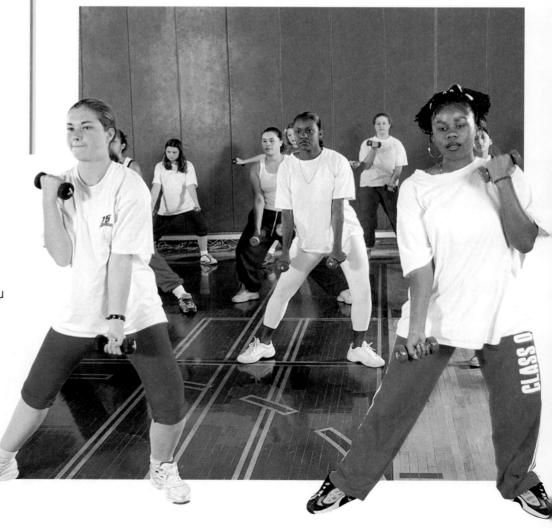

Your Exercise Prescription

In order to be effective, a medical prescription must be exact. It must include the name of the medicine, the dose needed, and how often the medicine should be taken. The same information needs to be present in an **exercise prescription.** This is *a breakdown of how often you need to work, how hard, the length of time per session, and the type of activity or exercise performed.* As shown in **Figure 3.8,** these factors of exercise prescription are often referred to as FITT: *frequency, intensity, time,* and *type.*

Like medications, exercise prescriptions are governed by three scientific principles: the overload principle, the specificity principle, and the progression principle. The **overload principle** states that *in order to improve your level of fitness, you must increase the amount of regular activity or exercise that you normally do.* You will learn more about the principles of specificity and progression in Lessons 3 and 4.

These principles are applied to an exercise program by adjusting any or all of the FITT factors in your prescription. These are:

- *frequency*—how often you work.
- *intensity*—how hard you work.
- *time*—the length of time, or duration, that you work.
- *type*—the specific type or mode of activity you choose.

Reading Check

Summarize List and describe the components of exercise prescription.

FIGURE 3.8

THE PARTS OF **FITT**
FITT stands for frequency, intensity, time, and type of activity. *How can each of these aspects of working out be adjusted to suit your goals and experience level?*

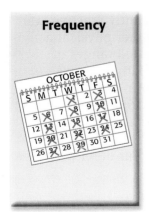
Frequency

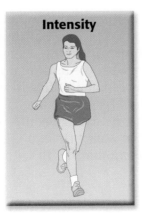
Intensity

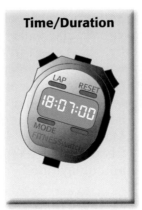
Time/Duration

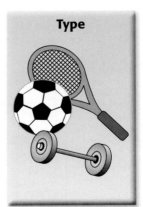
Type

FIGURE 3.9

FREQUENCY OF EXERCISES FOR VARYING FITNESS LEVELS

The frequency of your activity depends largely on your fitness level. *Based on this chart and your current level of activity, how often should you exercise in order to reach overload?*

Type of Activity	Frequency for Beginners	Frequency for Those of Average- to High-Fitness Levels
Cardiovascular conditioning	3–5 days per week	4–6 days per week
Weight training	2–3 days per week	3–5 days per week

Frequency

Frequency refers to *the number of times per week you engage in physical activity or exercise.* Exercise that is infrequent results in limited progress. Exercising too often can increase the possibility of injury.

How frequently do you need to do a particular activity or exercise in order to achieve overload? The answer to that question will depend on the intensity of your workouts, how much time you invest in each, and the type of activity you do. Other considerations include:

- **Your specific fitness goals.** Do you want to raise your levels of health-related fitness? Do you want to improve your performance on the playing field? One basic goal that should be part of every teen's fitness program is cardiovascular conditioning. This consists of *exercises or activities that improve the efficiency of the heart, lungs, blood, and blood vessels.*
- **Your current level of fitness.** Are you currently inactive? Do you regularly play sports or take part in other physical activities? The chart in **Figure 3.9** shows suggested ranges of workout frequency for people at different fitness levels.
- **Other priorities and responsibilities in your daily life.** As a teen, one of your chief responsibilities is school—getting an education. You probably also have after-school activities. Maybe you hold down a part-time job. You will want to set a frequency for exercising that fits in with your other priorities and obligations.

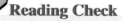

Reading Check

Explain What is the result if exercise frequency is limited?

Intensity

Intensity refers to *the difficulty or exertion level of your physical activity or exercise.* If the intensity is too low, progress is limited. If you work too hard, you fatigue quickly and increase your risk for injury.

How intense your workouts are will depend partly on the other three factors in the FITT formula: *frequency, time,* and *type.* Several additional methods can help you determine your intensity needs. These are explained in the sections that follow. The "Active Mind—Active Body" in Lesson 3 will help you to understand how increasing intensity affects your heart rate.

Percentage of Maximum Heart Rate. For cardiovascular conditioning, a reliable measure of intensity is a percentage of your maximum heart rate. The term **heart rate** refers to *the number of times your heart beats per minute.* Another name for heart rate is pulse. You will learn how to take your pulse in the "Active Mind—Active Body" activity on page **86.**

To compute your *maximum heart rate,* subtract your age from the number 220. (If you are currently 15, for example, your maximum heart rate is 205 beats per minute.) Once you know your maximum heart rate, you can refer to the chart in **Figure 3.10** for conditioning guidelines. As with the other components of exercise prescription, you need to take into account your current level of fitness. Beginners should work at a lower level of intensity than those with average-to-high fitness levels.

FIGURE 3.10

INTENSITY OF EXERCISES FOR VARYING FITNESS LEVELS

Your heart rate can help you determine the intensity of your workout. ***Using your maximum heart rate, how many times should your heart beat per minute if you are 16 years old and just beginning cardiovascular training?***

Type of Activity	Intensity for Beginners	Intensity for Those of Average- to High-Fitness Levels
Cardiovascular conditioning	60 to 70 percent maximum heart rate	70 to 90 percent maximum heart rate
Weight training	60 to 70 percent maximum strength	70 to 90 percent maximum strength

As noted, your heart rate, or pulse, can help you figure out your intensity needs for physical activity or exercise. In this activity, you will learn how to measure your heart rate.

What You Will Need

- Pen or pencil
- Paper
- Stopwatch, wristwatch, or clock

What You Will Do

1. Using two fingers on one hand, find the carotid (kuh-ROT-id) pulse on *one side* of your throat. Do *not* use your thumb, which has a pulse of its own.
2. *Press lightly* until you feel a slight throbbing sensation.
3. Using a clock or watch, count the number of throbs, or beats, in six seconds.
4. Record the number of beats. Add a zero to get your heart rate for one minute.
5. Now find your radial pulse on the thumb side of your wrist.
6. Repeat steps 3 and 4.

Apply and Conclude

What reading did you get for your carotid pulse? Was it the same as for your radial pulse? Try taking a partner's pulse. To get your true resting pulse, you will need to perform one of these techniques the instant you wake up in the morning. Why would taking your pulse then make a difference?

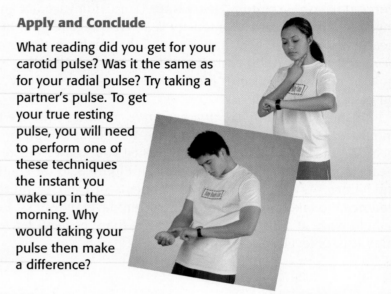

Perceived Exertion. Another method of determining intensity is using **perceived exertion.** This is *a measure of how hard you feel you are working during physical activity or exercise.* This rating is usually used to determine intensity of cardiorespiratory workouts. **Ratings of perceived exertion (RPE)** are based on your awareness of specific body "cues." These cues include how hard you are breathing, your heart rate, your body temperature, and any muscle or skeletal discomfort.

The perceived exertion scale in **Figure 3.11** assigns numerical values to different levels of perceived exertion. Notice that the range is from 6 ("no exertion at all") to 20 ("maximum exertion"). What rating would you assign to yourself at this moment?

Talk Test. A fourth method for monitoring your intensity uses the perceived exertion scale. It is also used in cardiorespiratory evaluations. This method is the **talk test.** It is *a measure of your ability to carry on a conversation while engaged in physical activity or exercise.* For example, if you are able to talk with some slight effort during a workout, your RPE is probably between 11 and 16 (light to vigorous). This is an appropriate intensity level for your fitness program.

RPE
For more on using the RPE scale, see Chapter 7, page **209.**

If talking is very difficult or impossible, you are overdoing it. If you are able to talk effortlessly, you are not working hard enough to derive benefits.

Percentage of Maximum Strength. For weight training, a useful gauge of intensity is a percentage of your **maximum strength.** *Maximum strength* is a measure of how much weight you can lift one time for a given exercise. Suppose, for example, that for a particular exercise you were able to lift 100 pounds just once. Then your maximum strength for that exercise would be 100.

Once you know your maximum strength, you can use the guidelines in **Figure 3.10** (on page 85) to determine a recommended intensity.

hot link

maximum strength
For more on maximum strength, see Chapter 10, page **308.**

FIGURE 3.11

PERCEIVED EXERTION SCALE
This scale reflects how hard a person feels he or she has worked during physical activity or exercise.

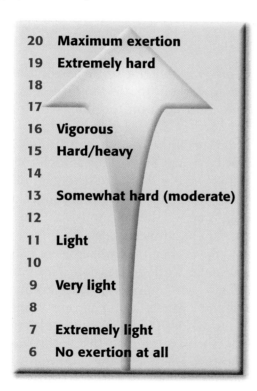

20	**Maximum exertion**
19	**Extremely hard**
18	
17	
16	**Vigorous**
15	**Hard/heavy**
14	
13	**Somewhat hard (moderate)**
12	
11	**Light**
10	
9	**Very light**
8	
7	**Extremely light**
6	**No exertion at all**

Source: Borg's Perceived Exertion and Pain Scales, 2002[1]

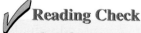

Reading Check

Identify What are the three methods for evaluating intensity that are used in cardiorespiratory conditioning?

FIGURE 3.12

EXERCISE TIME BASED ON FITNESS LEVEL

Based on this chart, how long should your exercise sessions last if you are just beginning cardiovascular conditioning? How long should sessions last if you are an experienced weight lifter?

Type of Activity	Time for Beginners	Time for Those of Average- to High-Fitness Levels
Cardiovascular conditioning	20–30 minutes	35 minutes to 1 hour
Weight training	20–30 minutes	45 minutes to 1 hour

Time

Time refers to *the duration of a single workout, usually measured in minutes or hours.* A workout that is too brief may result in limited progress. A workout that goes on too long will increase your risk for injuries.

Once again, your specific goals, current fitness level, frequency, intensity, time, and type will play a role in determining how much time to devote to a particular workout. The goal of weight loss, for example, is best accomplished by working longer at a lower intensity. Weight-training time will be determined by the number of exercises done and time spent between sets.

As **Figure 3.12** shows, beginning exercisers should do 20 to 30 minutes of cardiovascular work per session. This pace will allow you to progress slowly and safely and to increase gradually.

You may accumulate your minutes in one, continuous workout, or you may choose to work out in two or three shorter intervals per day. For example, you may choose to take a brisk walk for ten minutes in the morning, another in the afternoon, and again in the evening.

If you already have an average-to-high fitness level, you may find that the length of your workouts needs to be longer. One way to gradually increase your time is by alternating days with longer workouts (45 minutes to 1 hour) with days having shorter workouts (20 to 30 minutes).

The beginning weight trainer should spend 20 to 30 minutes per workout. How does this compare with the time needs of individuals with average to high fitness levels?

Type of Activity

The final component of the FITT formula is type. Type refers to *the particular type of physical activity or exercise you choose to do.* As a teen, you should be physically active on a daily basis. You should also engage in three or more sessions per week of activities that last at least 20 minutes and require moderate-to-vigorous levels of exertion. However, the choice and type of activity you participate in are up to you.

You should consider your personal fitness goals when choosing your activities. For example, if your goal is to improve your cardiovascular fitness, you should select activities that rate highly in that area, such as swimming, jogging, or cycling. Reviewing **Figure 3.1** in Lesson 1 can provide you with suggestions about the types of activities you may want to include in your program, depending on your personal goals.

The type of activity and the particular activity you do should be guided by several considerations. These include:

- What you enjoy doing
- How much time you have for the activity
- How much money you can afford to spend on needed equipment

 Reading Check

Describe What does *type* refer to in an exercise prescription?

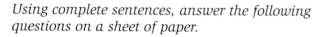
Lesson 2 Review

Using complete sentences, answer the following questions on a sheet of paper.

Reviewing Facts and Vocabulary

1. **Vocabulary** What is an *exercise prescription?*
2. **Vocabulary** Describe *overload principle.*
3. **Recall** What is the talk test? How and when should you use it?

Thinking Critically

4. **Compare and Contrast** What is the difference between frequency and time in a fitness program?
5. **Evaluation** Mike and Bill are both age 15. Mike is beginning a cardiovascular training program. Bill, who runs every day, wants to increase his cardiovascular fitness level. What tips can you give Mike and Bill about how long they need to work to improve or maintain their cardiovascular fitness levels?

Personal Fitness Planning

Applying Physiological Principles Review the plans you made in Lesson 1 to improve your performance in health-related and skill-related activities. Schedule a fitness workout for yourself to practice some of your weaker activities over the next month. How would you apply overload, frequency, intensity, time, and type to your plan?

The Principle of Specificity

What You Will Do

- Describe the specificity principle and how it applies to a fitness program.
- Design goals for your fitness program.

Terms to Know

specificity principle
short-term goals
long-term goals

Sophia wanted to improve her overall grade point average. She came up with a plan that focused specifically on improving her grades in English and then biology, her two weakest areas. After a few months of concentrated effort in those classes, Sophia succeeded.

In the last lesson you learned about the principle of overload in exercise prescription. Sophia's story is an example of another important component of any plan: *specificity*. Not only did she work harder, she worked harder in specific areas that would help her reach her goal.

Specificity and Fitness

The specificity principle states that *overloading a particular component will lead to fitness improvements in that component alone.* Every exercise or physical activity works at least one component. For example, cardiovascular conditioning works a component, the heart muscle.

Any component or muscle that is not involved in the exercise or activity will remain unchanged. If you lift weights, for example, muscles that are not required to help move the weights will not become stronger.

▼ Targeting specific areas can help you achieve your overall goal. *What specific area of your personal fitness would you like to target?*

Specificity and Change

The specific improvements that result from conditioning or training depend on the activity or exercise in which you engage. Suppose, for example, your goal is to become a better in-line skater. You will get the best results by focusing on conditioning and skill while you actually skate. Other activities, such as cycling on a regular basis, may lead to some improvements. However, these changes will not be as noticeable as they would be if your conditioning were *specific* to in-line skating.

To apply the specificity principle effectively, you need to evaluate your personal fitness goals and design a plan that will target specific areas of your fitness.

Goal Setting

Setting goals is essential to the success of any effort. Some goals are short-term goals. These are *goals that can be accomplished relatively easily and quickly.* Other goals are long-term goals. They are *goals that are more complex and require considerable time and planning.* Fitness goals require both short-term and long-term planning. The **behavioral-change stairway,** discussed in Chapter 1, is a good strategy for achieving your fitness goals.

Note that high-performance goals require more specific and detailed fitness plans than those for moderate levels of fitness and health. Consider Rita's goal: to take a 50-mile mountain-bike trip. Rita's short-term preparation includes mountain-bike riding on hilly courses. She is also doing a good deal of cardiovascular conditioning. This is because she understands that her long-term goal requires more cardiorespiratory fitness than strength and flexibility fitness.

Whatever fitness goal you choose for yourself, it should follow at least the minimum recommendations for teens spelled out in *Healthy People 2010.* You should also keep these recommendations in mind.

- Keep your goals simple, specific, and realistic.
- List ways that will help you reach your goals.
- Seek help from others (friends, family, and teachers) who can help you achieve your goals.
- Be flexible in case you need to reevaluate your progress.
- Keep records to monitor your progress.
- Be positive. Avoid being negative about yourself.
- Reward yourself in a healthy way as you achieve your goals.

Special Situations

Your personal fitness program should be designed to optimize your health and well-being. This means that you should be prepared to adjust your personal fitness plan and/or activities as the need arises. Two situations that require such adjustments are injury and illness. Imagine, for example, that while jogging to improve cardiovascular fitness you twisted your ankle. You would probably have to stop jogging until your leg healed. In the meantime, you could engage in other activities such as rowing. This would enable you to adhere to your conditioning goals without placing added stress on your leg.

behavioral-change stairway
For more on the steps of the behavioral change stairway, see Chapter 1, page **26.**

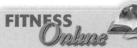

Keeping track of your personal fitness program is easy at **fitness.glencoe.com**.

Activity Set your personal fitness goals and record your progress in Glencoe's Online Fitness Journal.

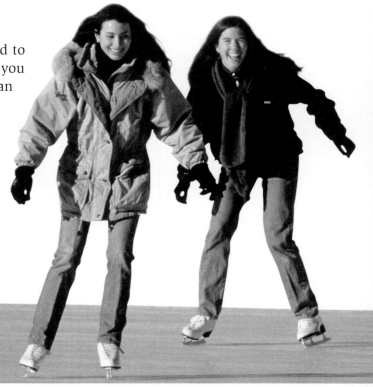

▶ The variety of physical activities that can be part of a personal fitness program is virtually limitless. *Which physical activities do you enjoy doing?*

Active Mind Active Body

The Effect of Intensity on Heart Rate

Imagine taking your pulse after completing moderate to vigorous physical activity. Would you expect this measurement to differ from your resting pulse rate? Why? In this activity, you'll find out.

What You Will Need

- Pen or pencil
- Paper
- Stopwatch, wristwatch, or clock

What You Will Do

1. Sit or lie down and remain still and quiet for five minutes. Then record your pulse. Note that this is an estimate of your resting pulse.
2. Now perform each of the following activities in the order shown. Allow one to two minutes of recovery time between each activity. After each, record your pulse:

   a. Stand in place for two minutes.
   b. Walk around the track for one minute.
   c. Jog slowly around the track for one minute.
   d. Bound, jump, or hop around the track for forty seconds.
   e. Do thirty jumping jacks.
   f. Sprint for forty seconds. (As you run, be careful and leave space between you and your classmates.)
   g. Walk around the track for three minutes.
   h. Sit and stretch in place for two minutes.
3. Copy the following graph from **Figure 3.13** onto a separate sheet of paper. Make a dot to indicate the heart beats per minute for each activity. (Steps *g* and *h* both correspond to *Recovery*.) Then connect the dots with a thin line.

Apply and Conclude

Which activity generated the highest pulse? The lowest pulse? Which activity was the easiest? The most difficult? What is the relationship between pulse and intensity? Which of these activities would be the best choice for a daily 20-minute cardiovascular training session? Why?

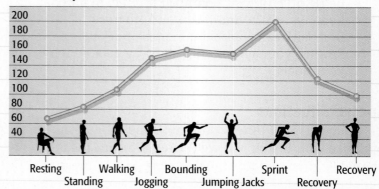

Sample Effects of Different Exercises on Your Heart Rate

Resting · Standing · Walking · Jogging · Bounding · Jumping Jacks · Sprint · Recovery · Recovery

Figure 3.13

Choosing Activities

As you plan the steps for meeting your goals, the types of activities you choose are especially important. You need to consider several factors when selecting physical activities for your fitness program.

- **Where you live.** You will most likely reach your fitness goals if you have a local and convenient place to participate in physical activities. For example, if cycling is part of your fitness plan, make sure you have a location that is safe and easy to access.
- **Time and place.** Schedule your program into your daily routine in a way that suits your needs and personality. Do not plan on jogging at 6:00 A.M. if you are not a morning person. The more thought you put into designing a schedule that

Marion Jones

On the Fast Track

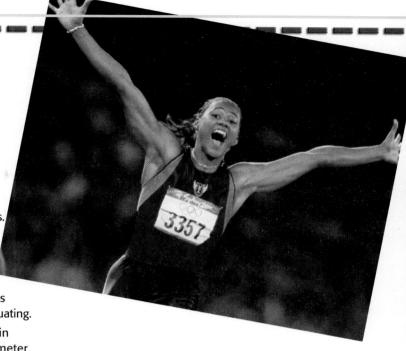

What must it feel like to win an Olympic gold medal, or even a bronze? Just ask Marion Jones. She's won both. In fact, she's won several of each!

Marion Jones was born on October 12, 1975, in Los Angeles, California. She was an excellent basketball player in high school, averaging 22.8 points per game during her senior year. Her first love, though, was track. She won several state competitions before graduating.

Marion entered the University of North Carolina in 1993. During her freshman year, she won the 100-meter dash and long jump in the ACC Conference Track Meet.

Marion burst onto the world track-and-field scene in 1998 and was named *Track and Field's* Athlete of the Year. Her best times were 10.65 seconds in the 100 meters, 21.62 in the 200 meters, and 50.36 in the 400 meters.

In the 2000 Olympic games, Marion represented the U.S. track team. She claimed three gold medals—one each for the 100 meters, 200 meters, and 4×400 meters relay. She won bronze medals in the long jump and 4×100 meters relay. She was named Athlete of the Year by the Associated Press, ESPN, and the International Amateur Athletic Federation (IAAF).

Marion Jones has become an international hero. Although not everyone has the talent and athletic resilience of Marion Jones, anyone can learn to develop his or her levels of health- and skill-related fitness. It's true: Any Body Can!

Research

Marion Jones has excelled in many track-and-field events as well as in basketball. Learn about another international figure, using print or online resources, who has excelled in different sports or physical activities. Share your findings with your physical education classmates.

---

works with your weekly routine, the easier it will be to accomplish your goals.

- **Personal safety.** Always consider your personal safety. If you exercise outdoors, such as running, make sure you choose a safe, well-lit area. Use appropriate safety equipment and procedures for all activities. Avoiding injury is important to keeping your fitness plan on track.
- **Comprehensive planning.** Try to participate in activities that benefit all five areas of health-related fitness. You may want to focus on different aspects of health-related fitness, but it is important to consider all five areas as you vary your activities.

Participating regularly in various physical activities is the short-term goal that will help you achieve your long-term fitness goals. Choosing and scheduling these activities wisely will make your fitness program more effective.

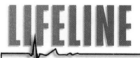

Applying Rules
When choosing physical activities that you would like to try, be sure you apply rules, procedures, and etiquette appropriately. For example, find out about rules and procedures that should be followed when using local facilities such as public basketball or tennis courts. Discuss your findings with the class.

Record Keeping

Record keeping is just as important to the beginning exerciser as it is to the high-performance athlete. Keeping records is critical to reaching your goals safely. It is convenient to keep records in a notebook or notepad. Your record-keeping book should include the following:

- Your goals (for example, to lose weight, get stronger, reduce stress, or run a marathon)
- The days you exercise
- Time, distance, and intensity (heart rate, amount of weight lifted on hard and easy days)
- Environmental conditions (temperature, smog, or humidity)
- Different routes you may have taken
- Places you exercised
- Specific activities or exercises you did
- Any injuries
- Foods and liquids consumed
- Weight loss or gain
- Progress

Reading Check

Identify List three items that should be included in your fitness record-keeping notebook.

Lesson 3 Review

Using complete sentences, answer the following questions on a sheet of paper.

Reviewing Facts and Vocabulary

1. **Vocabulary** Describe the *specificity principle*. What is its role in a personal fitness plan?

2. **Recall** List four factors to consider when setting personal fitness goals.

3. **Recall** How can record keeping contribute positively to your personal fitness program?

Thinking Critically

4. **Compare and Contrast** What is the relationship between the type of physical activity and exercise and your personal fitness?

5. **Extend** Jody and Megan are both age 15. Jody has been participating in her personal fitness program for 6 months. She is in the maintenance stage of the behavioral change stairway. Megan is just planning to start her program. What tips can Jody give Megan to develop a record-keeping book that will help Megan reach the maintenance stage of the behavioral change stairway? Develop a log sheet that Megan might use to record her fitness progress.

Personal Fitness Planning

Applying Specificity Review the fitness plan that you designed in Lesson 1. Explain how you can apply the specificity principle to your plan. Also, adjust your plan so that you can remain active in case any of these situations arise: injuries, illnesses, a condition that requires taking medication.

The Principle of Progression

So far you have learned about two scientific principles, overload and specificity, involved in exercise prescription. They govern fitness behaviors and outcomes. In this lesson, you will learn about a third principle: *progression.*

Progression

Have you learned to play a musical instrument or speak a second language? When acquiring any new skill, you start slowly, beginning with the basics. When you are ready, you progress to more advanced levels.

This same rule applies to fitness conditioning. It is known as the **progression principle.** The principle holds that *as your fitness levels increase, so do the factors in your FITT.* The work gets harder as you progress, and *you* are the best judge of when you are ready to move forward. You make this decision by "listening" to your body. You analyze how you feel as you adapt to new challenges.

It is important to note that you should never increase all the factors in your FITT at once. Neither should you increase any one factor too fast or too soon. If you do, you risk an **overuse injury.** This is a muscular injury that results from overloading your muscles beyond a healthful point.

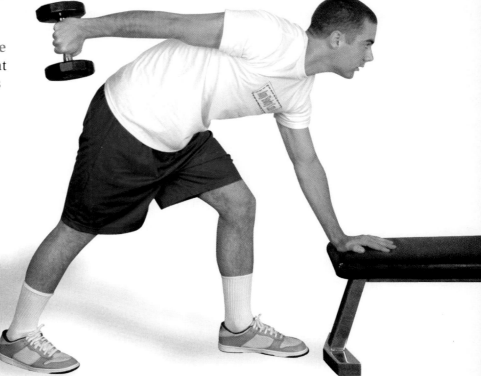

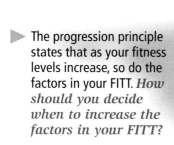

The progression principle states that as your fitness levels increase, so do the factors in your FITT. *How should you decide when to increase the factors in your FITT?*

What You Will Do

- Describe the progression principle and how it applies to your fitness plan.
- Recognize the relationship between progression and trainability.
- Explain how overtraining and detraining contribute to negative health problems.
- Identify ways of optimizing your recovery from physical activity or exercise.

Terms to Know

progression principle
overuse injury
trainability
training plateau
detraining
cross-training
overtraining
fatigue
insomnia
restoration

FIGURE 3.14

TYPICAL PROGRESS CHART

Progress in your fitness plan usually occurs in stages. *What factors do you think might affect the estimated time frames shown in this graph? What happens to the direction of the progress line at the various stages?*

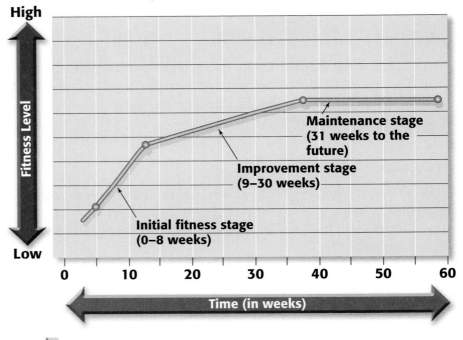

Stages of Progression

Progression in a personal fitness program usually occurs in three stages. Corresponding roughly to the steps of the behavioral-change stairway, these include:

- An initial stage
- An improvement stage
- A maintenance stage

Figure 3.14 shows how a person might typically advance through the stages of progression. The time frames shown are approximate. These will vary from person to person and program to program. Note how rapidly this person improved in the initial stage. This indicates that he or she probably was inactive at the start. Note also that as the program moves forward in time, the rate of improvement tends to slow. By the maintenance stage, the person's FITT levels off completely. It is important at this stage to continue your program to keep your FITT at this level.

✓ Reading Check

Summarize List and describe the stages of progression in a personal fitness program or exercise prescription.

Factors Affecting Progression. Remember that everyone's body and levels of fitness are different. Your rate of progress will depend on several factors:

- Your initial fitness level (the lower you start, the more quickly you usually improve)
- Your heredity
- The rate at which you overload your body or change your FITT
- Your specific goals (health or performance)

One additional factor that influences your rate of progression is your trainability. Trainability is *the rate at which an individual's fitness levels increase during fitness training,* discussed in the next section.

Trainability

Do you consider yourself a "quick study"? Do you tend to learn new physical skills quickly? Do you think of yourself as athletic? Your answers may be a clue to your trainability. Trainability is determined, to a large extent, by heredity. Heredity determines why "natural athletes" usually improve more quickly than nonathletes and enables an athlete to train at higher skill levels. **Figure 3.15** illustrates the trainability of five teens participating in the same conditioning program.

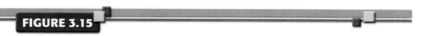

FIGURE 3.15

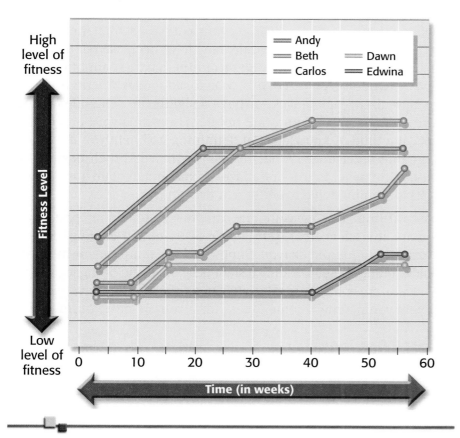

DIFFERENCES IN TRAINABILITY AMONG INDIVIDUALS
Different people train at different rates. *What is the difference in trainability for each of the individuals?*

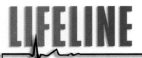

LIFELINE

Getting Help for a Friend

Not only can overtraining lead to serious health problems, it can also be a symptom of an even larger problem—an eating disorder. If someone you know displays any signs of overtraining, he or she may need professional help.

Begin by speaking with the person. Explain the health risks. If you don't seem to be getting through, share your concerns with a trusted adult.

Take a moment to study this graph. Which teen makes the most improvement over the course of a year? Which teen makes the least progress? Which would you describe as the least trainable?

Find the line on the graph corresponding to Andy's trainability. Notice that Andy improved rapidly for about twenty weeks, then leveled off. This leveling off is known as a **training plateau.** A training plateau is *a period of time during training when little, if any, fitness improvement occurs.* Plateaus are a natural part of training. Everyone experiences them at one time or another. Some people feel tempted to quit during plateaus. It is important to fight off this temptation and adhere to your fitness plan.

Detraining

Some people lose the battle of will when training plateaus occur and stop training altogether. These people will experience a phenomenon known as *detraining.* **Detraining** can be defined as *the loss of functional fitness that occurs when one stops fitness conditioning.* Some detraining will occur during relapses on the behavioral-change stairway. These relapses, as noted earlier, can arise from a number of causes, including illness and injury. In general, the longer the period of detraining, the greater the loss of fitness gains.

Take the case of Janean. Janean was forced to spend a month in bed as the result of an illness. Prior to her relapse, Janean was able to jog two miles in twenty minutes. Once she was back on her feet, she found it hard to jog one mile nonstop, let alone two miles in twenty minutes.

It is important to recognize that detraining affects different fitness modes at different rates. For example, if you detrain for four weeks, you may notice a drop in your cardiovascular fitness level. Your levels of strength, meanwhile, may have decreased only slightly. You should also realize that long-term fitness gains cannot be lost in a day, or two, or even three. It is wise to skip a day or two if you are unusually tired, feeling sick, or have a significant schedule conflict. At the same time, it is important not to discontinue your program for weeks at a time. A knowledge of detraining will help you *maintain* a reasonable level of personal fitness—which is much easier than *obtaining* the level in the first place. To maximize your fitness benefits, try to minimize your periods of detraining.

Cross-training. One measure that can prevent detraining, particularly if you are injured, is **cross-training.** Cross-training is *varying your exercise or activity routine or type.* Suppose, for example, you hurt your shoulder lifting weights. Riding a stationary cycle and lifting leg weights provides a cross-training solution. Doing these alternative exercises will help you maintain some fitness until you are past your injury.

 Reading Check

Infer In what way can cross-training be called a remedy for detraining for an individual with a training-related injury?

Overtraining and Health Problems

Look at the graph in **Figure 3.15** on page **97**. Note that the graph stops at about 56 weeks. If it were to continue, you would find Carlos's line dropping sharply over the next month. The reason for this sudden dip was an overuse injury resulting from overtraining, *exercising, or being active to a point where it begins to have negative effects.* Among these effects are abnormal levels of physical and mental stress or "burnout." Overtraining is also a leading cause of overuse injuries, as in Carlos's case.

Overtraining has a number of well-defined effects on health. Many of these are serious health problems. They include:

- Chronic fatigue—*the feeling of being tired all the time*
- Insomnia, or *sleeplessness*
- Constant muscle soreness
- Rapid weight loss
- Loss of appetite
- Elevated resting heart rate
- Elevated blood pressure
- Weakened immune system
- In females, absence of menstrual cycles, and possible infertility.

Overtraining itself can be a symptom of another serious health problem, **eating disorders,** such as bulimia and anorexia nervosa. Although an eating disorder is considered a psychological illness, people with bulimia or anorexia nervosa are likely to overtrain in an effort to fulfill their unhealthy desire to stay thin.

Sometimes people who overtrain suffer from an unhealthy physical and psychological dependence on exercise, often referred to as exercise addiction. These people exhibit all the classic signs of addiction. To them, exercise is more important than family, friends, work, or other commitments. They will exercise with excessive frequency and for extended periods of time, even if they are exhausted or injured. They become nervous and irritable if they are unable to work out.

Recovery from chronic overtraining can take weeks or months. People who are addicted to exercise may even require special counseling in order to recover.

h⊙t link

eating disorders
For more on eating disorders, see Chapter 6, page **176**.

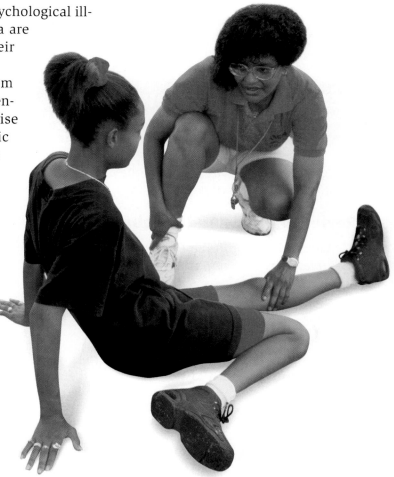

▶ Working hard is good, but be careful not to overtrain. *What are some risks of trying to do too much too soon?*

Restoration

Restoration refers to *ways in which you can optimize your recovery from physical activity or exercise.* The speed at which you recover depends upon your FITT. If you exercise daily, you will need to recover more quickly than you would if you worked out every other day. The same is true of working at very high versus lower levels of intensity. One of the most common conditioning mistakes is not allowing ample recovery time after physical activity or exercise.

Restoration is influenced by several factors. These include the following:

- **Age.** The older you are the slower you tend to recover.
- **Experience.** As a rule, the more experienced you are, the quicker you recover.
- **Environment.** The more extreme the environmental conditions, the slower the recovery.
- **Amount of rest.** Getting 8 to 10 hours of sleep a night will hasten recovery. Any less will lead to a slower recovery.
- **Nutrition, including fluids.** What you eat and drink is an important aspect of fitness training. You will learn more about how to make sound nutritional choices in Chapter 4.

 Reading Check

Identify Name four factors that affect the speed at which an individual recovers from physical activity or exercise.

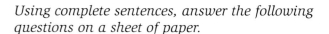

Lesson 4 Review

Using complete sentences, answer the following questions on a sheet of paper.

Reviewing Facts and Vocabulary

1. **Vocabulary** Describe the *progression principle.* Why is it important to your personal fitness program?

2. **Recall** What is a *training plateau?* What effect do plateaus have on an individual's fitness conditioning?

3. **Recall** Why do some individuals progress in their fitness level at faster rates than others?

Thinking Critically

4. **Explain** List the negative health problems associated with overtraining. What serious illness is associated with overtraining?

5. **Evaluate** Lisa and Debra are 14. Six weeks ago both girls started doing exactly the same conditioning. Lisa, however, has improved much faster than Debra. What factors might explain this difference? What tips can you give Debra to help her stay motivated?

Personal Fitness Planning

Identifying Risks Find out how overtraining contributes to negative health problems. Talk with an athlete on a school team. Ask if he or she has ever overtrained. If the answer is yes, ask if any of the symptoms described in the lesson were present. How did the person optimize recovery from exercise? Share your findings with the class.

Warm Up, Work Out, Cool Down

It was the first day of baseball practice, and Sean was excited. He couldn't wait to get out on the field and catch some flies. He was slightly annoyed, therefore, when the coach ordered the team to do two laps of the field. "Why do we have to run? I want to play ball," Sean grumbled to his teammate as they ran.

Sean didn't realize that running laps was a standard preliminary part of any workout: the warm-up. In this lesson, you will learn about the warm-up and other components of a complete workout.

What You Will Do

- Apply the physiological principles of warm-up and cooldown to a fitness program.
- Analyze the importance of warming up and types of warm-up in exercise and training.
- Analyze the importance of cooling down and phases of a cooldown in exercise and training.

Terms to Know

warm-up
active warm-up
passive warm-up
blood pooling
cardiovascular cooldown
stretching cooldown

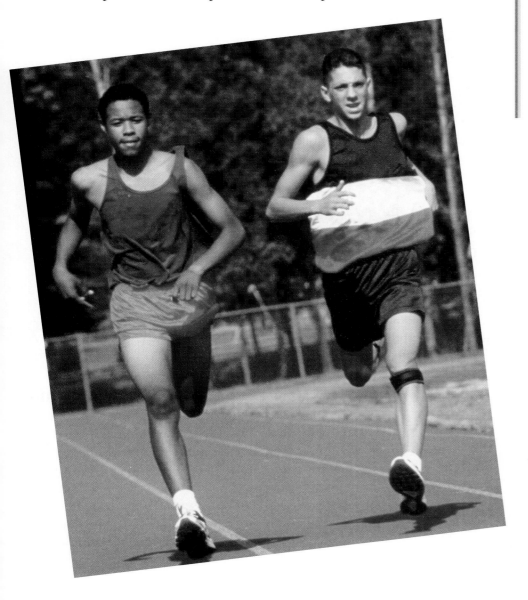

◀ A warm-up is one part of a complete workout. *Why do you think warming up is important prior to doing vigorous activity?*

FIGURE 3.16

COMPONENTS OF A COMPLETE WORKOUT

This chart contains components of one possible routine. *Is this workout similar to your own? How does yours differ?*

Component	Type of Activity	Time (in minutes)
Warm-up	Cardiovascular, stretch, low-level calisthenics, walking	10
Workout	*Cardiovascular Conditioning:* Walk, jog/run, swim, bike, cross-country ski, dance, stair step, in-line skating	20–50
	Muscular conditioning: Calisthenics, weight training	15–30
Cooldown	Walking, stretching	5–10

Components of a Complete Workout

A complete workout includes three main components: a warm-up, the workout itself, and a cooldown. **Figure 3.16** shows one possible approach to a complete workout. Note that the workout begins with a warm-up and ends with a cooldown. In the sections that follow, you will learn more about each of these components. You will also learn safe and healthy reasons for making them part of your workout routines.

The Warm-up

The warm-up is *a portion of a complete workout that consists of a variety of low-intensity activities that prepare the body for physical work.* A warm-up should always precede any moderate-to-vigorous activity. Unfortunately, many people warm up too quickly, or not at all. A well-designed warm-up will help you participate in a safe, successful, and enjoyable workout.

Why Warm Up? There are physiological principles related to the warm-up. The primary purpose of any warm-up is to raise your heart rate gradually before physical activity or exercise. This gradual increase causes a slight rise in muscle temperature. This in turn enables your muscles to work safely and more efficiently. In fact, your whole body benefits. Muscles, bones, and nerves perform better when the body temperature is slightly increased. Evidence suggests that warming up helps minimize physical-activity and exercise injuries. It may reduce some of the symptoms of muscle soreness.

STRESS BREAK

The Art of Planning

Your feelings about yourself—and what you believe others think about you—can influence the amount of positive and negative stress in your life. By organizing your daily routine, you can greatly improve your ability to deal with stress. Here are some tips:

- Plan your days in advance.
- Remember that fitness doesn't happen overnight.
- Set achievable goals.

Types of Warm-ups. There are two main methods of warming up, active and passive. An *active warm-up* *raises body temperature by actively working the body systems centering on the muscles, skeleton, heart, and lungs.* An active warm-up will have two phases:

- **A cardiovascular phase.** This phase is designed to gradually increase your heart rate and body temperature. A cardiovascular warm-up can include jogging slowly around a track, running in place or on a treadmill, or stationary cycling at low resistance.
- **A muscular-skeletal phase.** This phase is designed to loosen up the muscles and connective tissues. A muscular-skeletal warm-up is usually performed by doing static body stretches. These are stretches that are done slowly, smoothly, and in a sustained fashion. You will learn more about stretching in Chapter 11. You will also get some stretching practice in the "Active Mind—Active Body" activity on page **104.**

In contrast to the active warm-up, a *passive warm-up* *raises the body temperature through the use of outside heat sources.* These include blankets, hot baths, saunas, or skin creams. Obviously, the active warm-up is a far more effective way of preparing your body for physical work.

 Reading Check

Describe What types of physical activities might be included in each phase of the active warm-up?

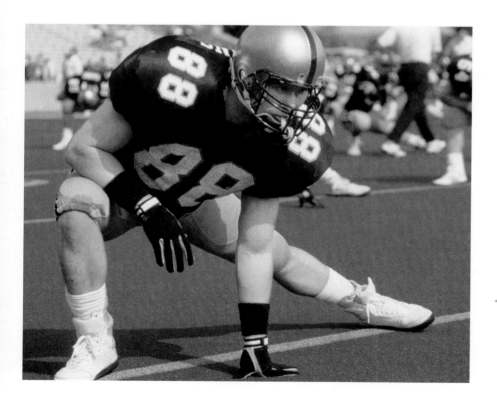

An active warm-up consists of a cardiovascular phase and a muscular-skeletal phase. *What phase of the warm-up are these athletes performing?*

Active Mind Active Body

Warm Up and Cool Down: Stretching Correctly

In this activity, you will apply the physiological principles related to exercise and training, including warm-up and cooldown. As you perform each stretch, concentrate on the muscle being stretched. See if you feel tension in the area of the body designated.

What You Will Need

- Your book (open to **Figures 3.17a–i** on page **106**)

What You Will Do

1. Before getting started, do a light cardiovascular warm-up as instructed by your teacher.
2. Study the picture and description of each stretching activity before trying it. Make sure you understand how the exercise is done.
3. Do each of the following slowly, holding a static position:
   a. **Side stretch**—stretches obliques:
      - From a standing position with feet at shoulders' width apart, raise your left hand over your head.
      - Place your right hand on your hip. Bend sideways (to the right) as far as possible.
      - Do not lean forward or backward.
      - Hold the position for 20 to 30 seconds. Then repeat on the other side.
   b. **Chest and arm stretch**—stretches pectorals and deltoids:
      - From a standing or sitting position, raise your arms out to the sides, to a shoulder-high position.
      - Straighten your arms, and place your hands palm down.
      - Try to touch your hands behind your back.
      - Hold this position for 20 to 30 seconds.
   c. **Trunk twist**—stretches back and hips:
      - Sit on the floor with both legs straight in front of you.
      - Bend the left knee far enough to place the left foot flat on the floor next to the right knee.
      - Now cross the left leg over the right leg, and place the left foot flat on the floor next to the right knee.
      - Place your right elbow on the left side of your left leg.
      - Place your left arm and hand on the floor behind you.
      - While pressing with your right arm, try to twist your body and head as far to the left as possible.
      - Hold this position for 20 to 30 seconds. Then change your leg and arm position and repeat.
   d. **Reverse hurdle**—stretches hamstrings and lower back:
      - Sit on the floor, with both legs straight in front of you.
      - Bend your left knee far enough to place the bottom of your left foot against the side of your right knee.

Specific and General Warm-ups. There are two types of active warm-ups: specific and general. A specific warm-up is structured primarily for skill or game-oriented activities. A specific warm-up for basketball, for example, might include layups, jump shots, and upper and lower leg stretches.

A general warm-up is less structured. It is usually used for individual physical activities. A general warm-up designed for swimming or jogging might include running in place, calisthenics, and various stretches.

Warm-up Guidelines. Like any other part of your workout, a warm-up should be done properly to reduce the risk of muscle injuries and

- Reach for your right ankle with both hands.
- Gently pull your body forward while trying to touch your head to your knee.
- Hold this position for 20 to 30 seconds. Then change your leg and arm position and repeat.

e. **"Yes," "no," "maybe"**—stretches head and neck:
- Tilt your head slightly back. Then bring your head forward and touch your chin to your chest. Return to normal. This is the "yes" stretch.
- Slowly turn your head as far to the right as possible, then back to the left as far as possible. Return to normal. This is the "no" stretch.
- Now pull both of your shoulders up toward your ears. Return to normal. This is the "maybe" stretch.
- Avoid using one continuous, circular motion for these stretches.
- Hold each position for 20 to 30 seconds.

f. **Side lunge**—stretches inner thigh and groin:
- From a standing position, step to the left with your left foot and leg.
- Bend your right knee, and balance most of your weight on your right leg.
- Keep your left leg straight out to the side.
- Balance yourself with one or both hands touching the floor.
- Hold this position for 20 to 30 seconds. Then change legs and repeat.

g. **Forward lunge**—stretches hip flexors:
- From a standing position, step directly to the front with your left leg.
- Bend your left knee to a 90-degree angle while keeping your right leg back and straight. Your right foot should be on its toes.

- Be sure not to let your left knee extend past your left foot.
- Balance yourself with one or both hands on the floor.
- Hold this position for 20 to 30 seconds. Then change legs and repeat.

h. **Butterfly**—stretches groin:
- From a sitting position, bend both knees, and place the bottoms of both feet against each other.
- Lean forward, and place both hands on your feet.
- Slowly pull the heels of your feet toward your body.
- You may lean forward slightly.
- Try to keep your knees out and down.
- Hold this position for 20 to 30 seconds.

i. **Calf stretch**—stretches gastrocnemius:
- From a standing position, face a wall. Place your feet 3 feet from the wall.
- Step forward with your left foot, and support your weight by placing your hands on the wall.
- Your right foot should remain in its position and should stay flat on the floor as you lean forward.
- There should be no weight on your left foot.
- Hold this position for 20 to 30 seconds. Then change legs and repeat.

Apply and Conclude

Were you able to isolate the muscle being stretched? Take note of any stretches you will need to retry. Practice these exercises as part of your warm-up and cooldown.

soreness. There are specific guidelines you can follow to make sure your warm-up is safe and effective.

- Remember to do a cardiovascular and muscular-skeletal phase in every warm-up.
- Start slowly, and gradually increase intensity.
- Warm up for five to fifteen minutes in temperate weather. When it is cold, you may want to take more time to warm up.
- Design a specific warm-up intended for your exercises or physical activities.
- Make your warm-up intensity high enough to produce an increase in heart and breathing rates and a light sweat.

FIGURE 3.17

RECOMMENDED WARM-UP STRETCHES

These stretches can help you meet flexibility goals safely.

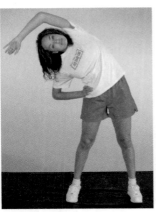

Figure 3.17a

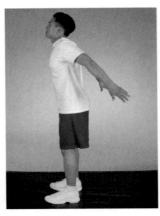

Figure 3.17b

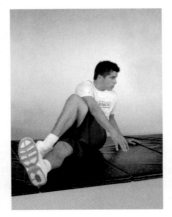

Figure 3.17c

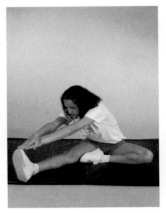

Figure 3.17d

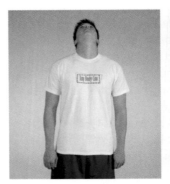
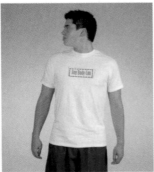
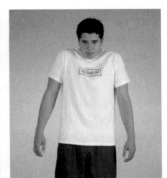

Figure 3.17e

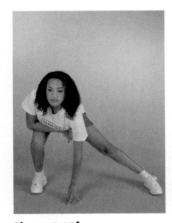

Figure 3.17f

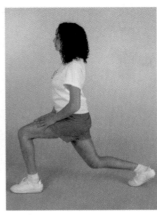

Figure 3.17g

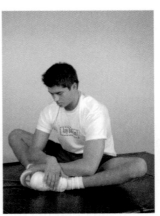

Figure 3.17h

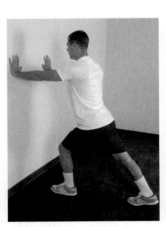

Figure 3.17i

FIGURE 3.18

Sample Fitness Prescription for a Teen

This is an example of a fitness prescription. *Does your exercise prescription look similar to this one? How does it differ?*

Frequency	3–5 days per week
Intensity	Moderate to vigorous and continuous, if possible
Time	Accumulate 20–60 minutes on each session
Type	Walk-hike, run-jog, bike, cross-country ski, dance, skip rope, row, stair climb, swim, in-line skate, endurance games
Resistance-Weight Training	8–10 exercises, 2–3 times per week
Flexibility	Include warm-up and cooldown stretches

The Workout

The workout phase of your fitness program is the period of time that you should spend daily, or almost daily, in physical activity or exercise. A well-designed workout phase should be based on scientific exercise principles. It should also be tailored to your personal fitness goals and experience level.

Figure 3.18 shows details of a sample "fitness prescription" designed for a teen. You might want to use this prescription in designing your workout. Note that the chart shows you how to combine the modes of your conditioning with FITT.

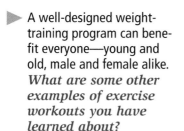

▶ A well-designed weight-training program can benefit everyone—young and old, male and female alike. *What are some other examples of exercise workouts you have learned about?*

The Cooldown

The cooldown portion of your routine is every bit as important as the warm-up. Yet, as with warming up, many people cool down too quickly or not at all. A well-designed cooldown after every workout will ensure a safe and more effective recovery.

The cooldown also follows physiological principles. The main job of the cooldown is the opposite of that of the warm-up: It is to lower your heart rate gradually. This gradual decrease will help you prevent **blood pooling** in the lower body. This is *a condition in which blood collects in the large veins of the legs and lower body* (see **Figure 3.19**).

Blood pooling can cause you to become dizzy and feel faint. That is because less blood is being pumped to your heart and brain. Blood pooling typically results from stopping abruptly at the end of an exercise or physical-activity session. Cooling down will prevent this.

Reading Check

Summarize Why is it necessary to cool down after participating in moderate to vigorous activity?

FIGURE 3.19

BLOOD POOLING

(a) Blood may pool around the one-way valves in the leg if you do not keep your legs moving during recovery. (b) During a proper cooldown, the muscles contract against the leg veins. Blood is squeezed back toward the heart.

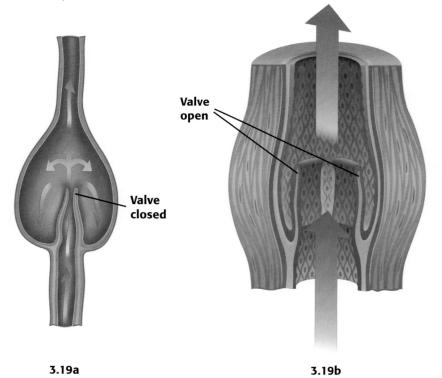

Valve open

Valve closed

3.19a

3.19b

Parts of the Cooldown. Like the warm-up, the cooldown has two phases. These are, in the order in which they should occur:

- **The cardiovascular cooldown.** A cardiovascular cooldown *consists of moving about slowly and continuously for three to five minutes following physical activity or exercise.* Variations include walking, standing in place and moving your feet up and down, or jogging slowly.

- **The stretching cooldown.** The stretching cooldown *involves three to five minutes of stretching.* This will minimize stiffness and muscle soreness. Cooldown stretches should use the same static stretching exercises you use to warm up.

▼ Cooldown is just as important as warm-up. Always be sure to include a cooldown in each workout session. *What are the elements of a proper cooldown?*

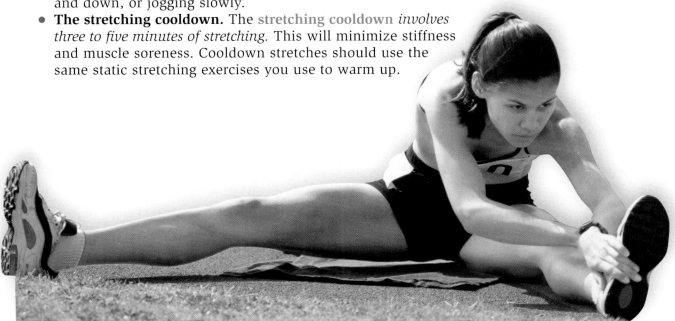

Lesson 5 Review

Using complete sentences, answer the following questions on a sheet of paper.

Reviewing Facts and Vocabulary

1. **Vocabulary** What is a *warm-up?* Why is it important?
2. **Recall** Name the two phases of an *active warm-up.*
3. **Recall** Name the two phases of a *cooldown.*

Thinking Critically

4. **Compare and Contrast** How do warm-up and cooldown activities differ? What common traits do the two share?
5. **Synthesize** Troy and Scott are both 16. Troy plans to try out for the basketball team. Scott wants to try out for football. What tips can you give each teen as to the specific types of warm-ups they should do in preparation for a workout in their sport?

Personal Fitness Planning

Applying Physiological Principles of Warm-up and Cooldown Design and apply a specific active warm-up or cooldown program for playing softball, volleyball, or another sport of your choice. Begin by thinking about or researching which body parts are used most often in the sport. Then write, draw, or demonstrate the kinds of stretches and activities that are involved in your warm-up.

TRUE OR FALSE

On a sheet of paper, write the numbers 1–10. Write True or False for each statement below.

1. Another name for skill-related fitness is cardiovascular fitness.
2. Power is a measure of performance fitness.
3. The three factors that can be adjusted to achieve overload are frequency, intensity, and type.
4. The number of times per week you engage in physical activity or exercise is known as time.
5. The principle of specificity states that overloading a particular muscle will lead to fitness improvements in that muscle alone.
6. Once you have developed a fitness plan, you should never alter it, even if you are injured.
7. If you work your muscles beyond a safe and reasonable point, you risk overuse injury.
8. Heredity is a factor that will affect your rate of progression.
9. Moderate to vigorous exercise sessions should always include a warm-up phase and a cool-down phase.
10. Blood pooling can be prevented by sitting down and relaxing after vigorous exercise.

MULTIPLE CHOICE

On a sheet of paper, write the letter of the word or phrase that best completes each statement.

11. The overload principle involves an increase in
    a. physical activity or exercise above what you normally do.
    b. the improvement you would normally expect.
    c. the changes that occur in your body.
    d. the negative effects that occur in your body.
12. Your exercise intensity is affected by your
    a. level of fitness.
    b. fitness goals.
    c. length of each workout session.
    d. all of the above.

13. Of the following, the piece of information that would NOT be recorded in personal fitness record book is
    a. a list of the foods you have eaten.
    b. the amount of progress made by a competitor.
    c. your goals.
    d. any changes in your body weight.
14. Potential differences in physical-fitness improvement between two people training the same way for the same length of time is due to
    a. overload.
    b. specificity.
    c. progression.
    d. trainability.
15. The principle which states that the factors in your FITT change as your fitness levels increase is
    a. specificity.
    b. progression.
    c. overload.
    d. mode.
16. All of the following are symptoms of overtraining EXCEPT
    a. constant muscle soreness.
    b. mental burnout.
    c. high performance.
    d. chronic fatigue.
17. A term that refers to optimizing your recovery from physical activity or exercise is
    a. restoration.
    b. detraining.
    c. overload.
    d. intensity.
18. All of the following are examples of active warm-up EXCEPT
    a. jogging slowly around a track.
    b. stationary cycling at low resistance.
    c. pitching in the bullpen.
    d. sitting in a sauna.
19. Of the following, the activity that would NOT be a specific warm-up for basketball is
    a. jumping jacks.
    b. layups.
    c. passing drills.
    d. free-throw shooting.
20. Blood pooling results from
    a. overtraining.
    b. detraining.
    c. failing to warm up properly.
    d. failing to cool down properly.

DISCUSSION

Using complete sentences, answer the following questions on a sheet of paper.

21. **Explain** Describe how the perceived exertion scale and your heart rate can be used to determine your exercise intensity needs.
22. **Identify** List some common signs of detraining. Tell how to avoid detraining.
23. **Describe** Explain the relationship between the four FITT factors.

VOCABULARY

On a sheet of paper, write the letter of the term in Column B that best fits the definition in Column A.

Column A

24. Frequency, intensity, time, and type.
25. The need to increase the amount of activity or exercise above what you normally do to improve your fitness level.
26. The kind of activity or exercise you do.
27. A loss of functional fitness resulting from a stoppage in fitness conditioning.
28. A condition in which blood collects in the large veins of the legs and lower body.
29. Your ability to use the five senses to determine and direct the movement of your limbs and head.
30. The amount of energy needed to perform different physical activities or exercises.

Column B

a. blood pooling
b. overload principle
c. FITT
d. type
e. energy cost
f. coordination
g. detraining

CRITICAL THINKING

Using complete sentences, answer the following questions on a sheet of paper.

31. **Explain** How can you influence your personal fitness progression by changing your FITT? Explain your answer.
32. **Evaluate** If a friend tells you that she started an exercise program to improve her physical fitness but quit after two weeks because she didn't see any improvements, what would you tell her?
33. **Synthesize** What advice can you give someone you know who becomes frantic over missing a single workout? Explain your answer.

CASE STUDY

GARY'S PERSONAL EXERCISE

Gary is a sixteen-year-old who has just transferred to your high school. He played soccer and baseball when he was younger but has since been sedentary. Although Gary likes athletics, he doesn't want to play sports in high school. He is interested in improving his health and personal fitness but hasn't had much experience with working out on his own.

Gary thinks that his personal fitness levels are about average, but he has noticed that he tires more easily than he did when he played sports. He doesn't have much energy left by the end of the school day. His goals are to lose 5 to 10 pounds, to improve his cardiovascular fitness levels, and to begin a regular weight-lifting program. Gary could use your personal fitness expertise.

HERE IS YOUR ASSIGNMENT:

Design a beginning physical-activity and exercise plan for Gary. Prepare a detailed two-week warm-up, workout, and cooldown program. Try to be as specific as possible when choosing activities and exercises. Use your knowledge and imagination to create a safe and effective personal-fitness program.

KEYS TO HELP YOU

The following tips may help you design Gary's program:
• Consider his history of personal activity and exercise.
• Consider his current fitness level.
• Consider his needs and goals.

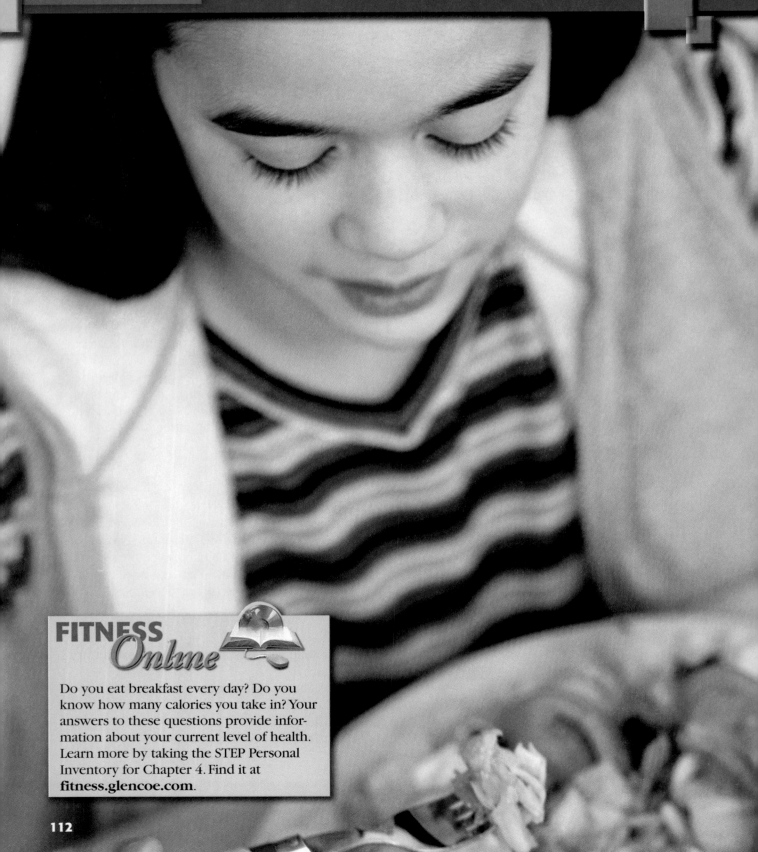

FITNESS
Online

Do you eat breakfast every day? Do you
know how many calories you take in? Your
answers to these questions provide information about your current level of health.
Learn more by taking the STEP Personal
Inventory for Chapter 4. Find it at
fitness.glencoe.com.

The Importance of Nutrition

Personal fitness requires a lifestyle that includes physical activity and several other positive lifestyle choices. One of those choices is healthful eating.

What does healthful eating mean to you? Does it mean living entirely on so-called "health foods" such as wheat grass? Does healthful eating mean saying goodbye forever to pizza, burgers, and candy bars? You may be relieved to find out that the answer to both of these questions is no.

Healthful Eating

From a scientific perspective, healthful eating means taking in the appropriate amounts of nutrients each day. Nutrients are *substances in food that your body needs for energy, proper growth, body maintenance, and functioning.* There are six classes of nutrients: carbohydrates, proteins, fats, vitamins, minerals, and water. Nutrient needs vary with age, gender, health, and activity level. *The study of food and how your body uses the substances in food* is known as nutrition.

In this lesson you will learn more about the importance of good nutrition. You will also see that there is room in a healthful eating plan for all your favorite foods.

A first step toward developing healthful eating habits is to examine the factors that influence your food choices.

Good nutrition involves eating a variety of healthful foods, including plenty of fruits and vegetables. *What are your favorite fruits and vegetables?*

What You Will Do

- Identify factors that influence your food choices.
- Explain the role of carbohydrates, proteins, and fats in your eating plan.
- Identify the recommended daily amounts of carbohydrates, proteins, and fats.

Terms to Know

nutrients
nutrition
culture
carbohydrates
proteins
fats
calorie
adipose tissue
dietary fiber
amino acids
vegetarian
saturated fatty acids
trans fatty acids
unsaturated fatty acids
cholesterol
LDL
HDL

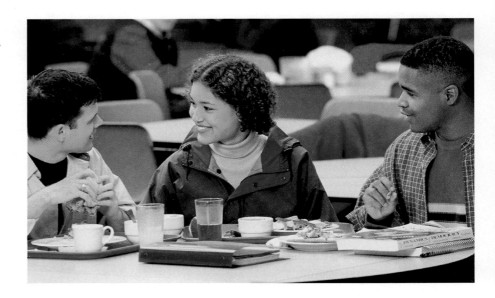

▶ Friends and peers can influence your food choices. *Give one example of how friends have a positive influence on your food choices and one example of how they might have a negative influence.*

Influences on Your Food Choices

Have you ever asked yourself why you choose to eat the foods you do? Several factors play a role in your food choices. These include:

- **Hunger.** Hunger is a natural, inborn drive that protects you from starvation. It is a physical need that drives you to eat.
- **Appetite.** Appetite is a personal desire, rather than a need, to eat. Appetite is psychological, not physical.
- **Culture.** *The shared customs, traditions, and beliefs of a particular group* make up a person's culture. Cultural or ethnic background may influence food choices. For example, rice is a staple in many Asian cultures.
- **Family and friends.** You may choose certain foods because you have grown up eating them. Friends and peers may also influence many teens' food choices.
- **Emotions.** Have you ever eaten just because you were bored? Have you ever been too upset to eat? Your feelings can have an enormous impact on your food choices.
- **Convenience and cost.** Due to busy schedules, many people, including teens, select foods that are easy to prepare and eat. For example, you may choose to buy foods from a vending machine because they can be eaten quickly. Cost is also a consideration for many people. For example, its low cost may make it easier to choose fast food.
- **Advertising.** Food advertising is a multibillion-dollar industry. Think about the food ads you have seen recently on TV. What products were these ads promoting? What eating decisions have you made based on food ads?

 Reading Check

Compare What is the difference between hunger and appetite?

Nutrients for Energy

What do running, taking a test, and sleeping all have in common? All these activities require energy. Even when you are asleep, your heart and lungs are hard at work, pumping blood and taking in air. Proper nutrition is necessary for your body to function at its best.

In a way, your body is like a car. Both need fuel in order to run. Your body's fuel comes from the energy sources in the foods you eat. There are three such energy sources, all of which are nutrients. They are carbohydrates, proteins, and fats.

- **Carbohydrates** are *the starches and sugars found in food.* They are the body's chief source of energy.
- **Proteins** are *nutrients that help build, maintain, and repair body tissues.* They also serve, when necessary, as a secondary source of energy.
- **Fats** *supply a concentrated form of energy and help transport other nutrients to locations in the body where they are needed.*

Your body's energy needs are measured in calories. A **calorie** is *the amount of energy needed to raise the temperature of 1 kilogram (about a quart) of water 1 degree Celsius.* You expend calories with everything you do.

It is important to note that your levels of physical activity and exercise have a direct bearing on your energy needs. As your activity level increases, so does your body's demand for more calories. **Figure 4.1** contains some general guidelines for daily calorie intake.

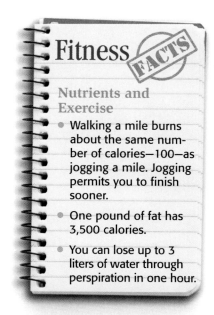

Fitness FACTS

Nutrients and Exercise

- Walking a mile burns about the same number of calories—100—as jogging a mile. Jogging permits you to finish sooner.
- One pound of fat has 3,500 calories.
- You can lose up to 3 liters of water through perspiration in one hour.

FIGURE 4.1

DAILY CALORIE INTAKE

Calorie intake depends on gender, age, and level of activity. *How many calories should you consume daily?*

2,800 Calories	2,200 Calories	1,600 Calories
Active Male Teenagers	Active Female Teenagers	Inactive Teenagers
Active Males	Active Females	Inactive Females
Many Athletes	Inactive Males	Some Older Adults

Source: USDA, 2002.[1]

Carbohydrates

Gram for gram, carbohydrates are more energy efficient than fat because they require less oxygen to be converted into energy. One gram of carbohydrates provides 4 calories of energy. Carbohydrates come mainly from plant sources of food and are classified as either simple or complex.

- **Simple carbohydrates.** These are sugars; they are found mostly in fruits, candy, cookies, and soda. Simple carbohydrates are absorbed quickly into the bloodstream and provide a quick form of energy.
- **Complex carbohydrates.** These are starches; they are found in certain vegetables such as corn and potatoes, as well as breads, cereals, pasta, rice, and dry beans. Complex carbohydrates are broken down more slowly by your body than simple carbohydrates and supply more vitamins. Thus, they are a better source of sustained energy than simple carbohydrates for endurance sports and activities such as running.

Between 45 to 65 percent of the calories you consume daily should come from carbohydrates, mostly complex carbohydrates. **Figure 4.2** lists carbohydrates from the various food groups.

FIGURE 4.2

SOURCES OF CARBOHYDRATES

Carbohydrates can be found in foods from many of the food groups. *How much energy does one gram of carbohydrate provide?*

Grains Group	Fruit Group	Vegetable Group	Milk Group
Bagels	Apples	Broccoli	Frozen yogurt
Breads	Bananas	Carrots	Milk (2% or skim)
Cereals	Fruit juices	Corn	Pudding
Crackers	Nectarines	Peppers	Yogurt
English muffins	Oranges	Potatoes	Cheese
Graham crackers	Pears	Green beans	
Pasta noodles		Tomatoes	
Popcorn			
Pretzels			
Rice			

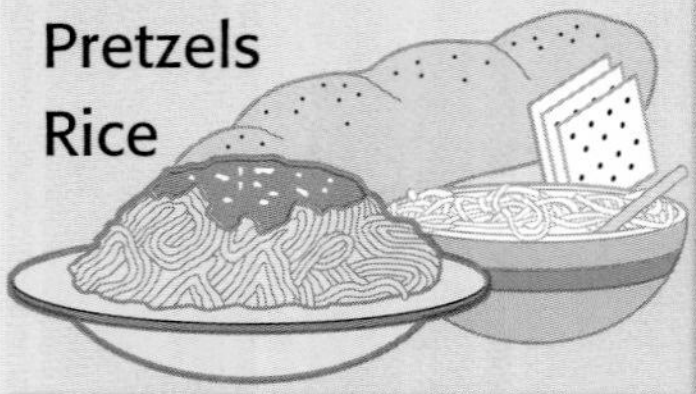

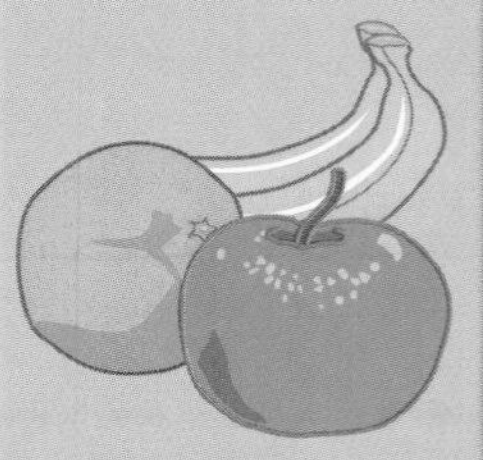

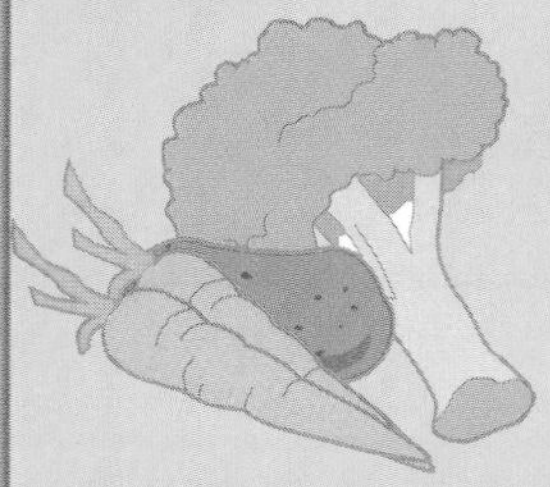

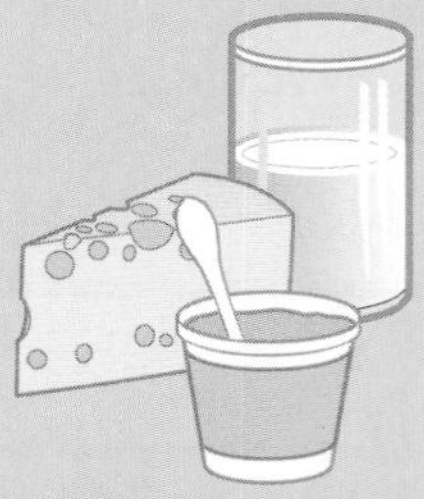

Carbohydrates in the Body

Before your body can use carbohydrates for energy, it must convert them to a simple sugar known as glucose. Excess glucose is also stored in the liver and muscles as a starchlike substance known as glycogen (GLY-kuh-jun). The body can convert glycogen back to glucose when more energy is needed. If a person takes in more carbohydrates than his or her body can use immediately for energy or store as glycogen, the excess glucose is stored as adipose tissue, or *body fat.*

People who engage in ultra-endurance training or competition lasting two hours or longer often deplete their glycogen stores. With careful training and eating practices, these athletes can make their bodies store more glycogen so that they have additional energy stores for prolonged physical performance. People who are regularly glycogen-depleted are at higher risk for overtraining and poor physical performance. To maintain normal glucose and glycogen levels, you must regularly replenish your carbohydrate stores.

Dietary Fiber

Dietary fiber is *a special subclass of complex carbohydrates that has several functions, including aiding the body in digestion.* Fiber is not digestible in humans and thus provides no calories.

Certain types of fiber may help reduce the risk of heart disease by lowering levels of cholesterol in the blood. Some types of fiber have also been useful in controlling diabetes by reducing blood glucose levels. For teens ages 14 to 18, the recommended amount of fiber is 38 grams per day for males and 36 grams per day for females.

Fiber-rich foods include whole-grain products, vegetables, and many fruits. These foods help you to feel full and satisfied while being low in calories. Fiber is best consumed in foods rather than supplements. Fiber-rich foods have many nutrients that supplements do not have.

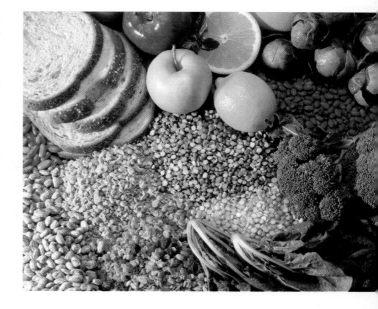

▼ These foods are good sources of dietary fiber. *Which of these foods are a part of your eating plan?*

 Reading Check

Explain What is the recommended daily amount of fiber for female teens? for Male teens?

Protein

Muscles are made up of 29 percent protein and 70 percent water. Protein is also a component of bones, connective tissues, skin, blood, and vital organs. Your body needs protein to grow, repair, and maintain itself. Daily living exposes body tissues to wear and tear. The proteins in the foods you eat help repair and maintain these body tissues. Protein helps fight disease, since parts of the immune system are also composed of protein. Protein also supplies your body energy in the form of calories.

The building blocks of proteins are called **amino** (uh-MEE-noh) **acids.** There are 22 different amino acids; your body can manufacture all but nine. These nine are called *essential amino acids* because you must get them from the foods you eat.

The total amount of protein in your eating plan should be between 10 and 35 percent of the calories you consume daily. In the United States, most people consume an adequate amount of protein with little effort. Be aware that if you eat more protein than you need, it will be stored as body fat if you already consume enough calories from carbohydrates and fat. **Figure 4.3** features a list of lean and low-fat foods that are high in protein and also gives examples of serving sizes.

Proteins can only do their job if you consume enough carbohydrates and fat to meet your energy needs. If you do not, the body will use protein for energy, rather than for growth, and for building and repairing cells and tissues.

Complete and Incomplete Proteins

There are two types of proteins found in foods: complete and incomplete. *Complete proteins* contain all nine essential amino acids. Animal products such as meats and dairy products are sources of complete proteins. With the exception of soybeans, plant foods contain *incomplete proteins*—that is, they lack one or more of the essential amino acids. This information is especially important for **vegetarians,** *individuals who eliminate meat, fish, and poultry from their eating plans.* If you are a vegetarian, make sure you eat a variety

FIGURE 4.3

PROTEIN IN VARIOUS FOODS

How many grams of protein would there be in taco filling that contains one serving of turkey and one serving of black beans?

Protein in Various Foods

Food	Protein (grams)	Serving Size
Turkey, roasted, diced	41	3 ounces
Cottage cheese, 2% fat	31	½ cup
Tuna, canned, water packed	30	3 ounces
Lean pork rib, roasted, boneless	21	3 ounces
Yogurt, plain, low-fat	12	8 ounces (1 cup)
Black beans, dry, cooked	15	½ cup
Eggs, hard-cooked	6	1 egg
Peanut butter	5	2 tablespoons

of plant-based foods and dairy products to ensure an adequate intake of complete proteins. Vegans (VEE-guhnz), vegetarians who also eliminate eggs and dairy products from their eating plans, need special nutritional guidance from a health professional to meet their protein needs.

 Reading Check

Compare What is the difference between complete and incomplete proteins?

Fats

Fats, or lipids, are another type of nutrient that provides energy. At nine calories per gram, fats supply more than twice the energy of a gram of carbohydrate or protein. Fats also

- transport and absorb vitamins A, D, E, and K.
- help regulate the hormone **testosterone,** which is used to build body tissues.
- enhance the flavor and texture of foods.
- help satisfy hunger because they take longer to digest.

Fats can be stored in the body as *triglycerides* (try-GLIS-uhr-idz) and used as energy for exercise or physical activity, especially for periods of exertion that last 30 minutes or longer.

Considering all the positive properties of fats, you may wonder why fats have such a bad reputation. Here's why: Eating too many fats is linked to many serious health problems, including heart disease and certain cancers. In addition, most fat that is not used by the body for energy is stored as adipose tissue. Excess body fat may lead to unhealthful weight gain and obesity, which increases the risk of health conditions such as type 2 diabetes.

Types of Fat

Fats are a mixture of different types of fatty acids, which can be classified into three basic types.

- **Saturated fatty acids** are *fats that come mainly from animal fats, including butter and lard, and are often solid at room temperature.* Fatty meats, cheese, ice cream, and whole milk contain saturated fats. Some oils, like palm oil and coconut oil, are also high in saturated fats.
- **Trans fatty acids** are *fats that are formed when certain oils are processed into solids.* Margarine and shortening are two examples of foods high in trans fats. The presence of trans fats in processed foods can often be identified by the words *partially hydrogenated* in the list of ingredients. Nutrition Facts panels may also contain information on trans fats.
- **Unsaturated fatty acids** are *fats that are usually liquid at room temperature and come mainly from plant sources.* Unsaturated fats include corn oil, soybean oil, olive oil, sunflower oil, and some fish oils.

testosterone
For more on testosterone and its role in building muscles, see Chapter 9, page **257.**

FIGURE 4.4

WHAT IS YOUR UPPER LIMIT ON FAT?

How many calories do you consume? How many grams from fat a day are recommended, based on your calorie intake? How many grams of fat do you consume?

Total Daily Calories	Recommended Daily Intake of Saturated and Trans Fat	Recommended Daily Intake of Total Fat
1,600	18 grams or less	53 grams
2,000	20 grams or less	65 grams
2,200	24 grams or less	73 grams
2,500	25 grams or less	80 grams
2,800	31 grams or less	93 grams

Cholesterol

Saturated fats and trans fats typically contain cholesterol. **Cholesterol** is *a fatlike substance that is produced in the liver and circulates in the blood.* Cholesterol is found only in foods of animal origin. Your body needs some cholesterol for certain processes. For example, cholesterol is used in the production of cell membranes and certain hormones. Your body can manufacture all the cholesterol it needs. Cholesterol can also be obtained from food, such as egg yolks, meat, and high-fat milk products.

High levels of cholesterol in the blood have been linked to an increased risk of heart disease, because excess cholesterol is deposited in the arteries. An eating plan that is high in saturated fats or trans fats raises blood cholesterol levels. Thus, it's important to limit intake of foods that contain these types of fatty acids. In addition, the American Heart Association recommends limiting dietary cholesterol to less than 300 milligrams per day.

Cholesterol in the Blood. Cholesterol circulates through the bloodstream in special fat-protein "packages" called lipoproteins (LY-poh-PROH-teenz). There are two major types of lipoproteins.

- **Low-density lipoprotein (LDL)** is *a type of compound that carries cholesterol from the liver to areas of the body where it is needed.* When too much LDL cholesterol is circulating in the blood, the excess amounts can build up inside arteries—blood vessels that carry blood away from the heart. This buildup increases the risk of heart disease or stroke. Thus, LDL cholesterol is sometimes referred to as "bad" cholesterol.

- **High-density lipoprotein (HDL)** is *a type of compound that picks up excess cholesterol and returns it to the liver.* Because it carries excess cholesterol to the liver before it can do any harm, HDL cholesterol is sometimes called "good" cholesterol.

Fat and Daily Calories

Fats should make up about 20 to 30 percent of your daily calories. Because of the link between excess consumption of saturated fats and an increased risk of heart disease, you need to keep your intake of saturated fats as low as possible. The chart in **Figure 4.4** provides some general guidelines for relative amounts of fats in your eating plan. Here are two other recommendations for reducing your fat intake.

- Limit your use of solid fats, such as butter, hard margarines, lard, and partially hydrogenated shortenings. Use vegetable oils as a substitute.
- Choose fat-free or low-fat dairy products, cooked dry beans and peas, fish, and lean meats and poultry.

Eating less fat overall may promote weight loss if calorie intake is less, too. However, restricting fat consumption to less than 20 percent of daily calories may be difficult to maintain over the long term and may not be healthful.

Reading Check

Evaluate Which types of fat increase blood cholesterol level?

Lesson 1 Review

Using complete sentences, answer the following questions on a sheet of paper.

Reviewing Facts and Vocabulary

1. **Vocabulary** What is *nutrition?*
2. **Vocabulary** List two categories of *carbohydrates.* Name two foods that are a good source of each type.
3. **Recall** What are the three types of fatty acids? Which two raise blood cholesterol levels?

Thinking Critically

4. **Analyze** Maya is considering following a vegetarian eating plan. However, she has heard that vegetarians do not get enough protein in their diets. What advice would you give her about proteins and vegetarianism?

5. **Compare and Contrast** What is the difference between saturated and unsaturated fatty acids? Between HDL cholesterol and LDL cholesterol?

Personal Fitness Planning

Evaluating Nutrition Make a list of your food choices over the past week. How many times did you eat fast foods or snack foods that contain saturated or trans fats? List four to five ways you can reduce the amount of foods you consume that contain saturated and/or trans fats. If you do not consume a lot of foods with saturated and/or trans fats, how would you advise a person who is trying to cut back on such foods?

What You Will Do

- Identify the two categories of vitamins and foods that provide them.
- List and describe the major minerals and their role in nutrition.
- Analyze the relationship between sound nutritional practices and physical activity.
- Explain the relationship between fluid balance and physical activity.
- Identify the importance of water to your body's functioning.

Terms to Know

vitamins
antioxidants
minerals
phytonutrients
dietary supplement

Vitamins, Minerals, and Water

Have you ever heard it said that good things come in small packages? This saying certainly applies to the nutrients known as vitamins and minerals. In this lesson, you will learn what these substances do for the body. You will also learn about another important nutrient, water.

Micronutrients

Because vitamins and minerals are nutrients needed in tiny amounts, they are known as micronutrients. Although you need only small amounts of these, they have very important functions. They help your body convert and release energy as well as protect your body's cells from certain types of damage.

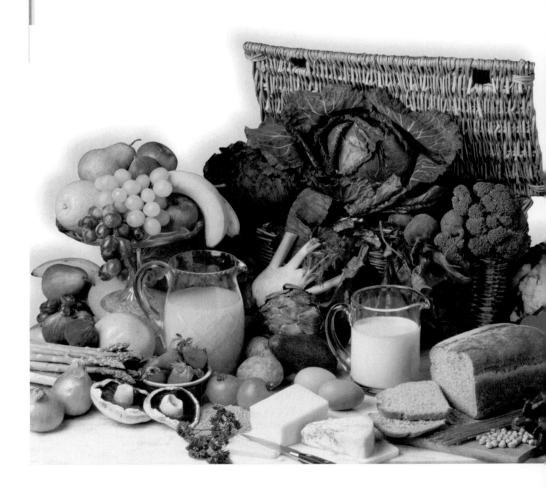

▶ You can get many of the vitamins your body needs from food sources instead of supplements. *What nutrients do these food sources provide?*

FIGURE 4.5

FAT-SOLUBLE VITAMINS

A variety of foods can provide you with the appropriate vitamins.
Which of the foods listed are a part of your regular eating plan?

Vitamin/Amount Needed Each Day	Function	Food Source
A Teen female: 800 mcg Teen male: 1,000 mcg	helps maintain skin tissue, strengthens tooth enamel, promotes use of calcium and phosphorous in bone formation, promotes cell growth, keeps eyes moist, helps eyes adjust to darkness, may aid in cancer prevention	milk and other dairy products, green vegetables, carrots, deep-orange fruits, liver
D Teen female: 5 mcg Teen male: 5 mcg	promotes absorption and use of calcium and phosphorous, essential for normal bone and tooth development	fortified milk, eggs, fortified breakfast cereals, sardines, salmon, beef, margarine; also produced in skin exposed to sun's ultraviolet rays
E Teen female: 8 mg Teen male: 10 mg	may help in oxygen transport, may slow the effects of aging, may protect against destruction of red blood cells	present in vegetable oils, nuts, seeds, whole grain breads and cereals, dark green leafy vegetables, dry beans, and peas
K Teen female: 55 mcg Teen male: 65 mcg	essential for blood clotting, assists in regulating blood calcium level	spinach, broccoli, eggs, liver, cabbage, tomatoes

Vitamins

Vitamins are *micronutrients that help control body processes and help your body release energy to do work.* Because vitamins do not contain calories, they don't provide your body with energy.

Vitamins may be classified as fat-soluble or water-soluble.

- **Fat-soluble vitamins,** carried by fat in food and in your body, can be stored in the body. The fat-soluble vitamins are vitamins A, D, E, and K. A list of fat-soluble vitamins and food sources for each may be found in **Figure 4.5.**
- **Water-soluble vitamins** are not stored in your body. They need to be replaced daily by eating nutritious foods. Vitamin C and the B complex vitamins (thiamin, riboflavin, niacin, folate, B_6, and B_{12}) are among these important vitamins. A complete list of water-soluble vitamins and food sources for each may be found in **Figure 4.6.**

Reading Check

Compare How do fat-soluble and water-soluble vitamins differ?

FIGURE 4.6

WATER-SOLUBLE VITAMINS

Many foods are a good source of more than one vitamin. *Name one food that is a good source of Vitamins B$_2$, Niacin, and B$_{12}$.*

Vitamin/Amount Needed Each Day	Function	Food Source
C (ascorbic acid) **Teen female: 60 mg** **Teen male: 60 mg**	protects against infection, helps form connective tissue, helps heal wounds, maintains elasticity and strength of blood vessels, promotes healthy teeth and gums	citrus fruits, cantaloupe, tomatoes, cabbage, broccoli, potatoes, peppers
B$_1$ (thiamine) **Teen female: 1.1 mg** **Teen male: 1.5 mg**	converts glucose into energy or fat, contributes to good appetite	whole-grain or enriched cereals, liver, yeast, nuts, legumes, wheat germ
B$_2$ (riboflavin) **Teen female: 1.3 mg** **Teen male: 1.8 mg**	essential for producing energy from carbohydrates, fats, and proteins; helps keep skin healthy	milk, cheese, spinach, eggs, beef liver
Niacin **Teen female: 15 mg** **Teen male: 20 mg**	important for maintenance of all body tissues; helps in energy production; needed by body to utilize carbohydrates, to synthesize body fat, and for cell respiration	milk, eggs, poultry, beef, legumes, peanut butter, whole grains, enriched and fortified grain products
B$_6$ **Teen female: 1.5 mg** **Teen male: 2.0 mg**	essential for amino acid and carbohydrate metabolism, helps turn the amino acid tryptophan into serotonin (a messenger to the brain) and niacin	wheat bran and wheat germ, liver, meat, whole grains, fish, vegetables
Folic Acid **Teen female: 180 mcg** **Teen male: 200 mcg**	necessary for production of genetic material and normal red blood cells, reduces risk of birth defects	nuts and other legumes, orange juice, green vegetables, folic acid-enriched breads and rolls, liver
B$_{12}$ **Teen female: 2.0 mcg** **Teen male: 2.0 mcg**	necessary for production of red blood cells and for normal growth	animal products such as meat, fish, poultry, eggs, milk, and other dairy foods; some fortified foods

Antioxidants. Some vitamins and minerals exhibit antioxidant (antee-OKS-uh-duhnt) properties. Antioxidants are *substances that protect body cells, including those of the immune system, from damage.* Cells can be damaged by by-products of cell energy production and by environmental factors, such as cigarette smoke and air pollution. Antioxidants protect cells from injury, thereby reducing the risk of cancer, heart disease, and premature aging. Vitamins C and E are both antioxidants.

Minerals

Minerals are *substances that the body cannot manufacture but that are needed for forming healthy bones and teeth and for regulating many vital body processes.* Like vitamins, minerals do not supply your body with energy. **Figure 4.7** lists several minerals, their key roles, and food sources for each.

Four minerals are addressed in detail here: calcium, potassium, sodium, and iron. The first three work as *electrolytes* because their electrical charges help maintain normal heart rhythm and control the body's fluid balance. **Fluid balance** is the body's ability to balance the amount of fluid taken in and the amount lost through perspiration or excretion. There is a direct relationship between fluid balance and performance during physical activity. Proper fluid balance prevents dehydration.

During vigorous physical activity or exercise, electrolyte levels can drop dangerously low if a person perspires heavily. Low potassium levels, in particular, can lead to muscle cramps or difficulties in the conduction of nerve impulses. You can avoid these problems through proper hydration. In some circumstances, athletes may benefit from consuming sports drinks that replenish electrolytes.

fluid balance
For more on fluid balance, see Chapter 2, page **41.**

FIGURE 4.7

MINERALS: KEY ROLES AND SOURCES

Minerals help your body function. *Which of the foods listed in the column on the right do you enjoy eating?*

Mineral/Amount Needed Each Day	Function	Food Source
Calcium Teen female: 1,300 mg Teen male: 1,300 mg	building material of bones and teeth (skeleton contains about 99% of body calcium), regulation of body functions (heart muscle contraction, blood clotting)	dairy products; leafy vegetables; canned fish with soft, edible bones; tofu processed with calcium sulfate
Phosphorus Teen female: 1,250 mg Teen male: 1,250 mg	combines with calcium to give rigidity to bones and teeth, essential in cell metabolism, helps maintain proper acid-base balance of blood	milk and most other dairy foods, peas, beans, liver, meat, fish, poultry, eggs, broccoli, whole grains
Magnesium Teen female: 360 mg Teen male: 410 mg	enzyme activator related to carbohydrate metabolism, aids in bone growth and muscle contraction	whole grains, milk, dark green leafy vegetables, legumes, nuts
Iron Teen female: 15 mg Teen male: 12 mg	part of the red blood cells' oxygen and carbon dioxide transport system, important for use of energy in cells and for resistance to infection	meat, shellfish, poultry, legumes, peanuts, dried fruits, egg yolks, liver, fortified breakfast cereal, enriched rice

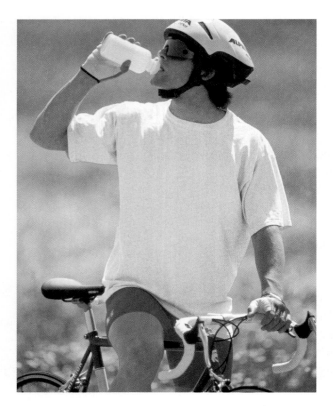

Calcium, potassium, and sodium help maintain the body's fluid balance. *What is fluid balance? How can you avoid dehydration during physical activity?*

ho**t** **l**i**n**k

hypertension
For more on hypertension, see Chapter 7, page **203.**

Calcium. Calcium helps build and maintain strong bones. It is particularly important to consume calcium during your teen years and young adulthood. During the teen years, bones continue to become more dense. After the age of 25, your body is no longer able to add to bone density and calcium stores on its own. Calcium must be replaced regularly since bones are constantly being maintained and repaired. Your muscles also use calcium when they contract. Eating calcium-rich foods, such as dairy products, dark green, leafy vegetables, and canned fish with soft, edible bones, is the best way to get the calcium you need. Taking calcium supplements is another way to make sure you are getting enough calcium. Weight-bearing and weight-lifting exercises can also help maintain and strengthen bones.

Potassium. Potassium aids in normal muscle contractions and in the sending of nerve impulses that control the movement of muscles. Bananas, many dried fruits, and many fruit juices are good sources of potassium.

Sodium. Sodium helps maintain the fluid balance inside and outside cells and helps in the transmission of nerve impulses. Many foods you eat are likely to contain sodium, which is one of the two minerals in table salt—*sodium chloride.* People with **hypertension,** or high blood pressure, need to monitor their sodium intake. Since hypertension is often hereditary, you may be at risk if a parent or grandparent has this health problem. See the *Dietary Guidelines* for specific suggestions on reducing your sodium intake.

Iron. Iron is part of the hemoglobin in red blood cells. Hemoglobin carries oxygen from the lungs to all cells throughout the body. Meats are good sources of this mineral. Because vegetarians do not eat meat, they are at higher risk for iron deficiencies. If you are vegetarian, you need to eat plant foods that contain iron, such as legumes (beans), peanuts, and dried fruits. Iron from plant sources is absorbed better if consumed with a Vitamin-C rich food.

 Reading Check

Explain What is the role of electrolytes in maintaining fluid balance?

Water

Between 60 and 70 percent of your body weight is water. Water is an essential nutrient for life. Without it, death would occur in six to seven days.

Water helps regulate body temperature, carries nutrients to cells, aids in digestion and elimination, and is important for many chemical reactions in your body. You need to consume a total of

64 ounces (8 cups) of water or other fluids daily to maintain normal fluid balance. Certain foods, such as fruits, vegetables, and soup, are also sources of water.

As explained in Chapter 2, drinking adequate fluids is critical when exercising and perspiring heavily. It is often difficult to "catch up" on your fluid balance if you wait until you are thirsty before you begin to rehydrate. Instead, hydrate before, during, and after physical activity or exercise. **Figure 4.8** lists some general guidelines for drinking water or other fluids when you are active. Although water is often the most convenient fluid, you may prefer a sports drink for the taste.

Phytonutrients

Literally meaning "plant nutrients," phytonutrients are *health-promoting substances found in plant foods.* According to current estimates, a simple plant-based food may contain several hundred phytonutrients. So far, scientists have been able to isolate only a few.

Some phytonutrients are antioxidants. One well-known example is *beta carotene* (BAY-tuh KAR-uh-teen). This phytonutrient gives certain fruits and vegetables their bright orange color. Carrots and cantaloupe are good sources of beta carotene.

Lutein [LOO-tee-en] is a phytonutrient that may protect against blindness. Lutein is found in yellow-orange fruits such as mangoes, peaches, tangerines, and yellow and red bell peppers. It is also found in green leafy vegetables such as kale, spinach, and collard greens.

 Reading Check

Identify What are two examples of phytonutrients?

FIGURE 4.8

FLUID REPLACEMENT AND PHYSICAL ACTIVITY
Drinking water before, during, and after physical activity is essential. Explain the relationship to water and salt loss.

Before	During	After
Drink 10 to 14 ounces of water one to two hours before the activity or exercise.	Drink ½ cup (4 ounces) of cold water every fifteen minutes.	Drink 2 cups (16 ounces) of cold water for every pound of weight loss.

Source: Play Hard, Eat Right: A Parent's Guide to Sports Nutrition for Children, *1998.*[2]

Dietary Supplements

A **dietary supplement** is *a nonfood form of one or more nutrients.* Vitamins and minerals have long been available in supplement form. More recently, herbs and other substances that claim to enhance health or improve certain health conditions are also sold as supplements.

People with special dietary needs may be advised by health care professionals to use dietary supplements. One such group is pregnant females, who need extra amounts of iron and the B vitamin folate. Older adults and people who get little exposure to sunlight may need a Vitamin D supplement if they do not consume enough Vitamin D-fortified milk or spend enough time in sunlight. Vegans are often counseled to take Vitamin B_{12} supplements because this vitamin is found only in animal foods.

While taking dietary supplements may be useful in certain cases, it is no substitute for eating healthfully. In addition, taking supplements may increase the likelihood of getting too much of a particular nutrient or other substance. For example, fat-soluble vitamins are stored in the body and can build up to toxic levels if taken in large amounts. Always seek advice from a health care provider before taking any dietary supplement.

In Chapter 6, you will explore another group of dietary supplements—those marketed as aids to weight loss or weight gain.

 Reading Check

Explain Who might be advised to take a dietary supplement?

Lesson 2 Review

Using complete sentences, answer the following questions on a sheet of paper.

Reviewing Facts and Vocabulary

1. **Vocabulary** What are *vitamins?* Name three fat-soluble and three water-soluble vitamins.

2. **Recall** Describe the importance of water to health.

Thinking Critically

3. **Synthesize** Explain the relationship between physical performance and proper intake of each of the following: calcium, potassium, and sodium.

4. **Analyze** After her early morning workout, Allie is always in a rush and doesn't properly rehydrate. What would you tell Allie about the importance of water to convince her to hydrate before, during, and after her workout?

Personal Fitness Planning

Analyzing Nutrition Keep a fluid log for three days. Note each time you consume a beverage, including the amount in ounces consumed. Also write down any food sources of water that you consume. Determine whether you are meeting your needs for this nutrient. If not, plan how you can go about doing so.

Choosing Foods Wisely

W hat foods do you enjoy eating? Which nutrients do these foods provide? When it comes to making food choices, both these questions are important.

You already know the answer to the first question. In this lesson, you will learn more about the answer to the second.

The Foods You Eat

The good news is that foods that are good for you can also taste good. Do you eat any of the foods in the photo on this page? These and other popular foods have high nutrient content. The sections that follow will introduce easy-to-use tools to determine if your food choices are nutritious. These are the *Dietary Guidelines for Americans*, Food Guide Pyramid, and Nutrition Facts panel on food labels.

Dietary Guidelines for Americans: Aim, Build, Choose

The U.S. Department of Agriculture and the Department of Health and Human Services has released the *Dietary Guidelines for Americans*. These guidelines spell out in simple language the healthy-eating and active-living needs for all Americans as a whole, including teens.

This document identifies ten main guidelines for healthy eating and living. These ten guidelines are shown in **Figure 4.9.** Note that they are categorized into three groups, under the headings *Aim for Fitness*, *Build a Healthy Base*, and *Choose Sensibly*. These ABCs of good health make it even easier to eat healthfully and maintain an active lifestyle.

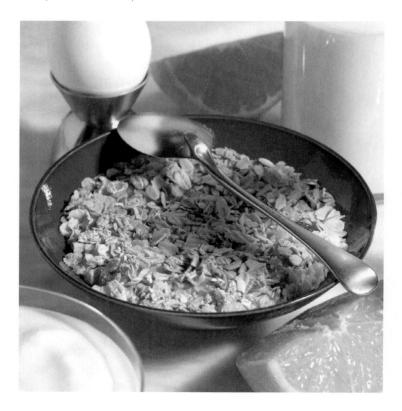

▶ The Food Guide Pyramid can help you determine a balanced eating plan for yourself. *To what food groups do each of the foods pictured belong?*

FIGURE 4.9

DIETARY GUIDELINES FOR AMERICANS

These guidelines can help you design a healthful eating plan.
Which of these guidelines do you already follow?

AIM FOR FITNESS	➤ **Aim for a healthy weight.** ➤ **Be physically active each day.**
BUILD A HEALTHY BASE	➤ **Let the Food Guide Pyramid guide your food choices.** ➤ **Choose a variety of grains daily, especially whole grains.** ➤ **Choose a variety of fruits and vegetables daily.** ➤ **Keep food safe to eat.**
CHOOSE SENSIBLY	➤ **Choose a diet that is low in saturated fat and cholesterol and moderate in total fat.** ➤ **Choose beverages and foods to moderate your intake of sugars.** ➤ **Choose and prepare foods with less salt.** ➤ **Avoid alcoholic beverages.**

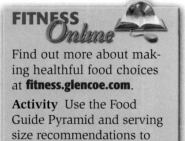

FITNESS *Online*

Find out more about making healthful food choices at **fitness.glencoe.com**.

Activity Use the Food Guide Pyramid and serving size recommendations to create a healthful meal plan.

The Food Guide Pyramid

Under the heading, "Build a Healthy Base," the *Dietary Guidelines for Americans* refers to the Food Guide Pyramid, a *visual guide to help make healthful food choices* (see **Figure 4.10**). You have probably seen it many times on cereal boxes, bread wrappers, and other food products. It shows a range of servings for the different food groups you need to eat each day to achieve and maintain good health.

The recommendations in the Food Guide Pyramid are based on Dietary Reference Intakes (DRI). Determined by nutrition and health experts, DRIs are *daily nutrient recommendations for healthy people of both genders and different age groups.*

What Is a Serving?

Take a moment to study **Figure 4.10**. Notice the Pyramid's structure. Observe that a range of servings accompanies each of the five food groups. The size of a serving and the number of servings varies from food to food and from group to group. **Figure 4.11** on page **132** gives examples of amounts of food that count as one serving within each group.

The base of the Pyramid—the Bread, Cereal, Rice, and Pasta (Grains) Group—is the largest. This means that most of your daily servings should come from this group.

You may have noticed that no specific serving range is given for the foods at the tip of the Pyramid—Fats, Oils, and Sweets. These foods should be consumed sparingly. An occasional soda, handful of chips, or piece of candy is fine but avoid eating too much of these types of foods too often.

For good nutrition, try to stay within serving ranges for each of the food groups. Eat at least the minimum number of servings to get enough nutrients. Be creative. A strawberry smoothie made from ½ cup of fresh strawberries, a cup of plain yogurt, and crushed ice makes a refreshing drink. It also gives you one serving from the Fruit Group and one from the Milk, Yogurt, and Cheese Group.

 Reading Check

Describe From which food group should most of your daily servings come?

FIGURE 4.10

THE FOOD GUIDE PYRAMID

This Pyramid is referred to in the *Dietary Guidelines for Americans.*
Have you seen this pyramid before? Where? Have you ever examined the information it contains? What does it tell you?

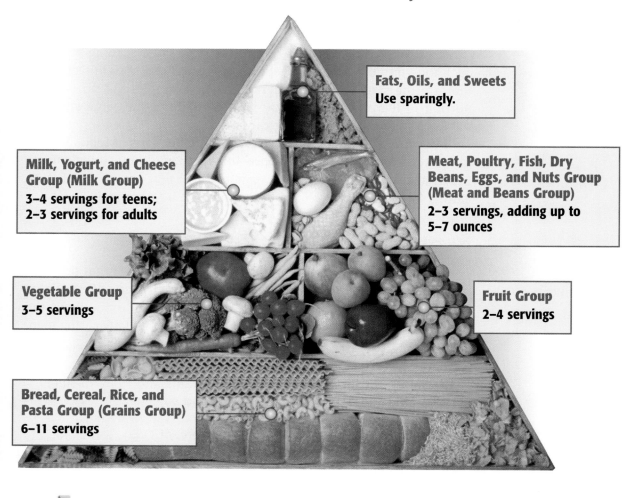

Fats, Oils, and Sweets
Use sparingly.

Milk, Yogurt, and Cheese Group (Milk Group)
3–4 servings for teens;
2–3 servings for adults

Meat, Poultry, Fish, Dry Beans, Eggs, and Nuts Group (Meat and Beans Group)
2–3 servings, adding up to 5–7 ounces

Vegetable Group
3–5 servings

Fruit Group
2–4 servings

Bread, Cereal, Rice, and Pasta Group (Grains Group)
6–11 servings

FIGURE 4.11

SERVING SIZES FOR EACH FOOD GROUP

Serving sizes for food groups vary. *How many cups of cooked or raw vegetables meet the recommended serving size?*

Grains Group	Vegetable Group	Fruit Group	Milk Group	Meat and Beans Group
• 1 slice bread • 1 tortilla • ½ small bagel • 1 cup dry cereal • ½ cup cooked cereal, rice, or pasta	• 1 cup raw leafy vegetables • ½ cup cooked or raw vegetables • ¾ cup vegetable juice	• 1 medium apple, orange, pear, or banana • ½ cup chopped, cooked, or canned fruit • ¾ cup fruit juice	• 1 cup milk or yogurt • 1.5 oz. natural cheese, such as Swiss • 2 oz. processed cheese	• 2–3 oz. cooked lean meat, fish, or poultry **Equivalents of 1 oz. of meat:** • ½ cup cooked dry beans/tofu • 1 egg • 2 tbsp. peanut butter • ⅓ cup nuts

Controlling Portion Size. Figure 4.11 shows the serving sizes for each food group. Learn to "eyeball"—to recognize by sight—portions that are the size of Pyramid servings. For example, a 2- to 3-ounce portion of lean meat or poultry would be about the same size and thickness as a deck of playing cards.

Many restaurants often serve extra-large portions of food. To control portion size, you might choose an appetizer as your main course. Learn also to pay attention to your body. When you feel full, stop eating. Take the leftover food home to eat at a later meal.

Nutrition Facts

All food product labels have a Nutrition Facts panel that provides *a thumbnail analysis of a food's calories and nutrient content for one serving* (see **Figure 4.12**). The *% Daily Value (%DV)* column shows the nutrients in one serving of the food to a 2,000-calorie daily eating plan.

- Serving size
- Calories per serving
- Calories from fat per serving
- Grams and %DV of total fat
- Grams and %DV of saturated fat
- Milligrams and %DV of cholesterol
- Milligrams and %DV of sodium
- Grams and %DV of total carbohydrate
- Grams and %DV of fiber and sugars
- Grams of protein
- Percent Daily Values for vitamins and minerals found in the food

By reading Nutrition Facts panels, you can compare different food products, make wise choices, and get an idea of what and how much you are consuming. Food labeling can help you balance your calorie intake and expenditure if you pay attention to serving sizes and know how much you're really eating.

 Reading Check

Summarize Identify two pieces of information found on a food label's Nutrition Facts panel.

FIGURE 4.12

NUTRITION FACTS PANEL
Reading the Nutrition Facts panel gives you valuable information about the food you eat. *What nutrients does this food provide and in what amounts?*

Nutrition Facts
Serving Size 30g (about 12 pretzels)
Servings Per Container 30

Amount Per Serving	
Calories 110	Calories from Fat 10

	% Daily Value*
Total Fat 1g	**2%**
Saturated Fat 0g	**0%**
Cholesterol 0mg	**0%**
Sodium 300mg	**13%**
Total Carbohydrate 23g	**8%**
Dietary Fiber 1g	**4%**
Sugars Less than 1g	
Protein 3g	

Vitamin A	0% •	Vitamin C	0%
Calcium	0% •	Iron	4%

* Percent Daily Values are based on a 2,000 calorie diet. Your daily values may be higher or lower depending on your calorie needs:

Total Fat	Less Than	65g	80g
Sat Fat	Less Than	20g	25g
Cholesterol	Less Than	300mg	300mg
Sodium	Less Than	2,400mg	2,400mg
Total Carbohydrate		300g	375g
Dietary Fiber		25g	30g

Calories per gram:
Fat 9 • Carbohydrate 4 • Protein 4

Serving Size and Servings Per Container
- Nutrient and calorie content is calculated according to serving size. The serving size on the label may differ from sizes in the Food Guide Pyramid. The number of servings in the package is also listed.

Calories and Calories from Fat
- The number of calories in one serving and how many of these calories come from fat is given here.

Nutrients (Top section)
- The amounts of total fat, saturated fat, cholesterol, and sodium per serving are listed in either grams (g) or milligrams (mg).
- The amounts of total carbohydrates, dietary fiber, sugars, and protein per serving are given.

Nutrients (Bottom section)
- Major vitamins and minerals are listed with their Percent Daily Values.

Percent Daily Value
- This section tells you how much the nutrients in one serving contribute to your total daily eating plan. The general guideline is that 20% or more of a nutrient is a lot and 5% or less isn't very much. Choose foods that are high in fiber, vitamins, and minerals and low in fat, cholesterol, and sodium.

The Footnote (Lower part of Nutrition Facts Panel)
- This information is the same from product to product. It contains recommendations about the amounts of certain nutrients that should be eaten each day.

Active Mind Active Body

Calculating Calories from a Sample Meal

In this activity, you will calculate the percentage of the calories you eat in a day that come from carbohydrate, protein, and fat. Understanding how much of each nutrient you consume is important for developing healthful eating habits.

What You Will Need
- Pen or pencil
- Paper
- Calculator (optional)

What You Will Do

1. List the food that you eat on a particular day. Add up the grams of carbohydrate, protein, and fat that you consume in the food you eat that day.
2. Calculate the number of calories in your food choices for that day. Use the following equivalents to determine calories:
   - 1 gram of carbohydrate = 4 calories
   - 1 gram of protein = 4 calories
   - 1 gram of fat = 9 calories)
3. Calculate what percentage of these calories comes from carbohydrate, protein, and fat. *Hint:* Divide the number of calories for each nutrient by the total number of calories from all the nutrients, then move the decimal point two places to the right.

Apply and Conclude

How many calories for the day are from carbohydrate? from protein? from fat? What percentages are they? Do you recall what percentage of your total daily calories should come from carbohydrate, protein, and fat? What are some ways to reduce fat calories in meals and snacks?

Developing Healthful Eating Habits

Whatever your food preferences might be, any food that supplies calories and nutrients can be part of a healthful eating plan. Good nutrition comes from an eating plan that has *variety, moderation,* and *balance.* Also remember that nutrition guidelines apply to all of your food choices all the time—even when snacking or dining out. However, healthful eating does not mean eliminating certain foods, or eating one particular kind of food all the time. By being aware of your serving sizes and nutrient needs, and with a little planning, you can eat the foods you like and have a healthy eating plan.

The Importance of Breakfast

Many nutritionists agree that breakfast is the most important meal of the day. Your body uses energy even while you sleep, and you need to replenish your body's energy supply once you wake up. A healthy breakfast can improve your physical and mental performance throughout the day. Eating breakfast is also important for maintaining a healthy weight. People who do not eat breakfast may have a tendency to overeat later in the day.

If you do not enjoy typical breakfast foods like cereal or eggs, try eating foods you like, even if they are not traditional breakfast foods. Just make sure you get enough Vitamin C from citrus fruit or juice. You may also want to include a high-fiber cereal, and get some calcium by having a serving of milk, cheese, or yogurt.

Snacking

Some people may believe that part of healthful eating means eliminating snacks. In reality, snacking is fine as long as you choose healthful snacks. Potato chips, soft drinks, and candy contain too many calories and not enough nutrients. They may also be high in fat, added sugars, or salt.

Try to plan your snacks and choose wisely. Healthful snacks can provide the extra energy you need during the growth years and provide nutrients that you might not have been able to eat at other meals. When choosing snacks, select whole-grain products, fruits, and vegetables. Also look for healthier alternatives offered by many companies, such as potato chips that are baked instead of fried. **Figure 4.13** lists the nutrition information for some sensible snacks. You will learn more about a healthful eating plan in Chapters 5 and 6.

✓ Reading Check

Summarize Why is it important to eat breakfast?

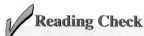

FIGURE 4.13

NUTRITIOUS SNACKS

A healthful eating plan includes nutritious snacks. *What healthful snacks do you enjoy? Explain the myth associated with snacking.*

Food	Food Group	Total Calories per Serving	Calories from Fat
Air-popped popcorn, 3 cups (plain)	Grains	23	0
Apple, 1 medium	Fruit	80	0
Bagel, ½ half (small, 2 oz.)	Grains	83	10
Bread stick, 1	Grains	42	6
Frozen juice bar, 4 oz.	Fruit	75	0
Skim milk, 1 cup	Milk	90	0
Sugar-free gelatin (½ cup) with ½ cup sliced banana	Fruit	76	0
Graham cracker squares, 3	Grains	80	15
Pretzel sticks, 50 small	Grains	60	9
Fat-free, sugar-free yogurt, 6 oz.	Milk	86	0

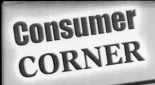
Dining Out: A Word to the Wise

More Americans are eating meals away from home than ever before. As a wise consumer, you can make smart choices and eat healthfully when you dine out. Here are some tips for eating wisely when dining out.

- **Pay attention to how your food is prepared.** For example, have your chicken grilled instead of fried. If possible, minimize use of high-fat sauces, sour cream, and butter.
- **Choose healthful side dishes.** For example, order a salad instead of french fries with your meal.
- **Watch portion sizes.** Ordering extra-large portions at fast-food restaurants may seem like a good value, but it probably provides more calories than necessary.

- **Estimate servings.** If you are served a large portion, try to estimate the true number of servings in that portion. Eat the equivalent of one serving, and take the rest home for a later meal.
- **Drink healthful beverages.** Choose low-fat milk or water instead of high-sugar soft drinks.

Investigate

Try implementing one or more of these suggestions the next time you dine out, either at a sit-down or fast-food restaurant. Report to classmates on the success of your efforts.

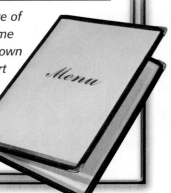

Keeping Food Safe to Eat

Eating healthfully means more than just choosing foods that meet your nutrient and calorie needs. It also means eating foods that have been handled and prepared safely. Otherwise, there is a risk of **food-borne illness**—*illness that results from consuming food contaminated with disease-causing organisms, the poisons they produce, or chemical contaminants.* You should discard any food that you suspect has spoiled. Never taste it to check. Remember: When in doubt, throw it out.

Anyone who handles food should use the following guidelines to help keep foods safe to eat.

- **Clean.** Wash your hands, cutting boards, and countertops with hot, soapy water before and after food preparation and after handling raw meat, poultry, or fish. This prevents **cross-contamination,** *the spreading of bacteria or other pathogens from one food to another.* Use cutting boards made of non-porous materials, such as plastic or glass, for preparing foods. Remember to wash fruits and vegetables before you eat them.
- **Separate.** Separate raw, cooked, and ready-to-eat foods while shopping, preparing, or storing. Use a separate cutting board for raw meats.

- **Cook.** Cook foods to a safe temperature: 160°F for ground beef, 170°F for roasts and poultry, and 145°F for fish. The juices of meat or poultry should run clear when properly cooked. Fish should be opaque and flake easily with a fork. Avoid eating dishes that contain raw or partially cooked eggs.
- **Chill.** Refrigerate perishable foods promptly. Foods should be at room temperature no longer than two hours—one hour on a warm day. Cold foods should be refrigerated at 40°F or less and frozen foods should be kept at 0°F. Defrost frozen foods in the refrigerator or microwave, or by running them under cold water—never on the kitchen counter.

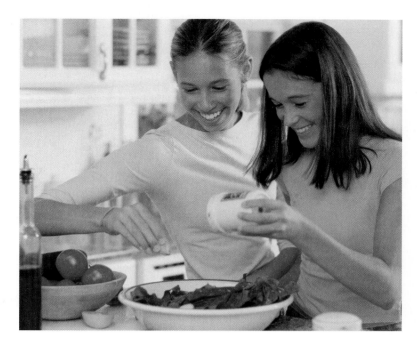

Handling and preparing food safely will prevent foodborne illness. *What are some tips to follow to keep food safe to eat?*

Reading Check

Identify What are four tips for handling food safely?

Lesson 3 Review

Using complete sentences, answer the following questions on a sheet of paper.

Reviewing Facts and Vocabulary

1. **Vocabulary** What is the *Food Guide Pyramid?*
2. **Recall** Why is eating breakfast important to your health?
3. **Recall** List three practices that can help prevent foodborne illness.

Thinking Critically

4. **Analyze** For lunch, Shauna had a turkey sandwich on whole-wheat bread, a glass of tomato juice, and a peach. Identify the group in the Food Guide Pyramid to which each food belongs. Then tell how many Pyramid servings of each Shauna had. What could she add to her lunch for more nutrition?

5. **Evaluate** Most restaurants do not list serving size and nutrition information on their menus. What can you do to make sure you maintain a healthy eating plan, even when dining out?

Personal Fitness Planning

Investigating Safety Inspect your kitchen at home. Write a list of ways you can help make the kitchen safer in terms of food preparation. In addition, check your refrigerator for any foods that might be spoiled or outdated. Share the results with your family members. Help them become aware of the dangers of foodborne illness and ways to prevent it.

What You Will Do

- Apply sound nutritional practices to physical activity and performance.
- Analyze the effects of performance-enhancing supplements on health and physical performance.

Terms to Know

pre-event meal
ephedrine
creatine
androstenedione

Nutrition for Peak Performance

Do you play a sport or participate in a competitive recreational activity? If so, you need to pay extra attention to what you eat before, during, and after physical activity. This lesson will provide some information about proper nutrition and physical activity.

Food for Performance Fitness

As noted in Chapter 1, athletics, sports, and competitive recreational activities all demand high levels of performance—or skill-related—fitness. One key factor to achieving high performance fitness levels is appropriate physical training. Another equally important factor is eating wisely to optimize your performance.

When you play hard, your body provides you with the energy you need by burning calories. **Figure 4.14** shows the relationship between physical activity and energy expenditure.

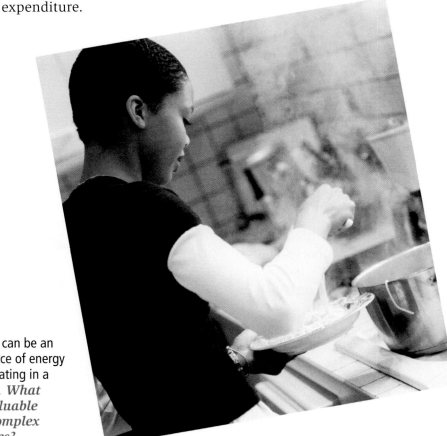

Carbohydrates can be an important source of energy before participating in a sporting event. *What foods are valuable sources of complex carbohydrates?*

FIGURE 4.14

CALORIES BURNED DURING PHYSICAL ACTIVITY

Analyze exercise as a method of weight control. Approximately how many calories would you burn in an hour of cycling?

Activity	Calories Burned in 30 minutes	Time to Burn 230 Calories
• Aerobics	211	33 minutes
• Bicycling 10–12 mph	158	44 minutes
• Frisbee	106	66 minutes
• Gardening	176	39 minutes
• Running at 6.7 mph, 9 min/mile	387	18 minutes
• Skateboarding	176	39 minutes
• Stretching (hatha yoga)	140	49 minutes
• Tennis doubles	211	33 minutes
• Walking at 4 mph	140	49 minutes
• Weight lifting (vigorous)	211	33 minutes

Pre-Event Meals

Proper sports nutrition begins *before* the competitive event. Eating the right variety and amounts of foods ensures a steady supply of energy during the event. It's important to choose foods wisely, not only on the day of the event but also in the days and weeks leading up to it.

Your **pre-event meal** is *the last full meal consumed prior to a practice session or the competitive event itself.* The pre-event meal should be eaten within one to three hours before the practice or event. This allows time for the food to fully digest. Eating any closer to the time of the event can result in nausea or stomach cramps.

The pre-event meal should consist primarily of foods high in complex carbohydrates. These include pasta, whole-grain breads, and rice. Foods high in protein or fat take longer to digest. Foods such as candy bars and other foods with simple carbohydrates do not supply energy right away. For endurance sports, a small sugar snack or drink may be acceptable. However, too much sugar may affect how fast your body replaces fluids. This can slow your performance. **Figure 4.15** on page **140** lists foods that might be part of an effective pre-event meal.

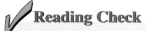

Reading Check

Explain What nutrient is most important to a pre-event meal?

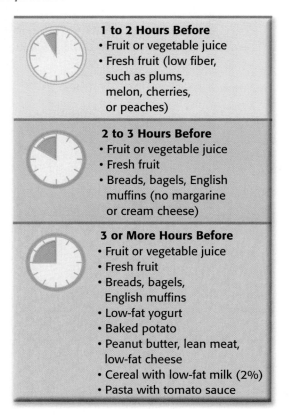

FIGURE 4.15

PRE-EVENT FOODS

Your pre-event meal supplies your body with enough energy for the event. *What main source of energy does each of these foods provide?*

1 to 2 Hours Before
- Fruit or vegetable juice
- Fresh fruit (low fiber, such as plums, melon, cherries, or peaches)

2 to 3 Hours Before
- Fruit or vegetable juice
- Fresh fruit
- Breads, bagels, English muffins (no margarine or cream cheese)

3 or More Hours Before
- Fruit or vegetable juice
- Fresh fruit
- Breads, bagels, English muffins
- Low-fat yogurt
- Baked potato
- Peanut butter, lean meat, low-fat cheese
- Cereal with low-fat milk (2%)
- Pasta with tomato sauce

Source: Play Hard, Eat Right: A Parent's Guide to Sports Nutrition for Children, *1998.*[3]

rehydrate

For more on proper ways to rehydrate before, during, and after exercise, see Chapter 2, page **42.**

restoration

For more on restoration and factors that influence recovery, see Chapter 3, page **100.**

Foods During Day-Long Events

Some competitions are day-long events or a series of events that span several hours, for example, track meets, basketball tournaments, and wrestling meets. When participating in this type of event, you need to eat at intervals during the day to renew energy. You also need to prevent dehydration, which will have a negative effect on your performance and may be dangerous to your health.

The best advice is to choose foods that have complex carbohydrates, such as bread, cereals, and pasta. Also include vegetables and fruit. Avoid simple sugars such as soft drinks, cookies, and candy. Make sure also to **rehydrate** throughout the day. Drink plenty of fluids to replace those lost through perspiration.

Post-Event Eating: Restoration

Following a high-intensity workout or competition, you need to eat foods that will promote **restoration.** Doing so is especially important if you plan to train or compete again the next day or shortly thereafter.

Foods rich in complex carbohydrates and protein are the best choice for optimizing recovery. These foods will renew your glucose level and your glycogen stores. You also need to replace fluids lost in the form of perspiration during physical activity.

There are three phases to post-event eating:

- **Phase 1: Drink Fluids.** Rehydrating with water or sports drinks should begin immediately after the event for proper restoration and continue for several hours until normal body weight is regained.
- **Phase 2: Have a Snack.** This should occur as soon after the event as possible, within the first 30 minutes. This phase consists of consuming a snack or beverage to begin the restoration process. The chart in **Figure 4.16** shows some possible food choices for this phase of recovery. A good guideline is to consume 1.2 to 1.5 grams of carbohydrate per kilogram of body weight and between 0.3 and 0.5 grams of protein per kilogram of body weight. For example, a 154-pound—or 70-kg—male (154/2.2 = 70) would need to consume between 84 and 105 grams of carbohydrates and 21 and 35 grams of protein.
- **Phase 3: Eat a Meal.** This should occur two hours after competition. This phase consists of a full meal, rich in carbohydrates. Small amounts of protein and fat can be added to the post-event meal for calories and taste.

Reading Check

Summarize What are the three phases of restoration?

FIGURE 4.16

POST-EVENT FOODS

Explain how eating foods like these after an event makes it possible to work out or compete again the next day.

Food	Carbohydrate (in grams)	Protein (g)
Medium bagel	50	7.5
Cranberry-apple juice (1 cup)	43	0.1
Fruit yogurt (1 cup)	40	9.9
Large banana	40	1.3
Apple juice (1 cup)	30	0.1
Orange juice (1 cup)	28	1.7
Pretzels (10)	23	5.5

Source: Play Hard, Eat Right: A Parent's Guide to Sports Nutrition for Children, *1998.*[3]

Understanding the Energy Equation

To maintain weight, the calories you take in from food must equal the calories you burn. The equation of calories consumed relative to calories burned varies from person to person. In this test, you will perform a 20-minute walk/jog evaluation to learn more about energy intake and energy demands.

Before you attempt this activity, perform a warm-up. Practice the test before you try it. Allow 5 to 10 minutes to cool down after taking the test. *If you feel dizzy or become overheated at any point during the test, stop immediately.*

Following your warm-up, begin walking or jogging. Try to reach a moderate-to-vigorous level of intensity that you know you can maintain for 20 minutes. If you are not used to walking or jogging, make sure you choose a pace that will keep you at a moderate intensity for the 20-minute duration. Review the guidelines for determining intensity level on pages **28–29,** Chapter 1, and for using the Borg scale on page **87,** Chapter 3.

Estimating Calories Expended

1. Determine if you have walked/jogged at a moderate-to-vigorous level. Then estimate how many calories you burned in 20 minutes by using the following guide:

Intensity Level	Average Calories Burned
Moderate intensity for 20 minutes	120 calories
Vigorous intensity for 20 minutes	160 calories

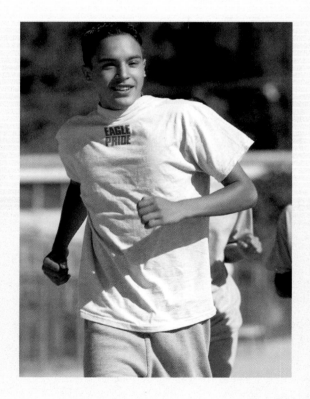

2. Now estimate how many calories you would have burned if you had kept walking/jogging for two hours and record that total.
3. Once you have that estimate, develop an eating plan for how to replace that same number of calories with nutrient-rich foods. Then make a plan to optimize your recovery if you had to walk or jog for two hours the next day.

Risks of Supplements

Dietary supplements are dangerous if used to enhance athletic performance. These include:

- **Ephedrine.** Also called ephedra or ma huang, ephedrine (eh-FED-ruhn) is *a compound that increases the rate at which the body converts calories to energy.* It increases resting heart rate and body temperature. Ephedrine may lead to heat-related injury, heart problems, and even death.
- **Creatine.** Creatine (KREE-uh-teen) is *a supplement that increases muscle size while enhancing the body's ability to use protein.* It is especially risky for teens because the long-term effects on growth and development are unknown.
- **Androstenedione.** Androstenedione (an-DROS-tuh-NED-ee-ohn) is *a chemical agent that aids the body in its production of testosterone.* Like anabolic steroids, this chemical promotes muscle growth. Its use may increase the risk of heart disease.

These supplements involve serious health risks for adults and teens. In addition, they may give the user an unfair advantage over fellow competitors. Athletes who choose to use such substances are putting their health and their athletic careers at risk.

Reading Check

Discuss Why should a person avoid performance-enhancing supplements?

Lesson 4 Review

Using complete sentences, answer the following questions on a sheet of paper.

Reviewing Facts and Vocabulary

1. **Vocabulary** What is a *pre-event meal?*
2. **Recall** Describe the three phases of post-event restoration through food.

Thinking Critically

3. **Compare and Contrast** Compare any two of the performance-enhancing supplements in terms of (a) what they claim to do and (b) their effect on health and physical performance.
4. **Analyze** Kim is on the school track team. Kim is not concerned about her pre- and post-event meals. Pretend you are Kim's coach and advise her about what she should eat before and after the event. Explain to Kim the relationship between sound nutritional practices and physical activity.

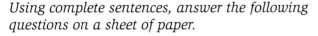

Personal Fitness Planning

Evaluating Products Visit a local pharmacy, food supplement store, or health food store. Review the labels on various herbal or food supplements the store carries. List any claims on product labels about improving personal fitness performance. Then access reliable print and online resources to evaluate the validity of these claims. Share your findings with the class.

TRUE/FALSE

On a sheet of paper, write the numbers 1–10. Write True or False for each statement.

1. Nutrient needs vary with age, gender, and activity level.
2. Hunger is a personal desire, rather than a need, to eat.
3. Dietary fiber is easily digestible and is high in calories.
4. Of your total calories, 20 to 35 percent should come from fat.
5. Vitamin K is an example of a water-soluble vitamin.
6. Antioxidants may help protect against cancer, atherosclerosis, overtraining, and premature aging.
7. DRIs are daily nutrient recommendations for healthy people of both genders and different age groups.
8. An example of the size of one serving of fruit is one medium apple.
9. If you are eating to compete, you should consume simple carbohydrates for quick energy right before the contest.
10. Taking the supplement ephedrine before engaging in intense physical activity may increase the risk for heat-related injuries.

MULTIPLE CHOICE

On a sheet of paper, write the letter of the word or phrase that best completes each statement.

11. Before your body can use carbohydrates for energy, it must convert them to
    a. fiber.
    b. glucose.
    c. fats.
    d. electrolytes.
12. Candy bars, cookies, and soft drinks all contain a category of nutrients known as
    a. simple carbohydrates.
    b. fiber.
    c. complex carbohydrates.
    d. fat.

13. Of the following, cholesterol is found only in
    a. plant foods.
    b. soft drinks.
    c. meats.
    d. corn and olive oil.
14. Of the following, the vitamin that is NOT fat soluble is
    a. Vitamin A.
    b. Vitamin C.
    c. Vitamin D.
    d. Vitamin E.
15. Of the following, the mineral that does not function as an electrolyte is
    a. sodium.
    b. iron.
    c. calcium.
    d. potassium.
16. The number of daily servings of fruit recommended by the Food Guide Pyramid is
    a. 2–3.
    b. 3–5.
    c. 2–4.
    d. none of the above.
17. The following are all tips for controlling portion sizes when dining out EXCEPT
    a. choosing an appetizer as your main course.
    b. ordering regular-size portions rather than bigger value sizes.
    c. noticing when you begin to feel full, then not eating any more.
    d. ordering more than you think you can eat.
18. A Nutrition Facts panel on a food label will contain all of the following information EXCEPT
    a. serving size.
    b. total grams of protein.
    c. the number of servings of vegetables you should eat daily.
    d. Percent Daily Values for some vitamins.
19. A pre-event meal should be eaten
    a. within 30 minutes of the competition.
    b. every day for several weeks leading up to the competition.
    c. 1 to 3 hours before the competition.
    d. none of the above.
20. Use by competitive athletes of performance-enhancing supplements such as ephedrine and creatine is
    a. legal.
    b. unfair.
    c. dangerous.
    d. all of the above.

DISCUSSION

Using complete sentences, answer the following questions on a sheet of paper.

21. **Discuss** Identify which factors identified in Lesson 1 have the greatest influence on your food choices. Be specific.
22. **Summarize** Make a checklist that could be used to evaluate food safety practices in any home or professional kitchen.
23. **Extend** If you were to train and compete in a 10-kilometer walk/run in your community, how could you modify your nutrition plan to optimize your performance?

VOCABULARY EXPERIENCE

On a sheet of paper, write the letter of the term in Column B that best fits the definition in Column A.

Column A

24. Fats that are formed when certain oils are processed into solids.
25. A nonfood form of one or more nutrients.
26. A fatlike substance that is produced in the liver and circulates in the blood.
27. A special subclass of complex carbohydrates that aids the body in digestion.
28. A natural inborn drive that protects you from starvation.
29. Substances that protect body cells from damage.
30. A personal desire, rather than a need, to eat.

Column B

a. antioxidant
b. hunger
c. dietary fiber
d. dietary supplement
e. appetite
f. trans fatty acids
g. cholesterol

CRITICAL THINKING

Using complete sentences, answer the following questions on a sheet of paper.

31. **Compare** What is the difference between water-soluble and fat-soluble vitamins?
32. **Explain** Why is it especially important for a physically active person to make sure that he or she is getting enough potassium?

33. **Compare** Compare your eating habits with those of a family member. Which one of you is making wiser food choices? Explain your answer.

CASE STUDY

JAVIER'S WEIGHT GOALS

Javier is an active fifteen-year-old male who is interested in gaining muscle mass. He has started lifting weights two times a week, but he knows that he also needs to create a nutritious and balanced eating plan in order to help him reach his goal safely and effectively. His current dietary habits include skipping breakfast, eating a light lunch, and having a large dinner. He doesn't snack between meals. Javier needs the help of someone knowledgeable about designing and implementing a fitness program that includes nutritional advice—someone like you!

HERE IS YOUR ASSIGNMENT:

Assume you are Javier's friend, and that he asks you for some assistance with his plans for gaining muscle by adjusting his nutrition and physical-activity routine. Make a list of things Javier should consider and do before beginning his program. Then list the recommendations you would give to Javier for the first two weeks of his program.

KEYS TO HELP YOU

- Consider Javier's current eating plan and nutrition habits.
- Decide how he should evaluate his current eating plan.
- Think about his needs and goals. For example, how should he go about changing his eating habits?
- Develop a reasonable eating plan for Javier.

FITNESS
Online

How often do you weigh yourself? Have you ever had your body composition measured to estimate your percentage of body fat? These questions can help you understand the importance of body composition. Complete the STEP Personal Inventory for Chapter 5. Find it at **fitness.glencoe.com**.

The Basics of Body Composition

There is no single ideal body weight or body type for everyone. Instead, there is an appropriate range of body weights that will help you to maintain your functional health and fitness. To understand the relationship among your weight, body composition, and health, you need to consider many factors. You will explore these factors throughout this chapter.

Your Body Type

If you look around your school, you will notice people of all sizes and shapes, or *body types*. Body type is determined by a number of characteristics. These include bone size, muscle size, muscle mass, and percentage of body fat. There are three general body types.

- **Ectomorph.** The ectomorph body type is *characterized by a low percentage of body fat, small bone size, and a small amount of muscle mass and size.* Ectomorphs exhibit a lean appearance, often with long, slender arms and legs.
- **Mesomorph.** The mesomorph body type is *characterized by a low-to-medium percentage of body fat, medium-to-large bone size, and a large amount of muscle mass and size.* Mesomorphs appear muscular and well-proportioned.
- **Endomorph.** The endomorph body type is *characterized by a high percentage of body fat, large bone size, and a small amount of muscle mass and size.* Endomorphs generally have a round face, short neck, and wide hips.

What You Will Do

- Identify various body types.
- Analyze how your body composition can influence your functional health and fitness.
- Determine your BMI.

Terms to Know

ectomorph
mesomorph
endomorph
lean body weight
body mass index (BMI)
body composition
overweight
essential fat
excessive leanness
overfat

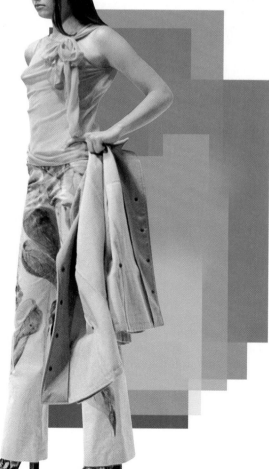

▶ The three basic body types are ectomorph, mesomorph, and endomorph. *What is the name for the body type shown in the picture?*

FIGURE 5.1

BODY TYPES: ECTOMORPH, MESOMORPH, AND ENDOMORPH

Body type is determined by heredity. *Do you have the same body type as someone else in your family?*

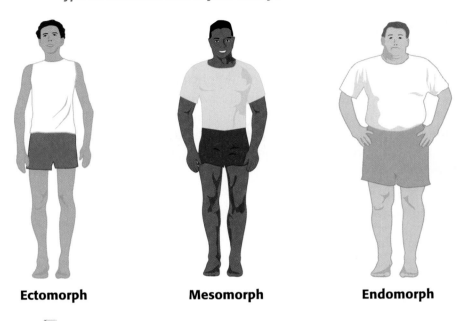

| Ectomorph | Mesomorph | Endomorph |

Mind OVER Matter

One Size Does Not Fit All

As a teen, you may feel inadequate because you don't look like one of the many models you see on television or in magazines.

Remember, however, that body type is hereditary. Models have been born with a body type that can't be achieved solely through any kind of eating plan or exercise.

Learn to accept your body type. It is part of who you are, like your hair color or eye color. It is part of your unique identity. Focus on exercise and eating habits as a way of maintaining your functional health and fitness—not a way to change who you are.

Figure 5.1 illustrates these three different body types. Body type is determined by heredity. Nevertheless, you still have some ability to control your body weight and composition as you age.

Your Body Weight

While your overall body type is determined by heredity, one aspect you can control is your weight. Although there is no one ideal weight, there are healthy ranges for each individual. These ranges are determined by several factors, including gender, age, height, body type, growth rate, metabolic rate, and activity level. For example, teens need more calories than adults because they are still growing. Active people need more calories than sedentary people because they burn more energy.

Many people place too much importance on weight. Weight by itself is not an accurate indicator of health. It tells you little about how lean or fat you are. In reality, when you compare two people of the same size, one may simply weigh more because he or she has more lean body weight than the other person. **Lean body weight** is *the combined weight of bone, muscle, and connective tissue.*

Body Mass Index

One way to determine if your weight is within a healthy range is by using **Body Mass Index (BMI)**. This is *a way to assess body size in relation to your height and weight.* **Figure 5.2** explains how to determine your BMI. Because BMI for teens varies according to age and gender, different charts are used for males and females. Adults also use a different chart for determining BMI. Notice that many different ratios of height and weight can be healthy. There is no single size and shape that's healthy for everyone.

Reading Check

Summarize How can a person determine if his or her weight is within a healthy range?

FIGURE 5.2

TEEN BODY MASS INDEX

BMI is a useful tool when evaluating your body weight.
What is your BMI?

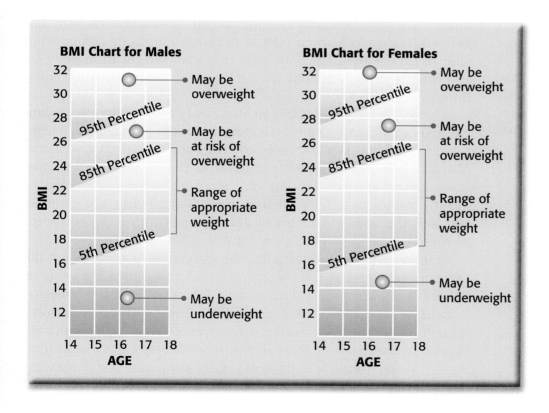

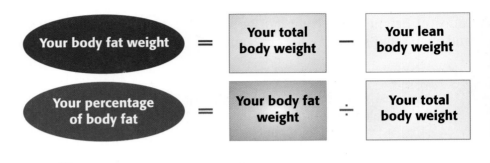

FIGURE 5.3

CALCULATIONS FOR BODY FAT

Lean body weight and body weight from fat are more relevant to understanding your health than total body weight. *Which tissues are included in lean body weight?*

obesity
For more information on obesity, see Chapter 2, page **36.**

Body Composition

Understanding body composition, *the relative percentage in your body of fat to lean body tissue, including water, bone, and muscle,* is important to understanding a person's overall health. Particularly important is the ratio of lean body weight to weight from body fat. You will learn more about how to evaluate your body composition later in the chapter. For now, note that your weight from body fat and your percentage of body fat can be calculated by using the equations in **Figure 5.3.**

Physical activity and nutrition affect body composition. For example, you can increase your muscle mass by weight training, and a high-calorie eating plan will increase body fat. The nutrients in your eating plan also influence your body composition. During adolescence, especially, certain nutrients become very important to the development of healthy, lean body tissues, such as muscles and bones. For example, zinc aids the body's growth and development. Iron is necessary for increasing muscles, and calcium for strengthening bones.

It is important to understand that amount of body fat is not the same as body weight. Overweight is *a condition in which a person is heavier than the standard weight range for his or her height.* **Obesity,** as defined in Chapter 2, is a medical condition in which a person's ratio of body fat to lean muscle mass is excessively high. Both conditions can be high-risk to your health, and overweight may lead to obesity. Being overweight, however, is not always the result of excess body fat, as is the case with some body builders. They may exceed the appropriate weight range due to their excess muscle tissue.

Body Fat

When asked which aspect of body type they would most like to change, most people mention body fat. However, eliminating body fat entirely is not possible, or desirable. Everyone needs some body fat. **Essential fat** is *the minimum amount of body fat necessary for good health.* It is necessary for several reasons. Essential fat

- insulates your body against the cold.
- cushions your internal organs, protecting them from injury.
- provides you with a valuable source of stored energy. This enables you to meet your body's need for fuel.

While there are no hard-and-fast guidelines on how much body fat teens need, various measures may be used to determine whether a person's body composition is *within normal limits* for good health. You may reasonably assume the following:

- Teen males need 7 to 19 percent body fat.
- Teen females need 12 to 24 percent body fat.

Body Composition and Your Functional Health and Fitness

Body composition has an impact on your overall health, as shown in **Figure 5.4.** If you carry too little body fat, you are excessively lean. **Excessive leanness** may be defined as *having a percentage of body fat that is below the acceptable range for your age and gender.* Being **overfat** means *carrying too much body fat for your age and gender.*

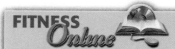

FITNESS *Online*

Find out what you can do to evaluate and control your body composition at **fitness.glencoe.com**.

Activity Calculate your BMI using the online tools. Then find out how to assess your risks and make healthful changes.

FIGURE 5.4

BODY COMPOSITION AND RISK FOR CHRONIC DISEASES

According to this graph, people with a high percentage of body fat are at the greatest risk for chronic diseases. *Which group is at second greatest risk?*

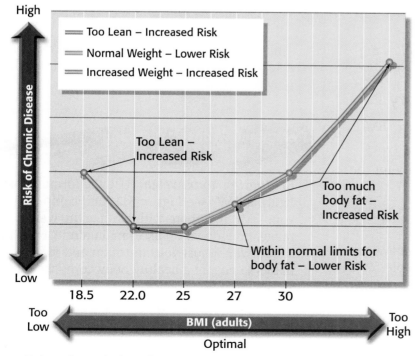

Source: Understanding Exercise for Health and Disease, 3rd Edition, 1997.[1]

Teen males are considered to be overfat and at risk for overweight when their body fat is greater than 20 percent. They are considered overweight when their body fat exceeds 25 percent. Teen males are excessively lean if their body fat is less than 7 percent.

Teen females are considered to be overfat and at risk for overweight when their body fat is greater than 25 percent. They are considered overweight when their body fat exceeds 32 percent. Excessive leanness for teen females is less than 12 percent body fat.

Overfat and excessive leanness place your functional health and fitness at risk for developing chronic diseases. In Figure 5.4 on page **151,** notice the *J* shape of the curve. This shape emphasizes the two population groups with the greatest risks for developing health problems. These are:

- People who weigh the least and are excessively lean
- People who weigh the most and have too much body fat

You will learn more about the risks associated with unhealthy weight and body composition in Chapter 6.

 Reading Check

Compare What is considered a healthy range for percentage of body fat for a female teen? for a male teen?

Lesson 1 Review

Using complete sentences, answer the following questions on a sheet of paper.

Reviewing Facts and Vocabulary

1. **Vocabulary** Define *Body Mass Index (BMI)*.
2. **Recall** Identify the three basic body types.
3. **Recall** Why is essential fat necessary for the health and functioning of your body?

Thinking Critically

4. **Compare** What is the difference between overweight and obesity? Is it possible for a person to be overweight, but not at risk for obesity? Explain.
5. **Extend** Jerry is 16 years old and has a BMI of 28. He is concerned because his family has a history of obesity. What advice can you give Jerry about whether he is at risk for being overweight?

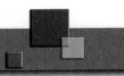
Personal Fitness Planning

Evaluating Your Weight Use the formula for figuring BMI (see **Figure 5.2**) and compute your BMI. If you are within a healthy weight range, how do you plan to maintain it? How should you adjust your nutrition and fitness habits to ensure a healthy body composition as you become an adult? If you are not within a healthy weight range, what goals can you set for achieving a healthy weight?

Influences on Your Body Composition

Body type, it was noted in Lesson 1, is determined by heredity. In this lesson you will learn about other factors that play a role in body size and shape. You will also learn which of them you can control and which you cannot.

Influences on Body Fat

After infancy, your teen years are the most dramatic growth period in your life. During these years, your body is rapidly transforming itself into an adult.

There is a common link between infancy and adolescence. They are the only times when the body develops new fat cells. The number of fat cells your body adds during adolescence depends in part on body type. Ectomorphs will acquire fewer new fat cells than mesomorphs or endomorphs. Endomorphs will acquire more new fat cells than mesomorphs or ectomorphs. This change is a fact of life—a fact of who you are. There is nothing you can do to change it. However, body fat percentage is both a function of the size of your body's fat cells as well as the *number*. Obese people, in other words, may have more fat cells than people who are within normal limits. Obese people also have larger fat cells.

Although you cannot control the number of fat cells in your body, you can control their size. The next section will discuss ways that can help.

▶ During the teen years, your body develops new fat cells. *What determines how many fat cells your body develops?*

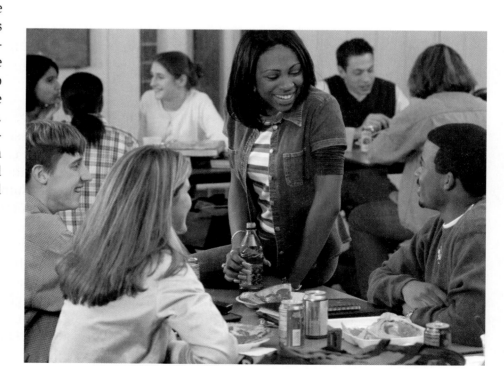

What You Will Do

- Identify influences on amount of body fat.
- Analyze the role of energy balance in maintaining body weight and body composition.
- Describe the importance of metabolism to the energy equation.
- Identify the role of exercise as a method of weight control.
- Calculate the calories expended during various physical activities.

Terms to Know

calorie intake
calorie expenditure
metabolism
resting metabolic rate (RMR)

Lifestyle Behaviors

Have you ever heard the saying, "You are what you eat?" There is some truth to this saying. Your body composition, in other words, is partly a function of your eating patterns. If you take in more calories from food than your body needs, the extra calories will be stored as fat. This stored fat will, in turn, increase the size of your fat cells.

Another lifestyle behavior that affects your body composition is activity level. The more physically active you are, the more calories you burn as fuel. The opposite, of course, is also true.

By eating healthfully and maintaining an active lifestyle, you can help control your body composition now and as you get older.

 Reading Check

Identify What are two lifestyle behaviors that can affect body fat?

The Energy Equation

The question of what percentage of your body weight is from fat comes down ultimately to energy balance. Do you recall reading about calories and energy in Chapter 4? To manage your weight and stay healthy, your body needs to maintain an energy balance. This means that it needs to expend, or use up, the energy taken in from food each day.

Energy balance is determined by calorie intake, *the total number of calories you take in from food*, and calorie expenditure, *the total number of calories you burn or expend.* If you take in fewer calories from food than you expend over a period of weeks or months, you will lower your percentage of body fat. The reverse is also true.

Calorie Intake

As explained in Chapter 4, three of the six nutrient classes provide calories—carbohydrates, proteins, and fats. **Figure 5.5** shows the number of calories supplied by each type. If you know the number of grams of these nutrients in the foods you eat, you can calculate the amount of calories you consume at meals and snacks. You can then use this information to determine if your daily calorie intake is appropriate for your energy needs.

Even if you have a healthy body composition as a teen, it will be necessary to adjust your eating habits and level of physical activity as you become an adult. This will help you maintain a proper energy balance as your body's needs change. The Daily Calorie Intake chart in **Figure 4.1** on page **115** shows estimates of calories needed by any given individual based on age and activity level. Remember that less active teens and adults require fewer calories than those who are physically active.

FIGURE 5.5

CALORIES PER GRAM OF NUTRIENT

All of these nutrients provide energy. *Which nutrient provides the most calories per gram? Which provides the most energy per gram?*

Nutrient	Calories per Gram
Carbohydrate	4
Protein	4
Fat	9

Calorie Expenditure and Metabolism

The process by which the body converts calories from food to energy is known as metabolism. Metabolism is an ongoing process. It occurs even when you are at rest. The rate at which the body uses energy varies from person to person and during different physical activities. Your resting metabolic rate (RMR) is *the amount of calories you expend for body processes while at rest.* Your calorie expenditure is determined by your RMR and how physically active you are each day.

Your RMR represents the energy needed for involuntary body activities. Among these are heartbeat, blood circulation, and breathing. For most young adults, such activities require between 1 to 1.5 calories per minute. You need to consume between 1,400 and 1,800 calories just to keep your body functioning.

Your Resting Metabolic Rate (RMR). Your RMR is shaped by several factors. These include:

- **Gender.** Males on average have higher RMRs than females, as illustrated in **Figure 5.6.** This is because male teens typically have a higher proportion of muscle mass to fat than do female teens. Muscle burns more calories than body fat.

FIGURE 5.6

YOUR METABOLIC RATE AS YOU AGE

Metabolic rate depends on several factors, including age and gender. *Describe the difference in the trends between male and female RMR.*

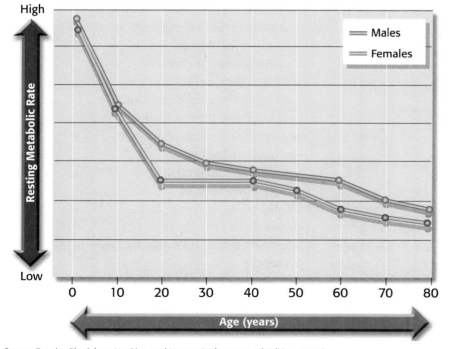

Source: Exercise Physiology, Nutrition, and Human Performance, 5th Edition, *2001.*[2]

Active Mind Active Body

Exercise and Calorie Expenditure

In this activity, you will determine the effect exercise and physical activity have on energy balance by determining the caloric expenditure for certain physical activities. This will help you analyze how exercise and physical activities you enjoy can influence your personal energy balance and affect body weight and composition.

What You Will Need

- Pen or pencil
- Paper
- Calculator (optional)

What You Will Do

1. Review **Figure 5.7** below. Select two physical activities or exercises that you do somewhat regularly.
2. Calculate and record how many calories you would expend for one week if you did each exercise or activity three times a week for the following durations:
   - 20 minutes
   - 40 minutes
   - 60 minutes

Apply and Conclude

What was the largest calorie expenditure you recorded? For what activity did you record this number?

Energy Demands of Activities

Activity	Cal/Lb/Min	Calculating Calories Expended
Aerobic dance (vigorous)	0.062	*Cal/Lb/Min* means *Calories per pound* of body weight *per minute*. In order to calculate the number of calories you would expend after several minutes of a particular physical activity, multiply the *Cal/Lb/Min* factor from this chart by your weight. Then multiply your answer by the number of minutes you spend on the activity.
Basketball (vigorous, full court)	0.097	
Bicycling (13 mph)	0.045	
Bicycling (19 mph)	0.076	
Canoeing (flat water, moderate pace)	0.045	
Cross-country skiing (8 mph)	0.104	
Golf (carrying clubs)	0.045	
Handball	0.078	
Horseback riding (trot)	0.052	
Rowing (vigorous)	0.097	For example, if you weigh 142 pounds, and you spend 30 minutes doing aerobic dance, you would do the following:
Running (5 mph)	0.061	
Running (7.5 mph)	0.094	
Running (10 mph)	0.114	0.062 Cal/Lb/Min × 142 = 8.8 calories per minute
Soccer	0.097	
Swimming (20 ypm)	0.032	8.8 Cal/Min × 30 = 264 calories expended
Swimming (45 ypm)	0.058	
Tennis (beginner)	0.032	
Walking (3.5 mph)	0.035	

Figure 5.7

Source: Nutrition Concerns for the Endurance Athlete.[3]

- **Age.** RMR decreases with age. As people grow older, they need fewer calories to meet their daily energy needs. If they fail to reduce their calorie intake or increase their energy expenditure levels, they will see a weight and fat gain.
- **Heredity.** Some people inherit much higher RMRs than others. This may explain, at least in part, why some people have an easier time losing weight than others.
- **Eating habits.** Your eating habits can stimulate or slow your RMR. For example, when you eat regularly (three to six small meals) throughout the day, you stimulate your RMR more often. This is because the act of digestion itself requires energy. However, if you eat only one meal per day (as many busy people do), your RMR may be slower. This can promote weight gain and increase your body fat.
- **Eliminating calories.** Restricting the number of calories taken in slows down your RMR. Suppose you reduced your daily calorie intake to 500 calories, which is well below daily recommendations. Over the course of several days, your RMR would drop as much as 50 to 75 percent. This would produce negative results. You probably would be tired, hungry all the time, and your energy would be low.
- **Physical activity and exercise.** Participation in regular physical activity or exercise stimulates metabolic rate. This is true not only during physical activity but also for a short while afterward. Thus, regular exercise or physical activity can increase your RMR.

Weight Control and Physical Activity

Obviously, the more physically active you are, the more calories you will burn. Yet, as with RMR, the number of calories you burn through physical activity will vary with respect to several factors. These include:

- **The number, size, and weight of body parts that you work.** If you work with your legs (by walking, for example), you will burn more calories than you would working your arms (by lifting weights, for example). The reason is simple: The leg muscles are larger than the arm muscles. The larger the muscle mass, the more energy needed to work it.
- **The intensity of your workout.** The more physically demanding, or intense, your workout is, the more calories you will burn. This is because harder work requires more fuel.
- **The duration, or time, of your activities.** If you engage in daily physical activities, you will burn more calories than someone who is sedentary. For example, Molly and her friend Nelda in **Figure 5.8** (page **158**) have the same RMR. Nelda burns more calories because she is physically active.

✓ **Reading Check**

Explain Describe the relationship between expending calories and physical activity or exercise.

FIGURE 5.8

ENERGY EXPENDITURE OF AN ACTIVE TEEN VERSUS AN INACTIVE TEEN

The chart shows a typical breakdown of the total energy needs of two different teens. *Why does Nelda burn 500 calories more than Molly? How many more calories will she burn in a week's time?*

Daily Energy Needs	Nelda (Active)	Molly (Sedentary)
Energy for RMR	1,600 calories	1,600 calories
Energy for physical activity	600 calories	100 calories
Total energy needs	2,200 calories	1,700 calories

Lesson 2 Review

Using complete sentences, answer the following questions on a sheet of paper.

Reviewing Facts and Vocabulary

1. **Vocabulary** What is *metabolism?*

2. **Recall** Explain the relationship among calorie intake, calorie expenditure, and amount of body fat.

3. **Recall** What are three factors that influence the amount of calories expended during physical activity or exercise?

Thinking Critically

4. **Synthesize** Marcus eats five small meals a day and gets at least 60 minutes of physical activity a day. Natasha eats two large meals a day and does not participate in regular physical activity. Which one most likely has the highest RMR? Explain your answer.

5. **Analyze** For exercise, Martin runs 60 minutes each day. His friend Jamel lifts weights for 45 minutes each day. Which teen expends more calories through these physical activities? Explain.

Personal Fitness Planning

Investigating Claims Some fitness equipment manufacturers claim that if you work out with their product you can easily burn 1,000 calories per hour. Using **Figure 5.7**, apply the physiological principles related to exercise. Calculate the type and intensity of activity a person would need to do to burn 1,000 calories in an hour. Do you think these claims are valid? Why or why not?

Evaluating Your Body Composition

In this lesson, you will learn about several ways to measure body composition. You will also learn how to perform some of these methods.

It is important to be aware that every method of measuring body composition has some degree of inaccuracy built in. If your body fat measurement is borderline for any test, you should consult a health care professional. You may need to make adjustments to your calorie intake and expenditure.

Body Circumference

Body fat is stored differently in males and females. In males, body fat accumulates primarily around the waist. In females, it gravitates toward the hips. The body-circumference test accounts for these differences by having separate procedures for males and females.

The body-circumference tests measure girth. This is *the distance around a body part.* For all of these tests, you will need a cloth tape measure and a ruler.

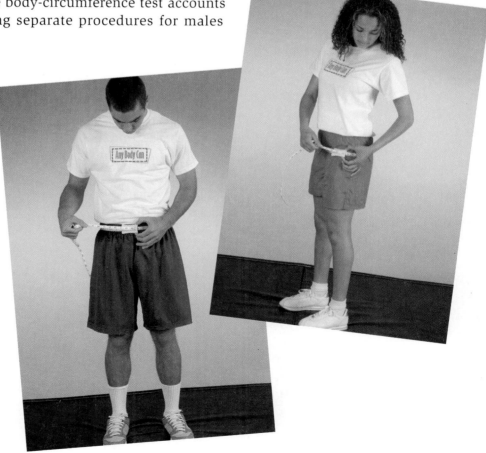

▶ Measuring body circumference is one way to evaluate body composition. *Why is body circumference measured differently in males and females?*

Body-Circumference Test for Males

For males, the body-circumference test has two steps. First, measure your weight in pounds. Then, measure your girth at the waistline.

Before weighing yourself, you should remove your shoes and dress in your exercise clothing. Measure your waist circumference with the tape measure pulled snugly, but not too tightly. Measure to the nearest half-inch. Once you have obtained your measurements, use the chart in **Figure 5.9** to help you determine your percentage of body fat. Using a ruler, connect the points from your body weight to your waist circumference. The point where the ruler crosses the scale in the center column is your approximate percentage of body fat.

Body-Circumference Test for Females

Females can estimate their percentage of body fat by measuring their height and the girth of their hips at the widest point. First, remove your shoes. Compute your height to the nearest half-inch. The hip circumference measurement should be taken with the tape measure pulled snugly, but not too tightly, and to the nearest half-inch.

Once you have obtained your measurements, you can use **Figure 5.9** to determine your percentage of body fat. Using a ruler, connect the points from your body height to your hip circumference. The point where the ruler intersects the scale in the center column is your approximate percentage of body fat.

FIGURE 5.9

BODY-FAT PERCENTAGE FROM CIRCUMFERENCE TESTS: MALE AND FEMALE

Body-fat percentages are calculated differently for males and females. *How are the two tests different?*

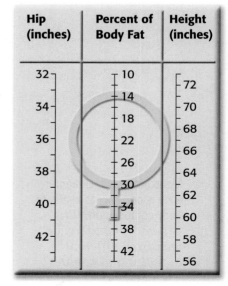

Males

Body Weight (pounds)	Percent of Body Fat	Waist (inches)

Females

Hip (inches)	Percent of Body Fat	Height (inches)

FIGURE 5.10

BODY-FAT RATINGS

Use your percentage of body fat to determine your health rating. *Where on this chart do you fall? What changes, if any, do you need to make to your body composition?*

% Fat (Males)	% Fat (Females)	Fitness Rating and Evaluation
25% or more	30% or more	Overfat – Too high *(A person in this range is at higher risk for chronic diseases.)*
20–24%	25–29%	Borderline High – Possible health risks *(A person in this range needs to lose weight.)*
10–19%	15–24%	Healthy – Most desirable level
7–9%	12–14%	Healthy Lean – Acceptable level
6% or less	11% or less	Too Lean – Possible health risks *(Acceptable only for a competitive endurance athlete)*

Evaluating Body Circumference

Once you have determined your percentage of body fat, you can use **Figure 5.10** to evaluate your body fat score. As mentioned in Lesson 1, males should carry 7 to 20 percent body fat. Females should carry 12 to 25 percent body fat. If you do not score in the *acceptable-to-most-desirable* health zones, try to improve your body composition.

Skinfold Measures

Another method used to evaluate body composition is skinfold measurement. The finger pinch test featured in the "Fitness Check" on page 8 is an example of a simplified skinfold test. More accurate skinfold measurements are made using calipers. This is *a tweezerlike device used to pinch a fold of skin surrounding adipose tissue.* The resulting fold is measured in millimeters.

A skinfold test is a good indicator of body composition because 50 percent of all body fat is between the muscles and skin, as shown in **Figure 5.11.** The other 50 percent is inside the body.

For adolescents, two skinfold measurements are typically taken: the back of the upper arm (triceps) and the inside of the calf at its widest part. See **Figure 5.13** on page **163** for percentages.

✔ Reading Check

Summarize What are the medical evaluations that can be used to measure body composition?

FIGURE 5.11

SKINFOLD TEST

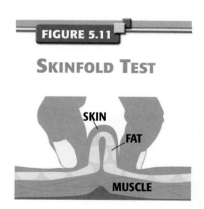

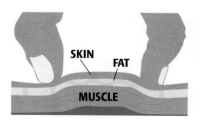

Measuring Body Composition

For your personal fitness assessments, skinfold evaluations of body composition are adequately reliable. In this activity, you and a partner will take turns performing a skinfold test on each other. Use a separate sheet of paper to record all calculations.

Procedure:

1. Use your left hand to grasp each skinfold. Avoid grasping the muscle or pinching too tightly.
2. For the triceps, use your thumb and index finger to pick up a skinfold in the middle of your partner's right arm exactly halfway between the shoulder and the elbow. Have your partner keep his or her arm relaxed at the side of the body. (See **Figure 5.12a.**)
3. For the calf, have your partner stand up and place his or her right foot on a bench or chair. Use your thumb and index finger to pick up a skinfold in the middle of the inside part of the lower leg at its widest part. (See **Figure 5.12b.**)
4. With your right hand, place the opened calipers one-half inch below the skinfold grasp and directly below the pinch, with the scale of the calipers visible.
5. Close the calipers on the skinfold. Hold it for two to three seconds. Read and record the measurement to the nearest millimeter. Repeat this step two more times.
6. Use the middle of the three readings as your skinfold score. (For example, if the three readings are 18, 16, and 15 mm, use 16 as your score.)
7. Add up your triceps and calf skinfold scores as follows:

   triceps (mm) + calf (mm) = sum of skinfolds

   Use **Figure 5.13** to determine your percentage of body fat. Read straight down from the sum of skinfolds to the "% fat" reading.
8. Calculate your body-fat weight by multiplying your weight by your percentage of body fat:

   weight × % body fat = body-fat weight
9. Calculate your lean body weight by subtracting your fat weight from your weight:

   weight − body-fat weight = lean body weight

10. For females, determine your ideal minimum weight by dividing your lean weight by 0.76. Determine your ideal maximum weight by dividing your lean body weight by 0.88.
11. For males, determine your ideal minimum weight by dividing your lean body weight by 0.81. Determine your ideal maximum weight by dividing your lean body weight by 0.93.
12. Refer to **Figure 5.10** on page **161** to evaluate your body-fat score. If you did not score within a healthy zone, try to improve your body composition by getting closer to your healthy body weight range.

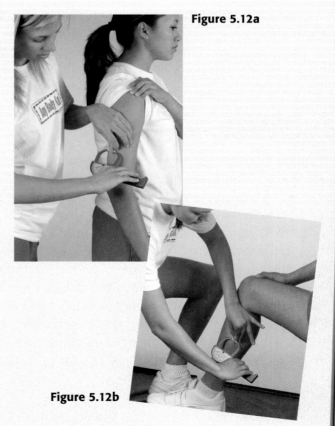

Figure 5.12a

Figure 5.12b

FIGURE 5.13

SKINFOLD MEASUREMENTS AND BODY-FAT PERCENTAGES

Skinfold measurements are one way to measure body composition. *Why is this a good indicator of percentage of body fat?*

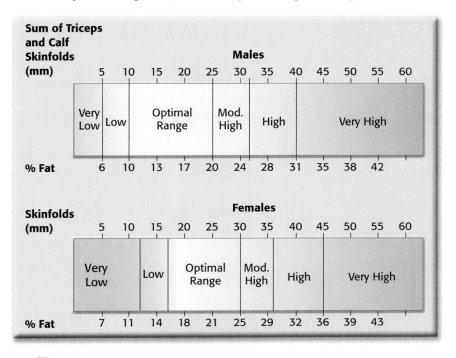

Lesson 3 Review

Using complete sentences, answer the following questions on a sheet of paper.

Reviewing Facts and Vocabulary

1. **Recall** Name two approaches for measuring body composition.

2. **Vocabulary** What are *calipers* used for?

3. **Recall** What is a healthy body-fat percentage for teen males? For teen females?

Thinking Critically

4. **Analyze** Emma wants to evaluate her body composition using the body-circumference test. Explain the procedure she should follow, including what she will need to evaluate her body-fat percentage.

5. **Evaluate** Harry had his skinfolds measured. The sum of his folds was 20. What would you tell Harry about his current level of health with respect to body-fat percentage?

Personal Fitness Planning

Evaluating Body Composition Using the body-circumference test described in this lesson, measure your body composition. Compare the results with your results from the "Fitness Check." Did you get the same results each time? What might account for the difference? Write a paragraph about how body composition impacts your personal fitness plan.

Maintaining a Healthy Body Composition

What You Will Do

- Identify strategies to manage weight.
- Explain the role of nutrition and physical activity in weight management.
- Analyze diet, exercise, physical activity, and a combination of both as methods of weight control.
- Evaluate consumer issues related to physical fitness such as choosing services for weight management.

Terms to Know

nutrient-dense foods

Now that you have learned to measure and evaluate your weight and body composition, you need to learn how to achieve and maintain a healthy weight and body composition. In this lesson, you will learn about various strategies and approaches to weight management. You will also learn how nutritional practices and physical activity combined contribute to a healthy body composition.

Healthful Strategies to Manage Weight

As with other parts of your fitness program, achieving and maintaining a healthy weight and body composition starts with you. By gradually adjusting your eating plan and physical-activity habits, you can begin to safely control your weight and body composition. The rate at which you modify your behaviors should be based on your personal fitness goals and your changing levels of body composition.

Do you recall the behavioral-change stairway in Chapter 1? It is a step-by-step procedure for achieving personal fitness goals. This stairway can be used to improve your eating habits and help you manage your body weight. Some other guidelines that can help you include:

- **Evaluate your needs.** Ask a health care professional to help you target your appropriate weight and identify your goals.
- **Be realistic.** For long-term success, a person should lose no more than 1 to 2 pounds per week for safe, effective results. If the goal is to gain weight, it's best to gain slowly—no more than $\frac{1}{2}$ pound per week.

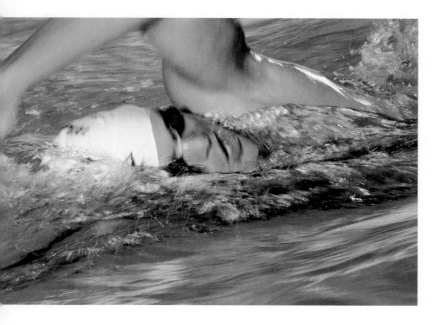

◀ Physical activity is a necessary component of maintaining body composition. *How does physical activity help a person maintain a healthy body composition?*

- **Design a personal plan.** Develop a plan in writing that includes healthful eating and regular physical activity.
- **Become physically active.** You should try to get 60 minutes per day of physical activity or exercise, or a minimum of 225 minutes per week. Engage in physical activities that are right for your goals. For example, aerobic exercise can help you burn calories and lose fat weight while activities like weight training can help you gain muscle mass and increase your RMR.
- **Keep track of your progress.** Monitor your body weight and body composition regularly (every three months).

Nutrition and Physical Activity

Where do you fit into the big picture? Are you happy with your current body composition? Do you want—or need—to make changes to your weight or body composition? To effectively do this, you need to understand the relationship between your eating plan and level of physical activity, and how each can be used to control weight and body composition.

Weight Control, Diet, and Exercise

To lose a pound of fat, you could reduce your calorie intake in your diet by 3,500 calories, or expend 3,500 more calories in physical activity. However, focusing on only one side of this energy equation is not healthful.

The best approach to weight loss or weight gain is a combination approach. The healthiest and most effective method is to combine a healthful eating plan with a program of regular physical activity or exercise.

Weight Loss. To lose weight, adjust your eating plan to reduce calorie intake while increasing calorie expenditure through physical activity or exercise.

When reducing calorie intake, be sure you are still getting the proper nutrients. Eat at regular intervals and get at least 1,700 to 1,800 calories per day to meet your daily needs. Use the Food Guide Pyramid and *Dietary Guidelines for Americans* to help you. Eat a variety of low-calorie nutrient-dense foods. These are *foods that are high in nutrients as compared with their calorie content.* These include vegetables, fruits, and whole-grain products. Remember to drink at least eight glasses of water daily to maintain your body's proper function.

In addition to proper nutrition, engage in physical activities or exercises that cause you to work for a longer period of time (45 to 60 minutes) at moderate-to-vigorous intensity. Those exercises are the most effective at burning fat and excess calories. This dual approach of diet and exercise enables you to build lean muscle mass and lower your percentage of body fat.

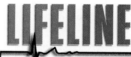

Practicing Safe Weight Management

Excessive weight loss over a short period of time can be a serious health concern. People who have a serious weight problem and are considering a diet plan that promises extreme, rapid weight loss should talk to their doctor or other health professional. As with any health issue, strict weight-loss programs like these must be followed only under the direction of a physician or other health care professional. Keep in mind that many unqualified individuals claim to have a wealth of knowledge about weight-loss procedures when they do not.

Do not accept the opinion of someone who is not professionally trained and qualified in nutrition and weight control. This can create unnecessary health risks, as well as a good way to get "ripped off." The best way to control your body weight and body composition is to speak to your doctor or other health care professional for advice. They can help you devise a plan that combines both exercise and diet to help you achieve total, personal fitness.

Interview

Speak to a doctor or other health care professional to evaluate how he or she would advise teen patients who are concerned with weight management and body composition. Ask about other qualified, licensed professionals who are good resources for advice about nutrition and weight management. Share your findings with your physical education classmates and your teacher.

"I Lost 100 Pounds Easy! Eating My Favorite Foods!!! This is the Greatest Diet Ever!"

Users Have Dropped Over 2 Million Pounds! TRY IT NOW!!

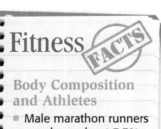

Fitness FACTS

Body Composition and Athletes

- Male marathon runners may have about 3.3% body fat; female runners about 10%.
- Male swimmers have about 6.8% body fat, female swimmers about 18.6%.
- Male gymnasts have about 4.6% body fat, females about 14%.

Source: Exercise Physiology: Energy, Nutrition, and Human Performance, *2001.[4]*

Weight Gain. If the goal is weight gain, a person should consume more calories and maintain his or her physical-activity level. Increase calorie intake by increasing complex carbohydrates, such as breads, pasta, and potatoes. Eat more than the minimum number of servings from each food group and choose healthy snacks.

It is healthiest for a person to gain weight slowly and steadily. This adds less body fat and more lean muscle. Also, a supervised resistance-training program will help a person gain weight by adding muscle mass without adding unwanted fat.

Weight Maintenance. If you are within an appropriate weight range and have a healthy body composition, you want to maintain it. If you maintain a healthful eating plan with the same amount of calorie intake, as well as continue to maintain a moderate level of physical activity, you will maintain your weight and body composition.

✓ Reading Check

Summarize Why are nutrient-dense foods necessary if a person is trying to lose weight?

Benefits of Achieving Your Goals

You will need to be persistent and patient in working toward your goals. Keep in mind that while you are young and growing, your body composition can change fairly quickly. As you get older, however, you may not experience much change for at least three to six months. When choosing types of activities, keep in mind that aerobic exercise can help you burn calories and lose body fat, while activities like weight training can help you gain muscle mass and increase you RMR.

Maintaining a healthy weight and body composition through proper nutrition and exercise has several benefits. It will

- increase your energy.
- increase your self-esteem.
- reduce your stress levels.
- reduce your risk for developing diseases.

The combination of diet and physical activity will help you look and feel your best.

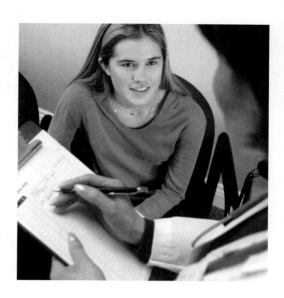

▲ Teens should always seek the advice of their parents and a health care professional when planning their weight maintenance program. *How will this help them in achieving their goals?*

 Reading Check

List What are the benefits of achieving your weight maintenance goals?

Lesson 4 Review

Using complete sentences, answer the following questions on a sheet of paper.

Reviewing Facts and Vocabulary

1. **Vocabulary** Define *nutrient-dense foods*.

2. **Recall** How many calories must you burn beyond what you consume to lose a pound of fat?

3. **Recall** What type of physical activity is effective for a person who needs to gain weight?

Thinking Critically

4. **Analyze** Explain why combining diet and exercise as a method of weight control is healthier and more effective than relying on diet or exercise alone.

5. **Evaluation** Tristan's goal is to gain 10 pounds over the next three months. He has adjusted his eating plan accordingly, but has decided to greatly reduce his level of physical activity. Explain why it is important for Tristan to maintain his physical activity.

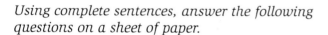
Personal Fitness Planning

Designing a Program Write a personal fitness plan to improve or maintain your body composition (depending upon your personal needs). Set a realistic goal for you to accomplish in the next month. Consider how your diet and exercise combined will help you achieve that goal. Include your eating plan and your physical-activity program. Explain how each will help you improve or maintain your body composition.

CHAPTER 5 Review

TRUE/FALSE

On a sheet of paper, write the numbers 1–10. Write True or False for each statement.

1. Your body type is determined by your genetic makeup.
2. Lean body weight equals body-fat weight divided by total body weight.
3. The graph showing the relationship between body weight and the risk for developing chronic diseases is J shaped.
4. There are no risks associated with excessive leanness.
5. The size of your fat cells will not increase after your teen years.
6. The energy balance includes energy input and energy expenditure.
7. RMR increases as you age and is higher for females than males.
8. Adopting a diet of less than 1,000 calories is a good way to lose weight.
9. One pound of fat is equivalent to 3,500 calories.
10. Teens should try to accumulate at least 225 minutes of physical activity and exercise per week.

MULTIPLE CHOICE

On a separate sheet of paper, write the letter of the word or phrase that best completes each statement.

11. What is the minimum recommended amount of essential fat for teen males?
    a. 1 percent
    b. 7 percent
    c. 12 percent
    d. 18 percent
12. What is the minimum recommended amount of essential fat for teen females?
    a. 1 percent
    b. 7 percent
    c. 12 percent
    d. 18 percent
13. Your body composition is influenced by which of the following?
    a. Genetics
    b. Age
    c. Gender
    d. All of the above
14. Your RMR is not influenced by which of the following?
    a. Age
    b. Height
    c. Gender
    d. Physical-activity level
15. If you want to lose weight, your eating plan should include
    a. mainly carbohydrates.
    b. mainly protein.
    c. nutrient-dense foods.
    d. vitamin-rich foods.
16. What percentage of your body fat is between your muscles and skin?
    a. 25 percent
    b. 50 percent
    c. 75 percent
    d. 100 percent
17. The body composition evaluation method of underwater weighing is based on what concept?
    a. Fat floats
    b. Fat sinks
    c. Fat neither sinks nor floats
    d. None of the above
18. What type of physical activity is especially important for you to include in your personal-fitness program if you are trying to lose body fat, but gain weight?
    a. Flexibility
    b. Plyometric
    c. Aerobic
    d. Weight-training
19. If you want to gain weight, how much in pounds per week would be healthful?
    a. $\frac{1}{2}$
    b. 1
    c. 2
    d. 5
20. If you want to lose weight, how many pounds per week maximum would be healthful?
    a. 1 to 2
    b. 3 to 5
    c. 5 to 7
    d. 10

DISCUSSION

Using complete sentences, answer the following questions on a sheet of paper.

21. Identify List and describe five factors that influence your body composition.

22. Identify List and describe three methods to evaluate your body composition.

23. Explain Tell how you can safely reduce your body weight, increase your body weight, or maintain your body weight.

VOCABULARY

On a sheet of paper, write the letter of the term in Column B that best fits the definition in Column A.

Column A

24. The process by which the body converts calories from food to energy.

25. The combined weight of bone, muscle, and connective tissue.

26. The minimum amount of body fat necessary for good health.

27. The total number of calories you take in from food.

28. The total number of calories you burn or expend.

29. The amount of calories you need and expend for body processes while at rest.

Column B

a. calorie intake
b. metabolism
c. calorie expenditure
d. essential fat
e. lean body weight
f. resting metabolic rate

CRITICAL THINKING

Using complete sentences, answer the following questions on a sheet of paper.

30. Analyze Why is body weight alone not an accurate indicator of total body composition? Explain your answer.

31. Identify What behaviors will slow down or speed up your resting metabolic rate?

32. Evaluate Analyze each of the following as methods of weight control: diet, exercise, and a combination of diet and exercise.

CASE STUDY

JACKIE'S ACTIVITY LEVEL

Jackie is a sixteen-year-old inactive female who has 32 percent body fat and would like to lose 20 pounds. However, she is unsure about how to lose the weight healthfully, reduce her body fat to 25 percent, and begin a regular physical activity or exercise program. Therefore, Jackie needs the help of someone knowledgeable about designing and implementing fitness programs—someone like you!

HERE IS YOUR ASSIGNMENT:

Assume you are Jackie's friend. She asks you for some assistance with her plans for improving her body composition. Make a list of things Jackie should consider and do before beginning a program to improve her body composition. Then list the recommendations that you would give to Jackie for the first two weeks of her program. Use the following keys to help you:

KEYS TO HELP YOU

- Consider Jackie's current body composition and percentage of body fat.
- Think about how her current body composition could be evaluated.
- Analyze her needs and goals. (For example, how should she go about improving her body composition?)
- Consider the importance of energy balance as you advise Jackie about her eating habits (calorie intake) and her level of physical activity (energy expenditure).

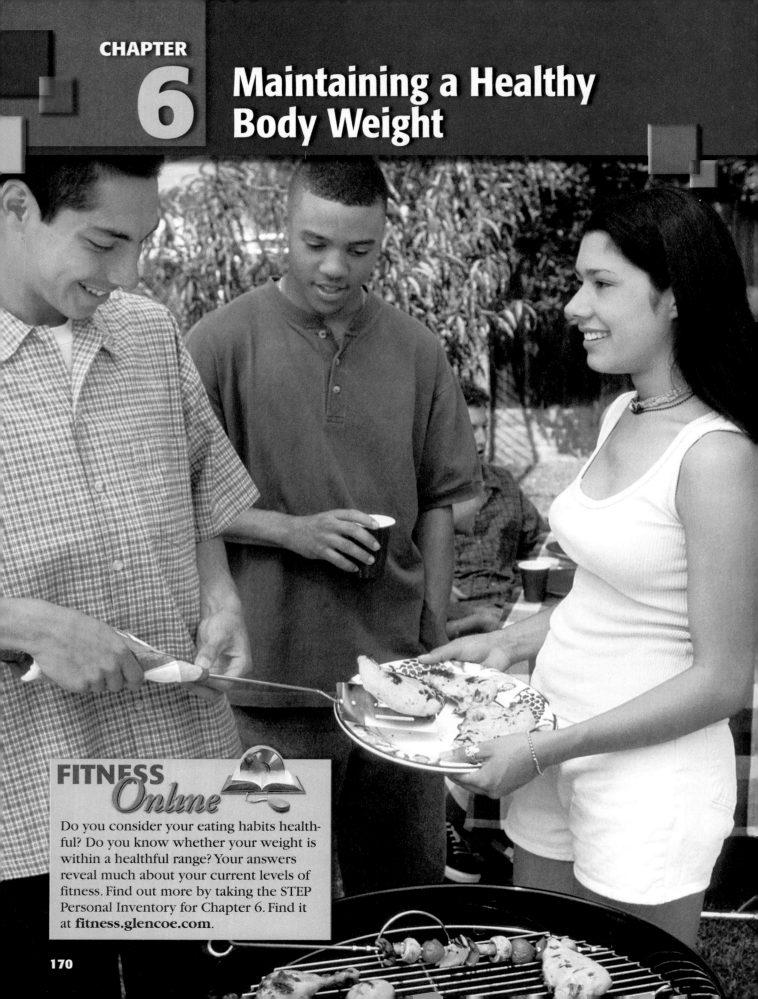

Maintaining a Healthy Body Weight

FITNESS Online

Do you consider your eating habits healthful? Do you know whether your weight is within a healthful range? Your answers reveal much about your current levels of fitness. Find out more by taking the STEP Personal Inventory for Chapter 6. Find it at **fitness.glencoe.com**.

Body Weight and Health Risks

In previous chapters, you read about the importance of being physically active and eating right. Both, as you have seen, can positively affect body composition. In this chapter, you will learn how to maintain a healthful body weight throughout your life. You will also learn how doing so relates to your functional health and fitness.

Overweight and Youth

In the last several decades, the number of teens in this country who are overweight has nearly tripled, as shown in **Figure 6.1.** This trend has become a major concern among health professionals.

As you learned in Chapter 5, overweight is a condition in which a person is heavier than the standard weight range for his or her height. This means a person with a **Body Mass Index (BMI)** that is above the 85th percentile for his or her age group is considered *at risk for overweight*. A person with a BMI above the 95th percentile for his or her age group is considered *overweight*. Remember that BMI changes with age.

What You Will Do

- Identify health risks related to overweight and underweight.
- Identify impaired glucose tolerance and its role in diabetes.
- Evaluate the effect of overweight on physical activity.

Terms to Know

excessive weight disabilities
sleep apnea
impaired glucose tolerance
  (IGT)
insulin
underweight

hot link

Body Mass Index
For more on body mass index (BMI) and how to evaluate it, see Chapter 5, page **149.**

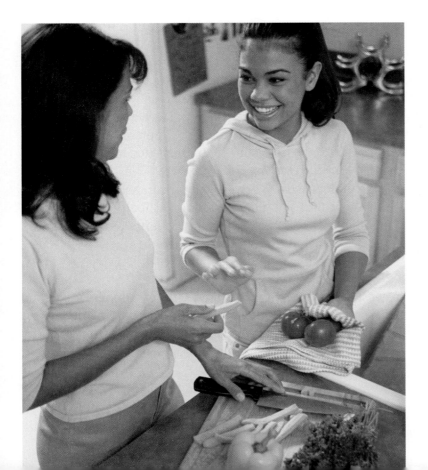

◀ Developing a healthy eating plan as a teen will reduce your risk of becoming overweight as you age. *How might learning to cook help you maintain a healthy eating plan?*

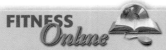
FIGURE 6.1

PERCENTAGE OF AMERICAN YOUTH WHO WERE OVERWEIGHT, BY AGE

The number of overweight teens has greatly increased over the past 40 years. *What percentage of teens (ages 12–17) were overweight in 1970? By how much has that percentage risen in recent years?*

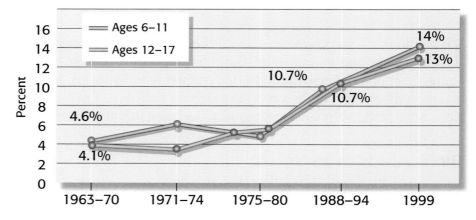

Source: Centers for Disease Control and Prevention, 2003[1]

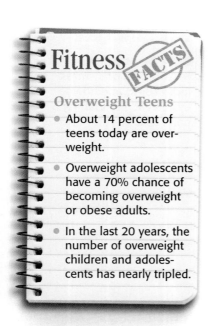

Fitness FACTS

Overweight Teens

- About 14 percent of teens today are overweight.

- Overweight adolescents have a 70% chance of becoming overweight or obese adults.

- In the last 20 years, the number of overweight children and adolescents has nearly tripled.

Source: The Surgeon General's Call to Action to Prevent and Decrease Overweight and Obesity.[2]

The Effect of Overweight on Health

Being overweight can affect a person's self-esteem and quality of life. This is especially true during the teen years. Adolescence is a time when the individual undergoes dramatic physical and social growth. Overweight can interfere with these natural and necessary growth processes.

Teens who are seriously overweight often have trouble taking part in physical games and activities. This can make these teens feel cut off from their peers. Simple everyday tasks such as walking up a flight of stairs become a physical challenge. Being overweight or at risk for overweight in adolescence can also prevent a person from developing positive eating and physical-activity patterns for his or her future functional health and fitness.

However, as you learned in Chapter 5, you can achieve and maintain a healthy weight and body composition. A healthy body allows you to stay physically active and enjoy the benefits personal fitness offers your physical, social, and emotional health.

Physical Health Risks

Being excessively overweight is linked with a number of chronic physical diseases and conditions. Overweight increases the risk of high blood pressure and high blood cholesterol. It also increases the risks of heart disease and some cancers.

Some conditions are grouped together under the heading **excessive weight disabilities.** This term refers to *health problems and diseases linked to or resulting directly from long-term overweight or obesity.* These disabilities include:

- **Breathing difficulties.** Accumulations of internal body fat may press against the **diaphragm.** This is the primary muscle involved in breathing. Even light physical activity may cause shortness of breath. Overweight people with asthma are at higher risk for more frequent and more severe attacks of this disease. They also may suffer from sleep apnea, *a condition in which a person stops breathing during sleep, due to obstructed or reduced air passages.* Individuals with sleep apnea often snore, wake up, and interrupt their normal restful sleeping patterns. Untreated, sleep apnea can cause high blood pressure and other cardiovascular diseases, memory problems, weight gain, and headaches.
- **Bone and joint problems.** Extra weight can put stress on the bones and joints. This, in turn, diminishes range of motion. It can also cause muscle aches.

Impaired Glucose Tolerance and Diabetes

Another especially serious condition related to overweight is impaired glucose tolerance (IGT). This is *a disorder in which blood glucose levels become elevated.* As noted in Chapter 4, carbohydrates from food are converted by the body into glucose, a simple sugar. This sugar is converted, in turn, into energy. The chemical in the body that is responsible for this process is insulin, *a hormone produced by the pancreas.* Often in people with IGT, the pancreas produces too little insulin to convert the glucose, which is then stored in the blood.

IGT is a major risk factor for type 2 diabetes. People with this disease develop infections more easily than healthy individuals. Other symptoms include blurred vision, nausea, muscle weakness, and fatigue.

At one time, IGT and type 2 diabetes were exclusively adult illnesses. With the rise of overweight in children and teens, however, childhood cases of these conditions are becoming more common. Teens with type 2 diabetes must remain under strict medical supervision and follow a restricted eating plan. Daily finger-stick tests to check blood glucose levels may become necessary. So may periodic injections of insulin. In short, diabetes can affect a teen's quality of life during adolescence.

hot link

diaphragm
For more on the diaphragm and its functions, see Chapter 7, page **194.**

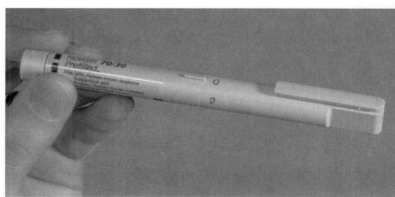

▼ Some people with type 2 diabetes must have regular insulin injections to help their bodies turn glucose into energy. *What are the symptoms of type 2 diabetes?*

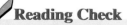

Reading Check

Explain What are excessive weight disabilities?

Exercise and Overweight

In this activity you will revisit two exercises from earlier Fitness Checks. This will permit you to experience what it would be like to exercise if you weighed more.

1. Insert schoolbooks into an empty backpack. Place the weighted pack on a scale. Aim for a total weight of 10 pounds, adding and subtracting books of different sizes as necessary.

2. Review the procedure for jumping jacks in **Figure 6.2**. Perform the exercise. Meanwhile, a partner should video-tape your performance.

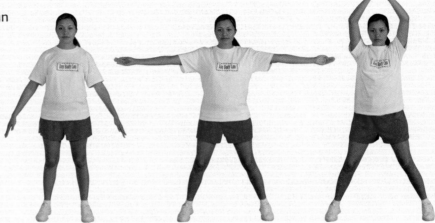

Figure 6.2

3. Next strap on the weighted backpack. Repeat the jumping jacks exercise, again while your partner videotapes your performance. (Note: If the weight feels too heavy, try subtracting five pounds. It is important that you avoid injuring yourself.)

4. Review the procedure for the Blind One-Leg Stand in **Figure 6.3**. Perform this exercise twice—once with and once without—the weighted backpack. Again your partner should videotape your performance.

5. Switch roles with your partner. Tape your partner performing the two exercises with and without the weighted backpack.

6. When each of you has completed all exercises described, review the videotapes. Determine whether your movement biomechanics changed while doing the tests with and without excess weight.

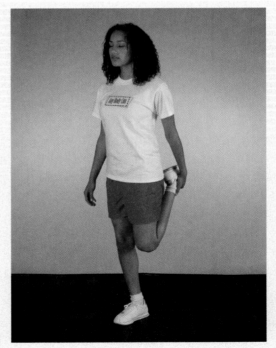

Figure 6.3

Underweight

In the face of the overweight epidemic, it is easy to lose sight of the reverse problem—being excessively lean, or underweight. **Underweight** may be defined as *having a Body Mass Index (BMI) that is below the 5th percentile for one's age.* Teens who are underweight usually have insufficient body fat. Since this fat stores protective nutrients, these teens are at greater risk of infection from cold viruses and other pathogens.

In addition, underweight teens may be undernourished. This means they fail to take in enough essential nutrients on a regular basis to ensure normal growth and body function. They also are not providing their bodies with a proper energy reserve, causing fatigue and irritability. Underweight teens also are at greater risk of anemia, a disease linked to a lack of iron. Undernourished female teens may experience irregular menstrual cycles. The risk of developing osteoporosis later in life also increases.

Underweight teens should eat three to four meals a day, consisting of nutrient-dense, high-calorie foods. They should also begin a resistance-training program to increase lean body weight.

Reading Check

Identify What are the health risks of being underweight?

Lesson 1 Review

Using complete sentences, answer the following questions on a sheet of paper.

Reviewing Facts and Vocabulary

1. **Recall** List and describe two health problems related to overweight.
2. **Vocabulary** What is *sleep apnea?*
3. **Vocabulary** Define *underweight.*

Thinking Critically

4. **Compare and Contrast** What is the relationship between impaired glucose tolerance and type 2 diabetes?
5. **Synthesize** Mackenzie is 16 years old and is underweight. What are some of the health problems Mackenzie might experience due to her low BMI?

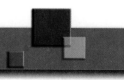

Personal Fitness Planning

Assessing Lifestyle Assess your current level of fitness in the area of nutrition and body weight. How does your eating plan and level of physical activity impact your ability to perform daily tasks? Do you generally feel healthy and energetic, or are there changes you would like to make? If so, make a list of changes you might make to your current behaviors, including your eating plan and daily physical activity, in order to improve your overall feeling of physical health.

What You Will Do

- Identify the symptoms and risks of eating disorders.
- Explain how to help a friend who may have an eating disorder.
- Explain how overtraining contributes to eating disorders.

Terms to Know

body image
eating disorders
anorexia nervosa
bulimia nervosa
exercise bulimia
binge eating disorder
bigorexia

Body Image and Weight Control

Have you ever glimpsed your reflection in a funhouse mirror? These mirrors are curved in a way that purposely distorts your image. *The way you see your body* is called your body image. Some people do not need a special mirror to have a distorted body image. They already see themselves as too fat or too thin. A distorted body image can lead to serious health risks.

Eating Disorders

Sometimes, a person's concerns about weight can become an obsession. Some teens develop eating disorders. These are *psychological illnesses that cause people to undereat, overeat, or practice other dangerous nutrition-related behaviors.* Although the exact causes of eating disorders are unknown, they are typically driven by mental or emotional factors, such as poor body image, social and family pressures, and perfectionism. Teens with a family history of weight problems, depression, or substance abuse may be at higher risk for developing an eating disorder.

People with these disorders wrongly view themselves as too heavy, too thin, or not bulked-up enough. To "correct" their perceived limitations, they will eat in an unhealthful manner that also disrupts their energy balance. This is particularly dangerous for a person whose body is still growing and developing.

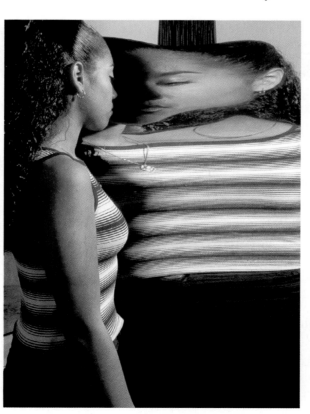

◀ Body image is the way you see your body. *Why is it important to have a positive body image?*

Anorexia Nervosa

Anorexia (an-uh-REK-see-uh) **nervosa** is *an eating disorder in which a person abnormally restricts his or her calorie intake.* More females than males suffer from anorexia, though the number of male cases is on the rise. People with this disorder have a fear of becoming fat or gaining weight. This belief persists even after the person becomes dangerously underweight.

People with anorexia can develop serious malnutrition. The loss of body fat can cause female anorectics to stop menstruating and can lead to sterility. Anorexia also causes reduced bone density, low body temperature, low blood pressure, slowed metabolism, and reduction in organ size. Anorexia can also lead to serious heart problems. In extreme cases, the disease can result in death.

Some common indicators of a person with anorexia include:

- Sudden, massive weight loss
- Lying about having eaten
- Denying feeling hungry
- Consuming minimal amounts of food in front of others
- Preoccupation with food, calories, and weight
- Signs of **exercise addiction**
- Withdrawing from social activities
- Belief that he or she is overweight

 Reading Check

Identify List three serious health risks of anorexia.

Bulimia Nervosa

Bulimia (boo-LEEM-ee-uh) **nervosa** is *an eating disorder in which people overeat and then force themselves to purge the food afterward.* This cycle is also called "bingeing and purging." The most common method for purging is self-induced vomiting. Laxatives may also be used. Excessive physical activity is another method used to purge food. **Exercise bulimia** is *an eating disorder in which people purge calories by exercising excessively.* These people will miss out on important events and appointments in order to work out, will work out even if they are sick or injured, and do not allow any days for recovery.

Like anorexia, bulimia has little to do with weight, calories, or being "thin." It is symptomatic, rather, of underlying turmoil or emotional problems. Unlike anorectics, bulimics often have normal body composition. This makes it harder to identify someone suffering with bulimia.

Bulimia can cause serious, negative long-term health effects. Health risks of bulimia include dehydration, osteoporosis, kidney damage, and irregular heartbeat. Frequent vomiting damages tissues of the stomach, esophagus, and mouth. It also erodes tooth enamel and leads to tooth decay. The use of laxatives interferes with proper digestion, causing nutrient deficiencies.

exercise addiction
For more on exercise addiction and the dangers of overtraining, see Chapter 3, page **99**.

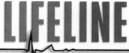

Helping an Anorexic Friend
People with anorexia may not know—or believe—that they need help. They will often refuse efforts to help them and deny they have a problem. You can still help a friend you suspect of being anorexic. If you know someone with several of the symptoms noted, talk to a trusted adult. Let him or her know your friend may be sick.

Many of the signs and symptoms of bulimia are the same as those for anorexia. Additional signs include:

- Malnutrition
- Excessive concerns about weight
- Eating large amounts of food without weight gain
- Use of laxatives and diuretics
- Visiting the bathroom immediately after meals. This is often a sign that the person is planning to induce vomiting.
- Practicing strict weight-loss programs followed by eating binges
- Excessive exercise

 Reading Check

Identify What are the long-term health risks of bulimia?

Binge Eating Disorder

Binge eating disorder is *an eating disorder where individuals eat more rapidly than normal until they cannot eat any more.* Binge eaters do not engage in purging, like bulimics. Yet, they have a poor body image. Binge eaters often have feelings of guilt, depression, lack of control, and frustration. Binge eaters may not necessarily become obese, but their habits can be addictive.

Bigorexia

Although it is not an eating disorder in the strict sense, bigorexia (by-guh-REK-see-uh) is a serious health condition nevertheless. Also known as "reverse anorexia," bigorexia is *a disorder in which an individual falsely believes he or she is underweight or undersized.* Bigorexia is more common in male rather than female teens. This disorder is closely associated with exercise addiction. Symptoms and signs of bigorexia include:

- Lifting excessive amounts of weight, even when not in sports training
- Using performance-enhancing **supplements**
- Checking their appearance in the mirror frequently
- Feeling ashamed to show their bodies in public, even when fully clothed

 Reading Check

Compare Discuss the difference between binge eating disorder and bigorexia.

Overtraining and Eating Disorders

Teens who engage in competitive athletics or in high levels of recreational competition may find that they can perform best when they are very lean. In certain cases, an athlete's desire to stay thin may result

supplements
For more on the dangers of performance-enhancing supplements, see Chapter 4, page **143**.

in overtraining, which has serious health risks, including insomnia, weight loss, weakened immune system, and infertility (in women).

If an athlete's desire to perform well becomes an obsession and is combined with certain other factors, such as poor body image, social and family pressures, or depression, he or she may not only be overtraining but may also have an eating disorder. A person with an eating disorder may overtrain, causing weight problems and health risks.

Help for Eating Disorders

People with eating disorders need professional help. If you believe a friend has an eating disorder, discuss the problem with a trusted adult, such as a parent, a counselor, or a teacher. Also speak to your friend and encourage him or her to seek professional help.

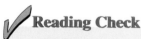

Reading Check

Identify What are the health risks of overtraining?

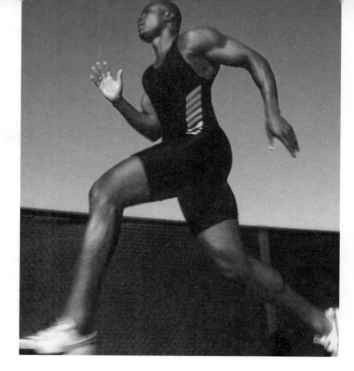

▲ Some competitive athletes may overtrain in an effort to perform well. *How is overtraining different from an eating disorder?*

Lesson 2 Review

Using complete sentences, answer the following questions on a sheet of paper.

Reviewing Facts and Vocabulary

1. **Vocabulary** Define *anorexia nervosa*.
2. **Recall** List three signs of *bulimia*.
3. **Recall** What are the symptoms of *bigorexia*?

Thinking Critically

4. **Evaluate** Explain the relationship between eating disorders and overtraining. How can overtraining contribute to eating disorders?
5. **Synthesize** Harrison is 16 years old and he hopes to have a massive body like those of the wrestlers he sees on television. He is 5 feet, 8 inches tall and weighs 145 pounds. He has begun drinking protein shakes and lifting weights every day. What disorder does he place himself at risk for if he tries to accomplish his goals? What advice would you give him?

Personal Fitness Planning

Analyzing Influences Although eating disorders are caused by a complex set of psychological and emotional factors, many believe that media images of thin and super-fit models and celebrities place added pressure on teens to be thin. Evaluate the degree to which images on television and in magazines impact your body image. Write a paragraph describing how you and other teens can avoid this pressure and have a positive body image.

Nutrition Myths and Fad Diets

What You Will Do

- Explain myths associated with physical activity and nutrition.
- Identify fad diets and risky weight-loss strategies.
- Evaluate consumer issues related to the safety of dietary supplements.

Terms to Know

fad diets

hotlink

RMR
For more on RMR, see Chapter 5, page **155**.

In our society, learning to achieve and maintain a healthy body weight is often complicated by misinformation about nutrition and physical fitness. In this lesson, you will explore several common myths associated with physical activity and nutrition, as well as identify fad diets and other risky weight-loss strategies.

Myths about Nutrition

With all of the information in the media about health and fitness, it is difficult to separate myth from reality. Many people lack the appropriate knowledge and expertise about fitness to know what is fact and what is fiction. The following section will help to clarify the truth behind several common myths about physical activity and nutrition.

Weight Control and Nutrition

Myth. *It is best to eat only one or two meals per day to control your body weight and composition.*

Fact. For most teens, it is best to eat several (three to five) smaller meals and snacks per day to control body weight and composition. Eating several small meals will also help you maintain a higher **Resting Metabolic Rate (RMR),** allowing your body to burn more calories through involuntary functions such as breathing and digestion. Eating more often also helps curb hunger and prevents overeating when you do get hungry.

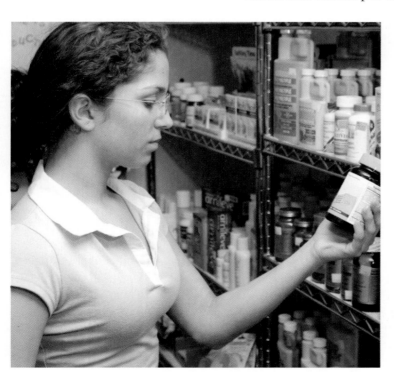

◀ Often, weight-loss products promote false ideas about health and fitness in an effort to sell their products. *What are some false claims you have seen on packages of weight-loss products?*

Myth. *It is reasonable to lose 10 to 20 pounds in one week.*

Fact. While some people can lose this much weight in one week, they usually lose mostly water weight, causing severe dehydration, and put themselves at risk for health problems because they are not eating enough calories or are exercising too much.

Myth. *Consuming large amounts of protein and lifting weights are the best ways to increase the size of your muscles and your muscular strength.*

Fact. Lifting weights is an excellent activity to help you increase the size of your muscles and your muscular strength. However, extra **protein** is not needed in your diet to increase the size of your muscles or your muscular strength. You can get all the protein you need by following the ABCs of nutrition.

Myth. *Consuming extra vitamins and minerals will help you feel better and perform better during exercise.*

Fact. Vitamins and minerals cannot give you extra energy because they do not supply your body with calories. Also, taking large amounts of vitamin and mineral supplements can cause health risks. You will learn more about dietary supplements later in this lesson.

Myth. *Vegetarianism is much healthier and better for exercise performance than a diet that includes animal sources.*

Fact. Vegetarians can be healthy and perform well during exercise. However, those who decide to become vegetarians may initially not get all the nutrients, vitamins, and minerals they need unless they eat a variety of foods, such as fruits, vegetables, leafy greens, whole grains, nuts, seeds, legumes, dairy foods, and eggs.

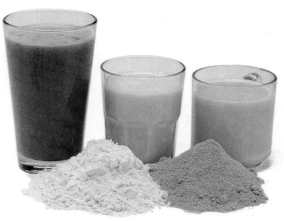

▲ Although protein powders and drinks are sold as supplements, it is not necessary to consume extra protein to build muscle mass. *What is the best way to build muscle mass?*

hotlink

protein
For more on protein, see Chapter 4, page **117**.

vitamins and minerals
For more on vitamins and minerals, see Chapter 4, pages **123** and **125**.

 Reading Check

Discuss Explain one myth associated with weight control and nutrition.

Physical Activity and Nutrition

Myth. *The best way to control your weight and body composition is by adjusting your exercise levels.*

Fact. While adjusting the amount of exercise you do will affect your weight, it is healthiest to combine exercise with a healthful eating plan for effective long-term weight control. This requires you to combine the ABCs of sound nutrition and to become physically active.

Myth. *It is easy to lose one pound of fat by burning 3,500 calories through exercise.*

Fact. Yes, you can burn 3,500 calories by exercising, but you must work at very high intensities. Even to burn 1,000 calories in one hour, you would have to run 8 to 10 miles in one hour, or cycle 25 to 30 miles in one hour. A more reasonable goal is to burn 400–600 calories in an hour by performing moderate-to-vigorous physical activity.

Myth. *Foods high in sugar, like candy bars and sodas, are good sources for quick energy if eaten 30 minutes before exercise.*

Fact. The energy you need for exercise comes from **pre-event meals** you have consumed the day or days before. Foods high in sugar consumed right before exercise can lower your glucose levels and leave you feeling tired.

Myth. *The best fluid you can drink after exercise to replace the fluids you have lost by sweating is water.*

Fact. The best fluid for your needs depends upon on how long you work, how dehydrated you were before you began exercise, how hard you work, and how quickly you need to recover before you exercise again. Sometimes sport drinks may actually be better than water for fast **rehydration.**

hot link

pre-event meals
For more on pre-event meals, see Chapter 4, page **139.**

rehydration
For more on rehydration, see Chapter 2, page **42.**

 Reading Check

Discuss Explain one myth associated with physical activity and nutrition.

Fad Diets

Many of the common misconceptions about nutrition and weight come from fad diets. These are *weight-loss plans that are popular for only a short time.* As their name implies, fad diets come and go. Information on them suddenly appears in the media and vanishes almost as quickly. Some popular fad diets that have appeared in recent years are listed in **Figure 6.4.**

FIGURE 6.4

SOME POPULAR FAD DIETS
Fad diets do not lead to healthy or effective weight loss.
What are some other fad diets you have heard of?

Diet	Claims	Health Risks and Problems
Liquid diets featuring fruit drinks	Simple to follow, rapid weight loss	Weight is quickly regained once normal eating habits are resumed
High-fiber diets	Rapid weight loss	Poor digestion, upset stomach, malnutrition
Fasting	Rapid weight loss; "detoxifies" body	Weight is quickly regained once normal eating habits are resumed

Active Mind Active Body

Analyzing Fad Diets

Understanding and evaluating marketing claims for fad diets are important skills. They can help you recognize false or misleading claims about weight-loss products or methods.

What You Will Need

- Pen or pencil
- Paper

What You Will Do

1. Working as a group, you and several classmates should each choose a different form of media, such as television programming (including the news), TV advertising (including infomercials), magazines, and so on.
2. For one week, each group member is to monitor his or her chosen medium. The group member should record the number of times he or she encounters information concerning weight-loss programs or products. Each member should take notes regarding
   a. the date on which the information appeared.
   b. the medium in which it appeared.
   c. the name of the diet or product.
   d. a brief description of the advertisement or program.
3. At the end of the week, the group should compile its findings. These are to be shared with the class in a round-table discussion.

Apply and Conclude

Which products or diets were featured in more than one medium? What claims were made about each product? What does this suggest about that particular product or diet? Was there any information about the product or diet that seemed to be left out (how it works, for example)? Which of the claims for a product or diet seemed to be the most misleading?

Although the theories behind fad diets often differ, the majority of them are based on faulty science. Some fad diets focus on one essential nutrient, excluding or ignoring others. Other fad diets assign some perceived fat-burning power to a single food, such as grapefruit or cabbage. Most of these strategies advocate taking in fewer daily calories than needed for proper energy and health. You may be aware of some of these, but others may be more difficult to identify. Be aware of any weight-loss plan or product that

- centers on eating one food.
- claims you can eat whatever you want.
- requires the purchase of a weight-loss aid, such as a supplement, appetite suppressant, or books and videos.
- does not include making changes to behavior and habits.

No matter what the angle, all fad diets have one thing in common. All place the unsuspecting consumer at risk of malnutrition or other health problems.

High-Protein Diets

One popular diet in recent years is one that involves an eating plan that is high in protein and eliminates carbohydrates. Some people also take protein supplements to increase muscle mass. However, these practices can be dangerous.

Following a high protein diet can have a negative impact on your physical performance. Such diets:

- increase the risk of dehydration, because they place extra stress on the kidneys.
- increase the risk of calcium loss from bone over time. This can eventually lead to osteoporosis, a disorder characterized by brittle bones.
- will not provide an adequate amount of carbohydrates, including fiber.

Consumer CORNER

Dietary Supplements

Dietary supplements may sound like an easy and safe way to lose weight or improve performance. However, they may not deliver what their ads promise, and they may pose a serious risk to your health.

Unlike other medicines and drugs, dietary supplements do not need approval from the Food and Drug Administration (FDA), and the FDA does not study the safety or effectiveness of the products before they are sold to consumers. The manufacturers themselves are responsible for accurately reporting the ingredients and testing the safety of their products. The FDA only studies supplements if there are reports of injury or illness. The FDA also does not regulate the advertising claims made by the manufacturers.

Many of the ingredients in dietary supplements marketed for weight loss have harmful effects. Some herbal supplements may have health effects, including dizziness, jitters, irregular sleeping patterns, and nausea. Even common supplements containing caffeine or protein can be harmful if taken in large doses.

Although they may seem like a convenient method of controlling weight, dietary supplements are not guaranteed to be effective or safe. Just because they are available for sale in many stores does not mean they are effective. If you have questions about weight loss and dietary supplements, ask your health care professional.

Analyze

With a partner, research more about dietary supplements and the role and responsibilities of the FDA. Find out why the FDA does not currently regulate dietary supplements, and establish a list of pros and cons regarding FDA regulation of dietary supplements.

Diet Pills

Many products claim to "burn" or "flush" fat from the body. Science has yet to devise such a medicine that is both safe and effective. Diet pills may help control the appetite, but they can have very serious side effects. Some cause drowsiness. Others may produce nervousness or anxiety. Some diet pills may even lead to addiction.

Risks of Dietary Supplements

As you learned in Chapter 4, a dietary supplement is a nonfood form of one or more nutrients. In an effort to avoid consuming too many calories, some people may try to get all the appropriate nutrients and vitamins from dietary supplements, or they may use dietary supplements as a method of suppressing their appetites and shedding unwanted pounds.

However, a person needs a healthful plan to meet the body's demands for nutrients. Also, as mentioned in Chapter 4, some vitamins can build up to toxic levels in the body if a person takes them in large amounts. Some supplements are marketed as "all-natural" weight-loss remedies, but they are not necessarily safe. A product's being natural is no guarantee against harm. For example, the leaves of the senna plant are a powerful laxative. Anyone who drinks senna tea in the hopes of purging weight should be aware of the potential health risks.

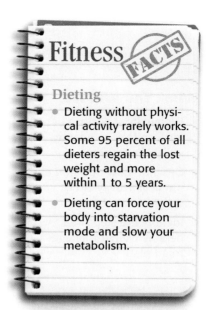

Fitness FACTS

Dieting

- Dieting without physical activity rarely works. Some 95 percent of all dieters regain the lost weight and more within 1 to 5 years.
- Dieting can force your body into starvation mode and slow your metabolism.

Lesson 3 Review

Using complete sentences, answer the following questions on a sheet of paper.

Reviewing Facts and Vocabulary

1. **Vocabulary** What are *fad diets?*
2. **Recall** What are the risks of a high-protein diet?
3. **Recall** List one myth associated with nutrition and weight control and one associated with nutrition and physical activity.

Thinking Critically

4. **Evaluate** Choose a fad diet discussed in this lesson. Explain why it is an ineffective method of weight loss and how it might put a person's health at risk.

5. **Analyze** Anna has recently started taking dietary supplements because she does not want to worry about counting calories in her eating plan. What are the risks associated with such a plan? What advice would you give her?

Personal Fitness Planning

Evaluating Information Make a list of any misconceptions you had about nutrition and fitness before reading this chapter. Write a paragraph explaining what you have learned and how understanding the realities behind these myths will impact your personal fitness plan in terms of your eating plan and physical activity.

What You Will Do

- Explain how positive behaviors can lead to healthy weight management.
- Describe how nutrition and physical activity affect weight control.
- Identify the steps in a healthy weight-management plan.

Terms to Know

weight cycling

Methods for Weight Control

In the last three lessons you have examined the many risks associated with body weight, body image, and myths about nutrition. However, achieving and maintaining a healthy weight should not put your health at risk. No matter what your current weight, everyone can achieve their fitness goals by making positive choices and practicing healthful behaviors.

By working with a health care professional to evaluate your current body composition and adjust your eating and physical activity habits, you can achieve and maintain a body weight and body composition that is best for you. This lesson will offer safe guidelines for achieving your goals.

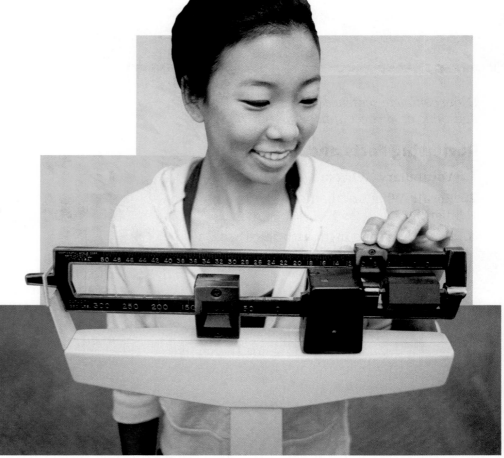

► Managing your weight in a healthy way will have a positive impact on your health and personal fitness. *How can maintaining a healthy weight benefit your mental and physical health?*

FIGURE 6.5

THE WEIGHT CYCLE

Positive fitness behaviors can help reverse the negative effects associated with weight problems. *What type of positive behaviors will help reverse this cycle?*

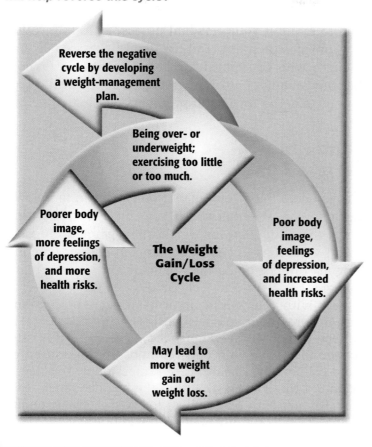

Reverse the negative cycle by developing a weight-management plan.

Being over- or underweight; exercising too little or too much.

Poorer body image, more feelings of depression, and more health risks.

The Weight Gain/Loss Cycle

Poor body image, feelings of depression, and increased health risks.

May lead to more weight gain or weight loss.

Achieving and Maintaining a Healthful Weight

A first step toward making behavioral changes that will lead to a more healthful weight is understanding the effect of unhealthful weight gain or weight loss. This cycle is illustrated in **Figure 6.5.** Take a moment to study this diagram. Notice that the arrows that point in a clockwise direction represent a cycle. Too much or too little weight, for example, can lead to a low self-image, or even depression. This in turn can lead to decreased levels of personal fitness and increased disease risks.

Now note the blue arrow containing the sentence "Reverse the negative cycle by developing a weight-management plan." This arrow points counter-clockwise. This shows that the cycle can be broken—that you can turn your behavior around.

Whether you adopt healthful behaviors and maintain a healthful weight is up to you. In this lesson, you will learn about ways of healthfully changing your weight and your overall level of personal fitness.

Healthy Weight Control

To manage your body weight, it is wise for you to develop a personal plan based on the guidelines listed below. It is important to be patient and consistent as you work to achieve your goals. This will help you avoid **weight cycling,** *the cycle of losing, regaining, losing and regaining weight.* To keep your weight within a healthy range, you need to monitor your personal fitness, including your BMI, eating plan, physical activity, and personal-fitness goals. You should always check with your physician or health care professional before you start any weight-control program. He or she will do a complete checkup, testing you for health problems relating to weight.

Diet and Physical Activity for Weight Control

Once you determine your goals, you can begin to follow a weight-management plan. Whether your BMI is high, low, or within the normal range, the basic plan for weight management is essentially the same, with variations in calorie intake and energy expenditure. The following list offers a guide for a realistic and healthy plan for managing weight.

- Check with your physician or health care professional if you are unsure about your weight-loss goals.
- Check your BMI (see **Figure 5.2,** page **149**). If it is too high or too low, have your body composition measured with skinfold calipers by a health care professional. You need to set a goal to bring your BMI within the healthy range (between the 5th and 85th percentiles) for your age and gender.
- Use the ABCs and the Food Guide Pyramid for healthy eating.
- Adjust calorie intake and energy expenditure, depending upon your needs. **Figure 6.6** offers specific guidance, based on BMI.
- Work 30 to 60 minutes per day of moderate-to-vigorous physical activity, or a minimum of 225–300 minutes per week for long-term success.
- Allow plenty of time (20–30 weeks) for long-term results.
- Retest body composition every three months.
- Keep a log of your progress and re-evaluate how your plan is working every three months.
- Reward yourself in a positive way as you meet your goals.
- Continue to make new short-term weight-loss goals every three months until you achieve your goal.

Your ultimate goal, in any case, should be to make permanent, positive changes in your eating habits. This approach will work far better than a series of short-term changes that can not be sustained.

 Reading Check

Explain How often should you evaluate your progress and make new goals?

FIGURE 6.6

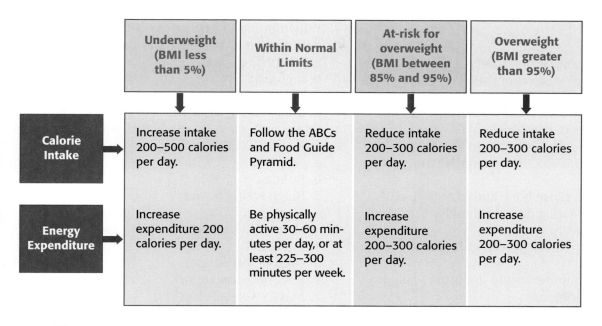

RECOMMENDATIONS FOR WEIGHT MANAGEMENT

To properly change or maintain body weight, it is best to adjust both calorie intake and energy expenditure. *What are some other important steps in a weight-management plan?*

	Underweight (BMI less than 5%)	Within Normal Limits	At-risk for overweight (BMI between 85% and 95%)	Overweight (BMI greater than 95%)
Calorie Intake	Increase intake 200–500 calories per day.	Follow the ABCs and Food Guide Pyramid.	Reduce intake 200–300 calories per day.	Reduce intake 200–300 calories per day.
Energy Expenditure	Increase expenditure 200 calories per day.	Be physically active 30–60 minutes per day, or at least 225–300 minutes per week.	Increase expenditure 200–300 calories per day.	Increase expenditure 200–300 calories per day.

Lesson 4 Review

Using complete sentences, answer the following questions on a sheet of paper.

Reviewing Facts and Vocabulary

1. **Vocabulary** What is *weight cycling?*

2. **Recall** Explain how unhealthful weight loss or weight gain can lead to further weight loss or weight gain.

3. **Recall** What is the first step in determining your weight goals?

Thinking Critically

4. **Analyze** Analyze methods of a weight control plan that includes diet and exercise.

5. **Evaluation** Dave is 16 years old. He has a BMI of 16 and 6 percent body fat. He wants to gain weight, but he is not sure what to do. What positive advice can you give him to gain weight in a healthful way?

Personal Fitness Planning

Designing a Plan Based on the information in this lesson, create a plan that states your goal for improving or maintaining your weight. For each step presented in this lesson, write a sentence or two explaining how and when you will implement each one.

TRUE/FALSE

On a sheet of paper, write the numbers 1–10. Write True or False for each statement.

1. A person whose BMI is between the 85th and 95th percentiles is considered overweight.
2. A person whose BMI is between the 85th and 95th percentiles is considered at risk for overweight.
3. Overweight can cause bone and joint problems.
4. Anorexia is an eating disorder in which an individual overeats.
5. Bigorexia occurs more in teen girls than in boys.
6. People who are underweight are more likely to get colds and influenza.
7. Fad diets are usually effective at helping you maintain weight loss over the long term.
8. To build muscle mass, it is necessary to consume large amounts of protein.
9. Eating foods high in sugar will provide your body with the energy it needs to perform well during exercise.
10. Teens should get 60 minutes a day or at least 225 minutes per week of moderate-to-vigorous physical activity.

MULTIPLE CHOICE

On a sheet of paper, write the letter of the word or phrase that best completes each statement.

11. A person with a BMI higher than the 95th percentile is
    a. within normal limits.
    b. underweight.
    c. overweight.
    d. at risk for overweight.
12. A person with a BMI lower than the 5th percentile is
    a. within normal limits.
    b. underweight.
    c. overweight.
    d. at risk for overweight.

13. Which of the following is not linked to obesity?
    a. Asthma
    b. Type 2 diabetes
    c. Bone and joint problems
    d. Anorexia nervosa
14. Which of the following terms is associated with the act of bingeing and purging?
    a. Anorexia nervosa
    b. Bigorexia
    c. Bulimia
    d. Binge eating disorder
15. Overtraining can be associated with all of the following EXCEPT:
    a. Anorexia
    b. Bulimia
    c. Binge eating disorder
    d. Bigorexia
16. Which of the following is not a symptom of anorexia?
    a. High blood pressure
    b. Poor body image
    c. Massive weight loss
    d. Excessive exercise
17. Bigorexia is also known as
    a. binge eating disorder.
    b. reverse anorexia.
    c. overtraining.
    d. weight cycling.
18. All of the following are examples of risky weight-loss strategies, EXCEPT
    a. high-protein diets.
    b. surgical procedures.
    c. the *Dietary Guidelines for Americans.*
    d. fasting.
19. The first step in any teen weight-control program is to
    a. reduce energy intake.
    b. increase energy intake.
    c. get 225 minutes of weekly physical activity.
    d. check with your physician if you are unsure about your weight-loss goals.
20. How often should you check your body composition during a weight-control program?
    a. Every 3 months
    b. Every 6–8 weeks
    c. Every 3 weeks
    d. Every 1–2 weeks

DISCUSSION

Using complete sentences, answer the following questions on a sheet of paper.

21. **Identify** What are three health risks associated with being overweight?
22. **Explain** How can overtraining contribute to an eating disorder?
23. **Evaluate** Why should you avoid fad diets?

VOCABULARY

On a sheet of paper, write the letter of the term in Column B that best fits the definition in Column A.

Column A

24. Health problems and diseases linked to or resulting directly from long-term overweight or obesity.
25. A disorder in which an individual falsely believes he or she is underweight or undersized.
26. Disorder in which blood glucose levels become elevated.
27. Weight-loss plans that are popular for only a short time.
28. Psychological illnesses that cause people to undereat, overeat, or practice other dangerous nutrition-related behaviors.
29. Hormone produced by the pancreas that helps convert carbohydrates into glucose.

Column B

a. insulin
b. impaired glucose tolerance
c. excessive weight disabilities
d. eating disorders
e. bigorexia
f. fad diets

CRITICAL THINKING

Using complete sentences, answer the following questions on a sheet of paper.

30. **Analyze** Why do you think the number of overweight teens has increased significantly over the past 25 years? Explain.

31. **Evaluate** You suspect a friend may have an eating disorder. What should you do?
32. **Describe** Explain one myth associated with physical activity and nutrition.

CASE STUDY

LOSING WEIGHT

Sandy is a 15-year-old active female. She participates in aerobic dance classes for 30 minutes, five times a week. However, even though she is physically active, she feels like she is overweight and has been thinking of going on a high-protein diet to lose more weight. She snacks on a candy bar or soda before dance class. Otherwise, she typically eats two meals a day.

HERE IS YOUR ASSIGNMENT:

Assume you are Sandy's friend, and she asks you for some assistance with her plans for losing weight. Make a list of things Sandy should consider and do before beginning her program. Then list the recommendations you would give Sandy for the first two weeks of her program. Use the following keys to help you:

KEYS TO HELP YOU

- Consider Sandy's current lifestyle habits and choices.
- List the possible health risks associated with her current eating habits.
- List the possible health risks associated with her future plan of a "high-protein" diet.
- Decide how she should evaluate her current diet.
- Think about her needs and goals. For example, how should she go about changing her diet?
- Determine a reasonable plan to give Sandy that covers the concepts of risky weight-loss strategies and recommended teen weight-control programs.

FITNESS
Online

Regular aerobic training allows the heart and lungs to work as efficiently as possible. Do you know the components of aerobic fitness? Are they part of your fitness plan? Find out by taking the STEP Personal Inventory for Chapter 7. Find it at **fitness.glencoe.com**.

Your Heart, Lungs, and Circulation

Josh loves to row and is a member of the school rowing team. Tina enjoys participating in a step aerobics class. Although Josh and Tina have very different interests, they have one thing in common. They both like doing aerobic activities and recognize the importance of doing them.

What are aerobic activities? How do they benefit the body? In this lesson, you will find out.

Aerobic Activities and the Body

The exercises that weightlifters do are targeted at certain muscles of the body. These include muscles of the arms, legs, chest, and back. The activities that Josh and Tina do are also targeted at a major muscle of the body. That muscle is the heart.

Aerobic activity is continuous activity that requires large amounts of oxygen. (The word *aerobic* means "with oxygen.") Like other aerobic activities, rowing and step aerobics temporarily raise the heart rate. Done regularly, aerobic activities strengthen the heart. They also strengthen another vital organ, the lungs. Aerobic activity also makes your working muscles more efficient at using oxygen. Before you can understand how aerobic activities work, you need to have some knowledge of the circulatory and respiratory systems.

What You Will Do

- Explain the importance of aerobic activity to your health and fitness.
- Recognize the role of the circulatory and respiratory systems in aerobic conditioning.
- Identify the physical benefits of aerobic activity.
- Evaluate your cardiorespiratory endurance level.

Terms to Know

aerobic activity
circulatory system
hemoglobin
stroke volume
arteries
capillaries
veins
respiratory system
diaphragm
cardiorespiratory endurance

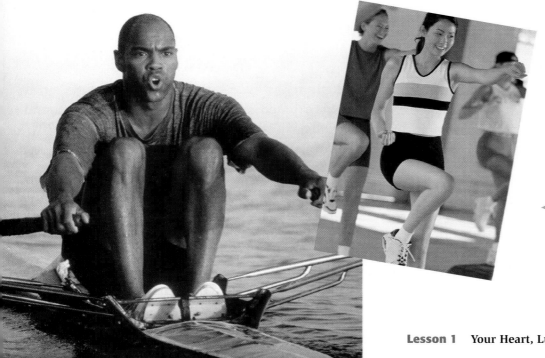

Participating in aerobic activities regularly will increase your cardiorespiratory endurance. *What are some aerobic activities that you enjoy doing?*

Your Circulatory System

The **circulatory system** *consists of the heart, blood, and blood vessels.* This system is also sometimes called the *cardiovascular system.* This system is responsible for circulating blood throughout the body.

The Heart

Figure 7.1 shows the heart, the main organ of the circulatory system. It is a muscle about the size and shape of your fist. The right side of the heart pumps blood to the lungs. There, the blood picks up oxygen and rids itself of carbon dioxide. The left side of the heart pumps oxygen-rich blood to the rest of the body. **Hemoglobin** is *an iron rich compound in the blood that helps carry the oxygen.* The oxygen helps your cells produce the energy you need to meet the demands of daily life.

The heart beats at different rates depending upon whether your body is at rest or at work. When resting, the heart beats an average of 72 times per minute. During strenuous physical activity, your heart rate—or *pulse*—increases, sometimes to twice or more its resting rate. *The amount of blood pumped per beat of the heart,* or **stroke volume,** also increases. This is because your working muscles demand more blood to supply them with oxygen and other nutrients.

The Blood Vessels

Blood is carried to and from the heart via a network of blood vessels. There are three types of vessels. *Vessels that carry blood from the heart to the major extremities—such as the arms, legs, and head—are known as* **arteries.** Smaller blood vessels called **capillaries** (KAP-uh-LAYR-eez) *deliver oxygen and other nutrients to individual cells.* **Veins** *deliver the blood back to the heart.* There it receives a fresh supply of oxygen and begins its journey again.

 Reading Check

Explain What are the main parts of the circulatory system and what is the function of each?

Your Respiratory System

The oxygen that your blood carries comes from the air around you. It is introduced into your body by means of your **respiratory** (REH-spir-uh-tor-ee) **system.** This is *the body system that exchanges gases between your body and the environment.*

The principal organ of your respiratory system is your lungs. Your lungs exchange oxygen and carbon dioxide. This process is known as *respiration.*

Unlike the heart, the lungs are not a muscle. Rather, they get their power from the **diaphragm,** *a muscle found between the chest cavity and abdomen,* as well as the intercostal muscles around the ribs

FIGURE 7.1

THE HEART

Your heart pumps about 5 liters of blood every minute when your body is at rest. During high levels of aerobic activity, the heart pumps 4 to 5 times as much blood. *Compute the number of liters of blood the heart pumps during 5 minutes of vigorous physical activity.*

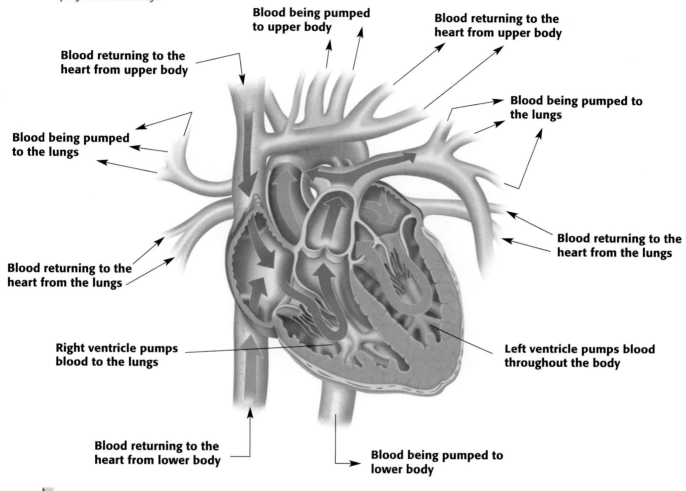

Blood being pumped to upper body

Blood returning to the heart from upper body

Blood returning to the heart from upper body

Blood being pumped to the lungs

Blood being pumped to the lungs

Blood returning to the heart from the lungs

Blood returning to the heart from the lungs

Right ventricle pumps blood to the lungs

Left ventricle pumps blood throughout the body

Blood returning to the heart from lower body

Blood being pumped to lower body

and the abdominal muscles in the lower stomach area. As shown in **Figure 7.2** on page **196,** when you inhale, the diaphragm contracts and moves downward. The chest cavity enlarges, allowing air into the lungs. When you exhale, the reverse happens.

Like your pulse, your breathing rate increases during vigorous physical activity. If your lungs are healthy, you can breathe about 6 liters of air per minute at rest and up to 100 liters of air per minute during vigorous exercise. The muscles involved in breathing become conditioned to make your breathing more efficient. This allows more oxygen to reach the heart, enabling it to pump more blood to the muscles and to remove carbon dioxide from your body more effectively.

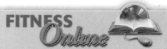

FITNESS *Online*

Gather information about asthma and fitness at **fitness.glencoe.com**.

Activity Investigate the site to find asthma triggers and treatments. Create a poster or brochure using information from the site.

FIGURE 7.2

THE PROCESS OF RESPIRATION

Your lungs bring in oxygen from the environment and send out carbon dioxide. *Explain how the lungs aid the circulatory system during strenuous activity.*

EXHALATION

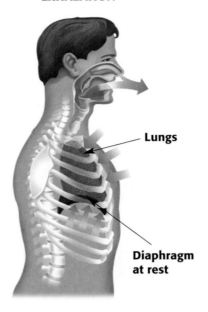

Lungs

Diaphragm at rest

INHALATION

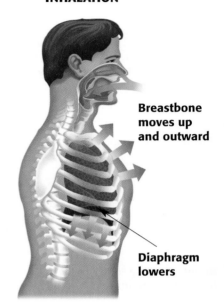

Breastbone moves up and outward

Diaphragm lowers

Benefits of Aerobic Activity

Regular aerobic activity strengthens the body in several ways. It increases stroke volume and lowers your resting heart rate. This means your heart is working more efficiently, resulting in a more effective delivery of oxygen to your body.

Aerobic activity also conditions the muscles used in breathing to function more efficiently. Such day-to-day tasks as climbing stairs require less effort because your muscles are more efficient. One of the most important benefits of aerobic activity is that it builds on itself. In other words, the more you condition aerobically, the more strenuous physical activity you are able to do.

▶ Jogging regularly is one great way to increase your stamina. *How can increased stamina benefit you in your daily life?*

Fitness Check

Evaluating Cardiorespiratory Endurance

In this activity, you will participate in one of two tests of cardiorespiratory fitness. The first is a 3-minute step test. The second is a 1.5-mile (2.5-k) run and/or walk. Warm up before you start either test. Stop if you feel dizzy or become overheated. After completing the test of your choice, allow between 5 and 10 minutes to cool down.

3-Minute Step Test

Procedure:

1. Begin stepping up and down on a 12-inch step at a rate of approximately 24 steps per minute.
2. At the end of 3 minutes, stop. Immediately take your pulse.
3. Use the Fitness Ratings Chart for the 3-Minute Step Test to determine your level of cardiorespiratory fitness.

Fitness Ratings: 3-Minute Step Test	
Pulse Rate	**Score**
84 or less	High
85 to 95	Good
120 or higher	Low

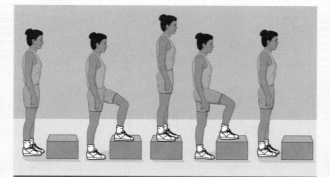

1.5-Mile (2.5-k) Run/Walk Test

Procedure:

1. Go to a local indoor or outdoor track or other flat course in your community. Select a day when the temperature is moderate—between 50 and 75 degrees F (11 and 25 degrees C)—and winds are calm.
2. Complete 6 laps or a distance of 1.5 miles (2.5 k) in as short a time as possible. You may walk, jog, or use a combination of both.
3. Use the Fitness Ratings Chart for the 1.5-Mile (2.5-k) Run/Walk to determine your level of cardiorespiratory fitness.

Fitness Ratings: 1.5-Mile (2.5-k) Run/Walk		
Males	**Females**	**Score**
9 min or less	11 min or less	High
9 to 14:30 min	11 to 15:30 min	Good
14:30 min or more	15:30 min or more	Low

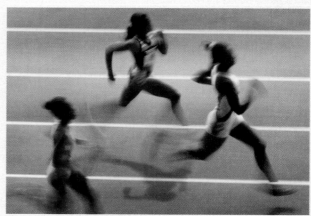

For many people, the hardest part of starting a program of aerobic conditioning is overcoming "inertia." A regular routine of inactivity can be a hard habit to break. But breaking out of such a routine yields great benefits to your cardiovascular system.

If you aren't physically active, make up your mind to take charge and begin a program of lifelong training today. There's no time like the present!

Long-Term Benefits of Aerobic Activity

One long-term result of regular aerobic activity is cardiorespiratory endurance. This is *the ability of the body to work continuously for extended periods of time*. Also known as *cardiovascular fitness*, cardiorespiratory endurance offers many benefits. People who have a high level of cardiorespiratory fitness have lowered risks of adult lifestyle diseases, such as cardiovascular disease, type 2 diabetes, and obesity. They also

- have increased energy.
- have less stress in their lives.
- look and feel better.

An Aerobic Lifestyle

Cardiorespiratory endurance increases your chances for living a longer and healthier life. The death rate from cardiovascular and other lifestyle diseases is much higher among adults who are inactive, or have low levels of cardiorespiratory endurance, than it is for those with higher levels.

As a teen, you may think that "heart health" is an adult concern. However, your adult years are just around the corner. A high level of fitness and health will be easier to maintain as an adult if you develop positive fitness behaviors and attitudes now. By engaging in regular aerobic activity now, you can reduce your risk of developing lifestyle diseases later.

 Reading Check

Summarize Make a list of both the immediate and long-term benefits of aerobic activity.

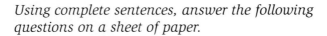

Lesson 1 Review

Using complete sentences, answer the following questions on a sheet of paper.

Reviewing Facts and Vocabulary

1. **Vocabulary** Define *aerobic activity*.
2. **Recall** What two body systems are most immediately involved in aerobic conditioning?

Thinking Critically

3. **Analyze** What is one benefit of aerobic activity to the heart? to the lungs?
4. **Synthesize** At what age do you think people should be encouraged to begin aerobic conditioning? At what age do you think people should be encouraged to stop? Explain your answers.

Personal Fitness Planning

Planning a Workout Design a walking or jogging course in or around your neighborhood that allows you to cover 2 miles in 20 to 30 minutes. When choosing your course, you should consider all safety issues and factors that will affect your intensity (hills, bridges, type of surface, and so on).

Problems and Care of Your Heart and Lungs

Y ou do not have to think about your heart beating because the process is automatic. So is the action of your lungs as you breathe. What is *not* automatic is care of these two organs and their body systems. Maintaining the health of these two systems requires both an awareness of health risk factors and a lifestyle that reduces your risks.

Risk Factors and Lifestyle Disease

Rolf and Ray are identical twins, although you might not know it to look at them. Rolf looks about 10 years older than his brother. He spends most of his time in front of the TV with a bowl of snacks. Ray, by contrast, works out at the gym regularly and maintains a healthful eating plan.

The more important difference between Rolf and Ray is one that is not plainly visible. That is because it is on the inside. The arteries leading to Rolf's heart have begun to close up, as a result of his unhealthful lifestyle. He is in the early stages of heart disease.

Heart disease, lung cancer, and other illnesses of the circulatory and respiratory systems are sometimes referred to as lifestyle diseases. These are *diseases that are the result of certain lifestyle choices.* Some lifestyles involve risk factors. Risk factors increase a person's

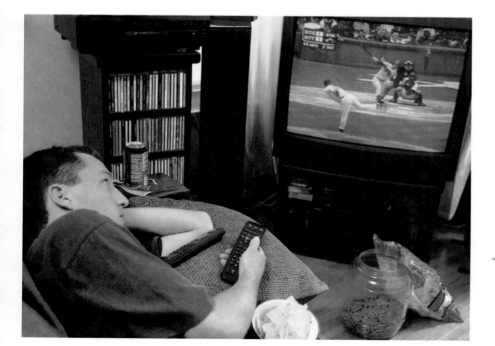

◀ Your lifestyle can affect your chances of developing certain diseases. *How does aerobic activity help to improve the health of your heart and lungs?*

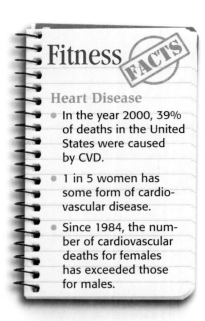

Fitness FACTS

Heart Disease

- In the year 2000, 39% of deaths in the United States were caused by CVD.

- 1 in 5 women has some form of cardio-vascular disease.

- Since 1984, the number of cardiovascular deaths for females has exceeded those for males.

Source: American Heart Association, 2002.[1]

hot link

cholesterol
For more on LDL and HDL cholesterol, see Chapter 4, page **120**.

▶ Being physically active helps reduce your risk of developing a lifestyle disease. *What other measures can you take?*

chances of developing disease. Some risk factors for heart and lung disease are

- inactivity.
- being overweight.
- smoking and using other forms of tobacco.
- eating foods high in fat and cholesterol.

✓ **Reading Check**

Explain In your own words, tell what a lifestyle disease is, and name two behaviors that can lead to such a disease.

Cardiovascular Disease (CVD)

In addition to being a lifestyle disease, heart disease is also considered a cardiovascular disease, or CVD. This is *any medical disorder that affects the heart or blood vessels*. CVD is the leading cause of death in the United States, claiming some 950,000 lives each year.

One health condition that is present in virtually all individuals diagnosed with CVD is atherosclerosis (ath-uh-roh-skluh-ROH-suhs). This is *a condition in which a fatty deposit called plaque (PLAK) builds up inside arteries, restricting or cutting off blood flow*. **Figure 7.3** shows the progression of atherosclerosis. The cause of atherosclerosis is not known for sure, although it is linked to a person's cholesterol levels. Regular aerobic activity lowers LDL **cholesterol** and raises HDL cholesterol and helps to reduce the risk of developing atherosclerosis.

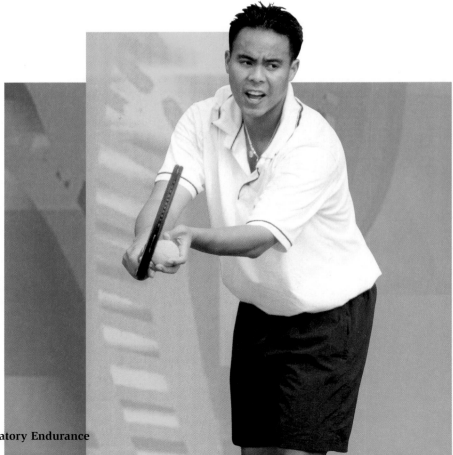

FIGURE 7.3

THE PROGRESSION OF ATHEROSCLEROSIS

As fatty deposits build up, the blood flow to the heart lessens.
Which of the artery cross-sections shown most likely belongs to someone who is physically active?

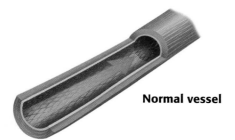
Normal vessel

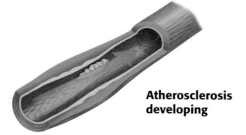
Atherosclerosis developing

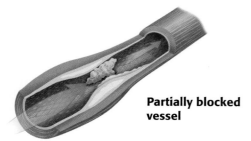
Partially blocked vessel

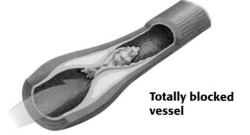
Totally blocked vessel

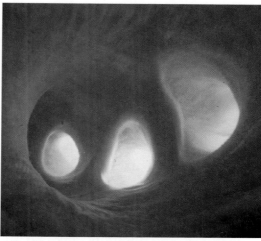
A healthy artery provides an open passageway for the flow of blood.

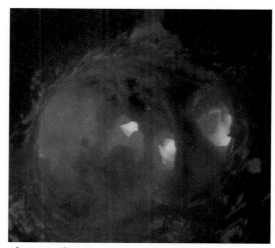
Plaques along an artery narrow its diameter and interfere with blood flow. Clots can form, making the problem worse.

Heart Attack

Each year 1 million people in the United States suffer heart attacks. Half of these people die. A heart attack results from blockage of a blood vessel that feeds the heart muscle. This causes damage to the heart muscle. Symptoms of heart attack include tightness in the chest, tingling or pain in the left arm, sweating, nausea, and

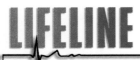

Helping Others

Would you recognize the signs of heart attack and cardiac arrest in others? Knowing them could save a life. They include:

- Tightness in the chest.
- Tingling or pain in the left arm.
- Abnormal or labored breathing.
- Loss of responsiveness.
- No signs of circulation.
- No movement or coughing.

If this occurs, call 911. Begin CPR immediately if you have been trained to do so.

shortness of breath. Anyone with these symptoms should get to a doctor or hospital quickly.

The loss of blood supply to the heart muscle during a heart attack may cause the heart to stop beating, referred to as cardiac arrest. However, all heart attacks are not fatal and a person who participates in regular aerobic activity has a reduced risk of suffering a fatal heart attack.

Sudden Cardiac Death

You may have read or heard stories about young athletes suffering cardiac arrest and dying suddenly during practice or a game. Sudden death from cardiac arrest is referred to as *sudden cardiac death.* Sudden cardiac death can occur in young and older people during strenuous activity.

Sudden cardiac death in people under age 35 is rare and usually is the result of a congenital (kuhn-JEN-ih-tuhl) heart defect (one occurring at birth). In the cases of people 35 and older, sudden cardiac death is usually associated with atherosclerosis. (**See Figure 7.4.**)

The best way to prevent this fatal CVD is to know the symptoms that precede it: a tight sensation in the chest, nausea, profuse sweating, and difficulty breathing. Another safeguard is to have a complete physical checkup before beginning a program of strenuous physical activity or exercise.

Stroke

The building up of deposits in the arteries poses a risk not only to the heart but to the brain. *When blood flow to a person's brain is interrupted or cut off entirely by the blockage of an artery, the individual is said to have suffered a* stroke. Some warning signs of a stroke include:

- Sudden numbness or weakness of the face, arm, or leg, especially on one side of the body
- Sudden confusion, trouble speaking or understanding
- Sudden trouble seeing in one or both eyes
- Sudden trouble walking, dizziness, loss of balance or coordination
- Sudden, severe headache with no known cause

A stroke, like a heart attack, can be minor or more major. A stroke usually results in damage to the brain and can leave a person partially or totally paralyzed. Sometimes when the damage from a stroke is minor, a person may be paralyzed only temporarily. However, a major stroke often results in death. If you perform regular aerobic activity or exercise, you will significantly reduce your risk for stroke.

Peripheral Vascular Disease

Peripheral (puhr-IF-uhr-uhl) vascular disease is *a CVD that occurs mainly in the legs and, less frequently, the arms.* It causes pain during physical activity or exercise. Primary risk factors for peripheral vascular disease include cigarette smoking and type 2 diabetes, which frequently occurs in overweight individuals.

FIGURE 7.4

CAUSES OF SUDDEN CARDIAC DEATH

The causes of sudden cardiac death vary with age. *Compare the percentage of individuals under 35 who died of enlarged heart with the percentage 35 and over who died of the same CVD.*

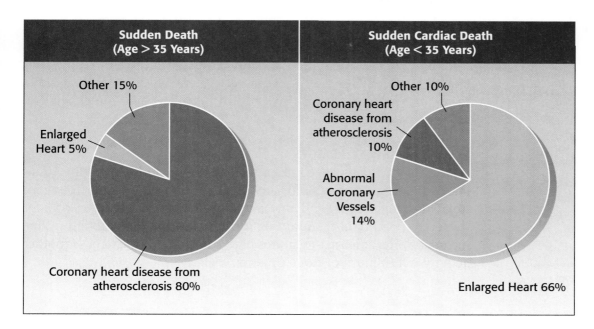

Sudden Death (Age > 35 Years)
- Other 15%
- Enlarged Heart 5%
- Coronary heart disease from atherosclerosis 80%

Sudden Cardiac Death (Age < 35 Years)
- Other 10%
- Coronary heart disease from atherosclerosis 10%
- Abnormal Coronary Vessels 14%
- Enlarged Heart 66%

Hypertension

High blood pressure, or **hypertension,** is a key risk factor in heart attacks, stroke, and heart failure. Because this CVD presents no symptoms, it is sometimes referred to as the "silent killer."

In 90 to 95 percent of all cases, the cause of hypertension is unknown. In fact, you can have the CVD for years without knowing it. Fortunately, hypertension can be treated effectively and safely under a doctor's supervision.

 Reading Check

Identify Select and describe one of the cardiovascular diseases mentioned in the previous sections.

Diseases of the Lung

Two lifestyle diseases of the respiratory system that deserve specific mention are lung cancer and emphysema (em-fuh-ZEE-muh). Of the 200,000 deaths from lung cancer each year, approximately half are directly linked to cigarette smoking. In fact, the American Cancer Society has singled out this deadly habit as the single most preventable cause of death in our society.

▼ Smoking is a dangerous habit—it kills more Americans each year than all other listed causes combined. *What are some other reasons people should avoid smoking?*

Smoking—*400,000*
Car accidents—*42,000*
Alcohol—*36,000*
Suicide—*30,000*
Homicides—*20,000*
Illicit Drugs—*20,000*
HIV/AIDS—*16,000*
Fires—*3,600*

Source: Centers for Disease Control and Prevention, 2003.[2]

Mind OVER Matter

Understanding Risks

People who smoke do serious damage not only to their lungs, but to their desire and ability to become aerobically fit. They are less likely to take part in aerobic activities because they have reduced lung capacity. This makes it harder for them to sustain aerobic activity. This begins a vicious circle.

The best way to avoid this circle is to make a decision to avoid cigarettes and other harmful substances, and focus on fitness!

Emphysema is *a disease in which the small airways of the lungs lose their normal elasticity, making them less efficient in helping to move air in and out of the lungs.* Once the lung tissues have been damaged, they can never be restored. People with emphysema have difficulty breathing and develop a chronic cough. In nearly all cases, the disease is caused by cigarette smoking.

Care of the Circulatory and Respiratory Systems

The diseases discussed in this lesson can be serious and even life threatening. The best treatment for cardiovascular and respiratory diseases is prevention and fortunately, there are steps you can take to prevent many of the serious health problems that affect the cardiovascular and respiratory systems.

Changeable Risk Factors

Although some of the risk factors related to problems of the circulatory and respiratory systems are inherited, many are within your control. One behavior that you have already learned about that can counter these risk factors is maintaining a program of aerobic activity. This includes doing at least 20 minutes of nonstop vigorous exercise or other activity a minimum of three times a week.

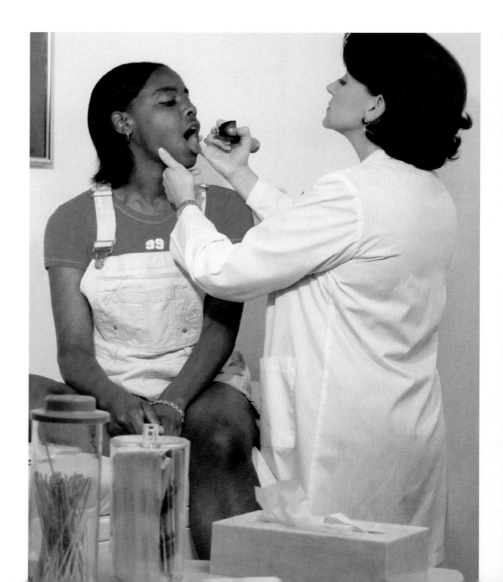

▶ Regular medical checkups are important for monitoring your risk factors for developing cardiovascular disease. *What is involved in a regular medical checkup?*

Any Body Can

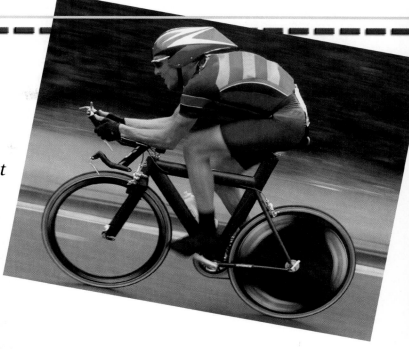

Lance Armstrong
The Champion Who Wouldn't Quit

Imagine receiving the news that you had cancer. What would you do? For an athlete named Lance Armstrong, the answer to this question was to work harder than ever.

Lance Armstrong was born on September 18, 1971, in Plano, Texas. At age 13, Lance won the Iron Kids Triathlon—a grueling athletic contest that combines swimming, bicycling, and running. After graduating from high school, Lance competed in national and international cycling competitions, including the 1992 Olympic Games.

Then in October of 1996, Lance was told he had advanced testicular cancer. Although he was given a 50-50 chance of surviving, Lance made up his mind he would not give in to his disease. After undergoing cancer treatment, he began to train again. He worked at improving his cardiorespiratory fitness until he was able to ride up to six hours (360 minutes) at a time.

In 1999, against all odds, Lance entered the ultimate bicycle race, the Tour de France, and came in first. He has since gone on to claim four more Tour de France titles.

Not everyone can win the Tour de France. However, anyone can regularly engage in aerobic activities for 150 minutes per week to improve his or her fitness. When it comes to improving cardiorespiratory endurance, Any Body Can!

Research

Lance Armstrong survived cancer and has won five Tour de France titles. Research another person who has overcome disease or poor health to lead a physically active life. Share your findings in a brief report.

Other activities that can keep your heart and lungs healthy include:

- **Avoiding tobacco.** Smoking puts added stress on the heart and lungs, and smokeless tobacco contains nicotine, a drug that increases blood pressure and heart rate. Exposure to secondhand smoke is also harmful.
- **Maintaining a healthy weight.** Being overweight has been linked to hypertension and heart disease.
- **Eating right.** This includes limiting your intake of foods high in fat and cholesterol. It also means eating foods high in **fiber**, which helps keep the arteries of the bloodstream clear.
- **Having regular medical checkups.** Seeing a health professional periodically for a **checkup** allows you to monitor the health of your circulatory and respiratory systems.

hot link

fiber
For more on fiber, see Chapter 4, page **117.**

medical checkups
For more on medical screenings, see Chapter 2, page **37.**

Blood Pressure

As part of a regular checkup, your health care professional checks your blood pressure. This is *the force of the blood in the main arteries*. Your blood pressure rises and falls as the heart and muscles of your body cope with varying demands, including stress and vigorous physical activity.

Each time the heart muscles contract, blood surges through the arteries with such force that the artery walls bulge. The pressure in the arteries, which is at its greatest at this point, is called *systolic* (sis-TOL-ik) *pressure*. As the muscles of the heart relax to refill with blood, pressure in the arteries drops to its lowest point. This is called *diastolic* (dy-uh-STOL-ik) *pressure*.

Blood pressure is reported as two numbers, such as 120 over 80, which is written 120/80. Your systolic blood pressure is the top number. Your diastolic blood pressure is the bottom number. Normal blood pressure should fall below values of 140/90 on average, when measured on a regular basis.

 Reading Check

Identify Describe three behaviors that contribute to a healthy heart and lungs.

Lesson 2 Review

Using complete sentences, answer the following questions on a sheet of paper.

Reviewing Facts and Vocabulary

1. **Vocabulary** What is *blood pressure*? Explain *systolic* and *diastolic pressure*.

2. **Recall** What are some symptoms of a heart attack?

3. **Recall** Explain sudden cardiac death from exercise. What can cause it in individuals under age 35? In those over age 35?

Thinking Critically

4. **Compare and Contrast** Compare the risk factors for CVD with the strategies for avoiding these illnesses. Make a list of five *do's* and five *don'ts* for healthy, disease-free living.

5. **Synthesize** How might you respond to the following argument? "So what if I smoke? I watch what I eat, and I get some exercise."

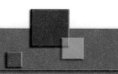 **Personal Fitness Planning**

Investigating Heart Disease Speak with a physician or learn through print or online resources about kinds of physical activity that are appropriate for someone recovering from a heart attack. Identify ways that inactivity is a changeable risk factor affecting health. Then design a walking/ stationary cycling program for such a person. Include a description of precautions that should be taken and of differences between this program and one for a completely healthy individual.

Influences on Cardio-respiratory Endurance

What You Will Do

- Describe how cardiorespiratory endurance is measured.
- Identify factors that influence cardiorespiratory endurance.
- Evaluate the effect of added weight on aerobic performance.
- Explain the physical, mental, and emotional benefits of cardiorespiratory endurance.

Dorothy, who is 81 years old, just completed her fourth marathon, a run of over 26 miles. Do you know any remarkable older adults like Dorothy? What permits some people to stay fit well into their later years? What are the advantages of staying aerobically fit? In this lesson, you will find answers to both these questions.

Terms to Know

maximal oxygen consumption
(VO_{2max})
fast-twitch muscle fibers
slow-twitch muscle fibers

Measuring Cardiorespiratory Endurance

As noted in Lesson 1, cardiorespiratory endurance is the ability of the body to work continuously for extended periods of time. Fitness experts generally measure cardiorespiratory endurance in terms of **maximal oxygen consumption**, or VO_{2max}. This is *the largest amount of oxygen your body is able to process during strenuous aerobic exercise.* Specifically, VO_{2max} measures the amount of oxygen (or O_2) in milliliters (ml) per kilogram (kg) of body weight per minute. In general, the more aerobically fit you are, the higher your VO_{2max} will be and vice versa.

hotlink

VO_{2max}
For more on VO_{2max} and how to estimate it, see Chapter 8, page **221.**

◄ It is possible to maintain high levels of cardiorespiratory endurance, regardless of age. *Why might a physically fit older person seem younger than his or her age?*

Factors Affecting Cardiorespiratory Endurance

Although Dorothy has managed to maintain a high level of fitness, her husband Arthur has fared less well. Even though Arthur is a year younger than Dorothy, he has suffered a stroke and is now confined to a wheelchair. Some people believe that such differences are a matter simply of genetics. Yet, there are other factors besides heredity at work. Among these are age, gender, body composition, and level of conditioning.

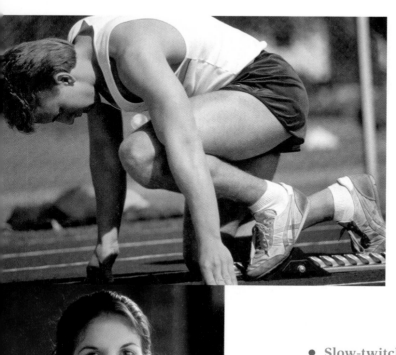

Age

As a person ages, he or she loses cardiorespiratory fitness. Generally, one's fitness level begins a gradual decline after age 25. The typical rate of decline in VO_{2max} is about 0.5 ml/kg/min. per year or 5 ml/kg/min. per decade. Part of this decline is due to a decrease in the heart's ability to work as efficiently as it once did.

Heredity

Your genetic makeup affects both your initial levels of cardiorespiratory endurance and your capacity to improve it. The amount of blood your heart can pump per beat is determined by your genetic makeup. Also, some people develop higher levels of cardiorespiratory fitness than others because they are born with a greater proportion of slow-twitch to fast-twitch muscle fibers.

- **Slow-twitch muscle fibers** are *muscle fibers that contract at a slow rate*, thus allowing for greater muscle endurance. Found in higher proportion in long-distance runners, these fibers are associated with an increased ability to do aerobic work.
- **Fast-twitch muscle fibers,** in contrast, *contract rapidly, thus allowing for greater muscle strength.* These muscle fibers, found in greater proportion in weight lifters, have little bearing on aerobic levels.

The skeletal muscles of young adults tend to consist of about 50 percent slow-twitch and 50 percent fast-twitch fibers. Adults who perform well at aerobic activity and have high levels of cardiorespiratory fitness have closer to 70 or 80 percent slow-twitch fibers.

Gender. After puberty, males on average retain higher cardiorespiratory fitness levels than females. The chief reasons for this difference is that males generally have higher hemoglobin levels and carry less body fat than females.

The individual's ratio of slow- to fast-twitch muscle fibers can make a difference in his or her fitness level. *Which of the teens pictured likely has a higher proportion of slow- to fast-twitch muscle fiber? Explain.*

 Reading Check

Describe What is the difference between slow- and fast-twitch muscle fibers?

Active Mind Active Body

The Effect of Added Weight on Aerobic Performance

Have you ever wondered what carrying excess weight or being obese does to your exercise heart rate? In this activity, you'll find out. You'll determine for yourself what effect added weight has on your heart rate and RPE (rating of perceived exertion) during aerobic training.

What You Will Need

- Backpack
- Textbooks or small weights
- 12-inch high step
- Stopwatch, clock, or wristwatch

What You Will Do

1. Fill a backpack with textbooks or small weights. The total weight of the loaded pack should be 20 lbs (9 kg).
2. Strap the backpack to your shoulders.
3. Begin stepping up and down on a 12-inch step at a rate of approximately 24 steps per minute. Continue for three minutes.
4. Stop and measure your heart rate for one minute and record your rating of perceived exertion using the RPE scale to the right.

20	Maximum exertion
19	Extremely hard
18	
17	
16	Vigorous
15	Hard/heavy
14	
13	Somewhat hard (moderate)
12	
11	Light
10	
9	Very light
8	
7	Extremely light
6	No exertion at all

Source: Borg's Perceived Exertion and Pain Scales, *2002.*[3]

Apply and Conclude

How did your heart rate and RPE with the backpack compare to the results in the Fitness Check in Lesson 1? Why do you think the results were different? How do you think gaining weight influences cardiorespiratory endurance?

Body Composition

Your percentage of body fat also influences your cardiorespiratory endurance. Carrying high amounts of **body fat** reduces aerobic capacity because fat is just "extra baggage" that does not help you burn calories. By controlling your body composition—reducing body fat and increasing lean muscle mass—you can improve your fitness level.

Level of Conditioning

Your level of conditioning can affect your cardiorespiratory endurance. If you are currently doing no aerobic activity at all, you can improve your fitness level by beginning a personal fitness program that includes aerobic exercises. Your potential for fitness depends not only on your initial fitness level but also on genetics, trainability, your application of FITT principles, and your specific goals.

Reading Check

Identify Name five factors that affect your cardiorespiratory endurance.

hot link

body fat
For more on body fat see Chapter 5, page **151.**

FIGURE 7.5

BENEFITS OF AEROBIC ACTIVITY

Heart and Lungs:	• Lower resting heart rate • Increases in stroke volume at rest and maximal exercise • Decreases in heart rate at moderate levels of aerobic activity • Lower blood pressure during sub-maximal aerobic exercise • Better ability to maintain high breathing rates for longer periods of time	**Muscle Cells and Bones:**	• Increased ability to use oxygen in cells • Increased ability to store (energy) glycogen • Increased ability to use fat as a fuel • Increase number of red blood cells and capillaries • Can help increase bone strength which helps prevent osteoporosis
Blood and Arteries:	• Higher HDL "good" cholesterol • Lower LDL cholesterol and other "bad" blood fats • Higher hemoglobin levels • Decrease in blood stickiness • Lowered risk of athero-sclerosis • Better blood flow • Lower blood pressure at rest • Improved ability to deliver oxygen to tissues and organs	**Body Composition:**	• Helps burn calories and control body weight • Helps increase muscle mass
		Emotions:	• Reduces stress levels • Improves regulation of stress hormones
		Image and Lifestyle:	• Improves self-image • Improves personal appearance with weight control • Increases functional health and functional fitness as you age and can increase your longevity

Benefits of Cardiorespiratory Fitness

The physical and emotional benefits of aerobic activity are listed in **Figure 7.5**. Participation in regular aerobic activities can reduce your anxiety and improve your concentration and alertness. Working toward your fitness goals can provide you with positive feedback that can improve your self-image. In addition, regular physical activity and exercise are associated with better regulation of stress hormones. Regular aerobic workouts help you decrease the production of these hormones and reduce daily tensions. They enhance your ability to deal with daily challenges.

Extended aerobic activity promotes the brain's release of mood-elevating substances called *endorphins* (en-DOR-fuhnz). These chemicals produce a feeling of pleasure. The person experiences less fatigue and a sense of renewed energy.

Aerobic exercise reduces the risk of certain preventable cancers, including cancer of the colon and rectum. There is also evidence that exercise can lower the risk of breast and reproductive cancer in women.

Making the Most of What You Have

Several of the factors described in the previous sections are beyond your control. Among these are age, gender, and heredity. However, anyone can sustain a relatively high level of fitness, regardless of age, gender, and heredity. The strategy for doing so includes the following steps.

- **Start while you're young.** As a teen, your potential for cardiorespiratory fitness is greater than it will be at any time in your future. Begin a program of regular activity.
- **Stay active.** As **Figure 7.6** shows, an active 45-year-old female can achieve a VO_{2max} nearly as high as a less-active 15-year-old male. Highly trained female distance runners or cross-country skiers often have a VO_{2max} twice that of untrained males.
- **Pay attention to fitness factors you can control.** This includes your level of conditioning, your weight, and your body composition.
- **Make your body work *for* you, rather than *against* you.** A major source of muscle fuel is fat, and most body fat is lost by burning it in the muscle. Aerobic exercise conditions your muscles and burns more fat, helping to control your blood fat levels.

 Reading Check

Describe Explain in detail one of the benefits of maintaining a high level of cardiorespiratory fitness.

FIGURE 7.6

VO$_{2MAX}$

Activity level, gender, and age are all factors that affect VO_{2MAX}. *Over which factors do you have some control?*

Group	VO$_{2MAX}$ (ml/kg/min)
Inactive Female	35
Inactive Male	40
Active/Fit Female	45
Active/Fit Male	55
Elite Trained Female	70
Elite Trained Male	80
Inactive Female (Age 45)	32
Inactive Male (Age 45)	35
Active/Fit Female (Age 45)	38
Active/Fit Male (Age 45)	42
Cardiac Patient (Male or Female)	20

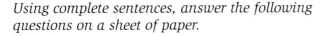

Lesson 3 Review

Using complete sentences, answer the following questions on a sheet of paper.

Reviewing Facts and Vocabulary

1. **Vocabulary** What is VO_{2max}?
2. **Recall** Explain why males on average have higher VO_{2max} levels than females.
3. **Recall** Name two factors that influence a person's cardiorespiratory endurance level. Name two benefits of maintaining a high cardiorespiratory endurance level.

Thinking Critically

4. **Compare and Contrast** How do slow-twitch fibers differ from fast-twitch fibers?

5. **Synthesize** Wilbur is 15 and has a VO_{2max} of 30 ml/kg/min. What does this reveal about him?

Personal Fitness Planning

Evaluating Your Environment Make a list of environmental factors in your community that might be used to build your cardiorespiratory endurance level. Possibilities might include a long flight of stairs or hill that you could climb without stopping. Try implementing this challenge with your personal fitness program. Note your pulse rate before and after the challenge in your Fitness Journal.

What You Will Do

- Compare aerobic and anaerobic fitness.
- Identify examples of anaerobic activities.
- Explain the benefits of interval training.

Terms to Know

anaerobic activity
anaerobic fitness
interval training

Aerobic vs. Anaerobic Physical Activities

Total fitness is like a coin. That is, it has two sides. In the previous lessons of this chapter, you learned about one of these sides, cardiorespiratory fitness. In this lesson, you will learn about the other—*anaerobic fitness*.

What Is Anaerobic Fitness?

Cardiorespiratory fitness, as noted earlier, is developed by engaging in aerobic activities. Remember, *aerobic* means "with oxygen" and oxygen plays a key role in helping the heart pump blood to the large muscle groups of the body. In order to do its job, aerobic activity must occur over a sustained period of time.

Anaerobic activity works differently. It is *activity that requires high levels of energy and is done for only a few seconds or minutes at a high level of intensity.* The term *anaerobic* itself means "without oxygen" because the energy produced in such exercises does not depend on oxygen. Participation in anaerobic activities leads to anaerobic fitness, which may be defined as *higher levels of muscular strength, muscular endurance, and flexibility.*

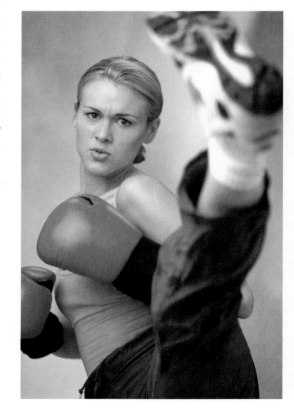

▶ Anaerobic fitness is defined by muscular strength, muscular endurance, and flexibility. *How are these three elements of health-related fitness necessary in kickboxing?*

Active Mind Active Body

Are You Working Aerobically or Anaerobically?

Is the physical work you do more aerobic than anaerobic? Is it the other way around? This activity will help you find out.

What You Will Need

- Weight room access
- Stopwatch, wristwatch, or clock
- Access to football or soccer field
- 1-mile (1.6-km) track or walking course

What You Will Do

1. Go to a weight room, warm up, and then do a bench press with a weight you can press six to seven times. Write down your RPE (rating of perceived exertion) score for the lift. *(Note: Make sure you have appropriate weight training, including a spotter, before attempting the bench press.)*
2. Warm up, and then do two hard 40-yard (38-meter) sprints. Have a classmate time you and record your RPE. Record the average of the two trials.
3. Finally, warm up and then walk one mile. Again, record your time and your RPE after five minutes.

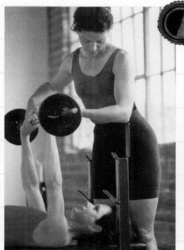

Apply and Conclude

Which of the activities you performed were aerobic? Which ones were anaerobic? Did monitoring your RPE help you understand which was which? Explain.

Anaerobic Activities

Examples of anaerobic activities include running up two flights of stairs, sprinting 40 yards, doing a fast break in basketball, or swimming 100 meters as fast as you can. These activities require large amounts of energy—a requirement that your body cannot meet for very long. This is because your heart cannot supply enough oxygen-rich blood to your tissues and organs to meet the high demand. Therefore, your ability to work anaerobically depends on the ability of your tissues and organs to function with limited amounts of oxygen.

Reading Check

Explain Tell the difference between aerobic and anaerobic activities.

hot link

talk test
For more on the talk
test and scoring, see
Chapter 3, page **86.**

Aerobic versus Anaerobic Work

When you can meet your energy needs by supplying large amounts of oxygen to your body, you are working primarily in an aerobic mode. If you cannot meet the oxygen demands of a high-intensity physical activity, your body is more conditioned to working anaerobically. To determine which mode your body operates in, try the **talk test** on page **86,** if you have not already done so. This test involves carrying on a conversation while working steadily. If you are unable to pass the talk test because you are breathless at a high work intensity, you are working anaerobically.

Many physical activities and sports are part aerobic and part anaerobic. For, example, tennis is played more or less continuously over a sustained period of time, which works the heart and lungs (aerobic). The sport also involves short bursts of intense activity—for example, sprinting and hitting the ball hard—mixed in with short rest periods (anaerobic).

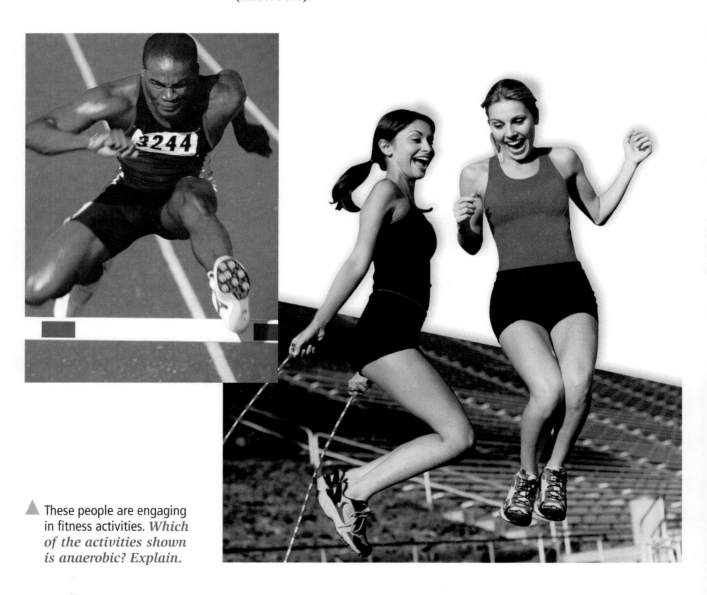

▲ These people are engaging in fitness activities. *Which of the activities shown is anaerobic? Explain.*

Interval Training

One way of achieving the best of both types of activity at once is through interval training. This is *a program in which high-intensity physical activities alternate with low-intensity recovery bouts for several minutes at a time*. Sprinting along the straight-aways on a track and walking or jogging around the curves for several laps is an example of interval training.

Advantages of Interval Training

For individuals just starting out, interval training has several advantages over activities and exercises that are exclusively aerobic or anaerobic. First, such training allows you to work at higher intensities for longer periods of time than you otherwise could in a continuous manner. By increasing intensity level for short periods during your work-out you enable your body to burn more calories than it would working at a constant intensity level. It also increases your ability to work at higher intensities. In addition, interval training improves skill-related fitness and health-related fitness simultaneously.

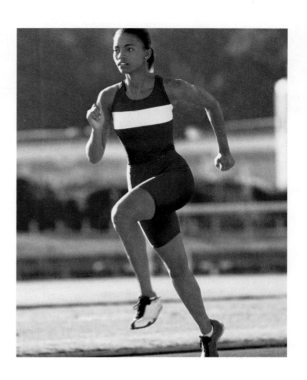

▲ Interval training can allow you to work aerobically and anaerobically in the same workout. *Why might interval training be a good way to start an overall fitness program?*

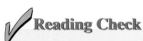

Reading Check

Explain What is interval training?

Lesson 4 Review

Using complete sentences, answer the following questions on a sheet of paper.

Reviewing Facts and Vocabulary

1. **Vocabulary** What is *anaerobic activity?*
2. **Recall** What is *interval training?*

Thinking Critically

3. **Analyze** Explain how a physical activity such as handball might be classified as both aerobic and anaerobic.
4. **Synthesize** Karen is interested in improving her anaerobic fitness level in order to participate in soccer. Is soccer primarily an aerobic or anaerobic sport? List three activities Karen can do to improve her anaerobic fitness level.

Personal Fitness Planning

Participating in Aerobic Activity Determine whether you can jump rope for three minutes at a rate of 120 skips per minute. If you can, you are working primarily in an aerobic mode. If not then you are working primarily in an anaerobic mode. Find two activities that will help you improve or maintain your cardiorespiratory endurance.

CHAPTER 7 Review

TRUE/FALSE

On a sheet of paper, write the numbers 1–10. Write True or False for each statement below.

1. The main organ of the circulatory system is the lungs.
2. The heart beats at different rates depending upon whether your body is at rest or at work.
3. Atherosclerosis is a condition in which a fatty deposit called plaque builds up inside arteries.
4. When blood flow to a person's heart is cut off by a blocked artery, the person has suffered a stroke.
5. Hypertension is a disease in which the small airways of the lungs lose normal elasticity.
6. VO_{2max} is the largest amount of oxygen your body is able to process during strenuous aerobic exercise.
7. Slow-twitch muscle fibers are associated with your ability to do anaerobic work.
8. One benefit of regular aerobic activity is reduced anxiety and improved concentration.
9. Anaerobic activity requires high levels of energy and is done very briefly at a high level of intensity.
10. Interval training is a program in which high-intensity physical activities alternate with low-intensity recovery bouts for several minutes at a time.

MULTIPLE CHOICE

On a sheet of paper, write the letter of the word or phrase that best completes each statement.

11. Of the following, the organ that is NOT part of the circulatory system is
    a. the heart.
    b. the diaphragm.
    c. the capillaries.
    d. the arteries.

12. Done regularly, aerobic activity does all of the following EXCEPT
    a. strengthen the heart.
    b. strengthen the lungs.
    c. strengthen the arm muscles.
    d. raise the heart rate.

13. The diaphragm is
    a. a muscle.
    b. part of the heart.
    c. part of the circulatory system.
    d. all of the above.

14. Of the following, the one that is NOT a benefit of regular aerobic activity is
    a. increased energy.
    b. less stress.
    c. immunity from disease.
    d. looking and feeling better.

15. Of the following, the one that is NOT a risk factor for heart and lung disease is
    a. inactivity.
    b. being overweight.
    c. smoking.
    d. avoiding foods high in fat.

16. A CVD is
    a. a disease of the circulatory system.
    b. a device for measuring cardiorespiratory fitness.
    c. a machine that increases anaerobic fitness.
    d. none of the above.

17. Another name for hypertension is
    a. cardiorespiratory fitness.
    b. high blood pressure.
    c. heart attack.
    d. cardiorespiratory endurance.

18. Factors affecting cardiorespiratory endurance include
    a. age.   c. heredity.
    b. gender.   d. all of the above.

19. All of the following are anaerobic activities EXCEPT
    a. running up a flight of stairs.
    b. sprinting 40 yards.
    c. swimming 100 meters.
    d. 30 minutes on a treadmill.

20. Interval training may best be defined as
    a. exercising on different days.
    b. alternating high-intensity work with low-intensity work.
    c. alternating high-intensity work with rest periods.
    d. exercising different body parts.

DISCUSSION

Using complete sentences, answer the following questions on a sheet of paper.

21. List and identify five different physical activities or exercises that will help you improve or maintain your cardiorespiratory fitness level.

22. List and describe five benefits of cardiorespiratory conditioning that a previously inactive young adult might realize after 8 to 30 weeks of training.

23. What are the benefits of anaerobic fitness?

VOCABULARY

On a sheet of paper, write the letter of the term from Column B that best fits the definition in Column A.

Column A

24. A disease in which the small airways of the lungs lose their normal elasticity.

25. The muscle between the chest cavity and the abdomen.

26. Arteries, veins, and capillaries.

27. Sprinting the straight-aways on a track and walking/jogging the curves for several laps.

28. An iron-rich compound in the blood.

29. The force of the blood in the main arteries.

30. Higher levels of muscular strength, muscular endurance, and flexibility.

Column B

a. hemoglobin
b. interval
c. diaphragm
d. blood pressure
e. circulatory system
f. anaerobic
g. emphysema

CRITICAL THINKING

Using complete sentences, answer the following questions on a sheet of paper.

31. Explain How can you reduce your risk of cardiovascular disease?

32. Discuss How can you use interval training in your personal cardiorespiratory fitness plan? Explain your answer.

CASE STUDY

DIANE'S FITNESS LEVEL

Diane, who is now seventeen, was very active earlier in her teens. She participated regularly in aerobic dance, walking, and swimming. However, in the past year she has become very inactive because she works at a part-time job after school and is taking several honors courses, which keeps her busy much of the time. Lately, Diane has begun feeling tired and has low levels of energy. Because she has never had a class that educated her in personal fitness, she needs the help of someone knowledgeable to design and implement a fitness program. That someone is you!

HERE IS YOUR ASSIGNMENT:

Organize a list of factors Diane should consider before beginning a moderate-to-vigorous personal cardiovascular fitness program. Then list the recommendations you would make for the first two weeks of her conditioning. Use the following keys to help you:

KEYS TO HELP YOU

- Consider Diane's history of personal aerobic activity and exercise.
- Consider how she should evaluate her current cardiorespiratory fitness level.
- Consider her needs and goals (for example, how she will find time to do physical activity or exercise).
- Determine a reasonable plan for Diane that covers the concepts of overload and FITT factors.

Developing Cardiorespiratory Endurance

FITNESS
Online

Did you take either of the endurance tests presented in Chapter 7? How did you do? Tests like these measure your cardiorespiratory endurance. To learn more about your level of cardiorespiratory fitness, take the STEP Personal Inventory for Chapter 8. Find it at **fitness.glencoe.com**.

Evaluating Your Cardiorespiratory Endurance

In Chapter 7 you learned about the basics of cardiorespiratory fitness. In this chapter, you will apply your knowledge. You will learn how to build and maintain healthful, lifelong levels of cardiorespiratory fitness. In this first lesson, you will learn how to evaluate your current fitness levels using a variety of physical activities, including running, swimming, and cycling.

Cardiorespiratory Fitness Tests

Several tests can be used to evaluate cardiorespiratory fitness. Two of these—the 3-minute step test and 1.5-mile run/walk test—were featured in the "Fitness Check" in Chapter 7 (page **197**). These tests, like the three that follow, measure cardiorespiratory endurance over time, distance, or both. They are:

- **Steady-state walk test.** This is *a test that requires you to pace yourself steadily as you briskly walk for 30 minutes and try to achieve a specific goal distance.*
- **Cooper's 1.5-mile run test.** This is *a test that requires you to jog/run as fast as you can to cover the distance of 1.5 miles.*
- **Steady-state jog test.** This is *a test that requires you to pace yourself steadily as you jog for 20 minutes and try to achieve a specific goal distance.*

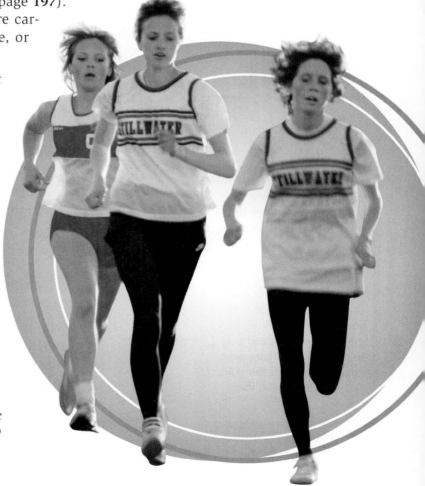

▶ Some cardiorespiratory-endurance evaluations involve running or jogging for a specific amount of time. *What other aerobic activities can be used to evaluate cardiorespiratory endurance?*

FIGURE 8.1

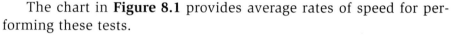

AVERAGE SPEEDS FOR ADULTS AND TEENS

At what speed should you walk when completing the steady-state walk test? Explain.

Test	Average Speed (Miles per Hour)
Walking	2 to 4 mph (30 to 15 minutes per mile)
Jogging	4 to 5 mph (15 to 12 minutes per mile)
Running	5 to 7 mph (12 to 8.5 minutes per mile)
Swimming	1.5 to 2 mph (30 to 40 minutes per mile)
Cycling	7 to 8 mph (8.5 to 7.5 minutes per mile)

The chart in **Figure 8.1** provides average rates of speed for performing these tests.

Your initial cardiorespiratory-fitness goal should be to complete these tests at good-to-better ratings for your age and gender. You will learn more about these ratings in the pages ahead. If you cannot meet the standards of these evaluations at first, keep trying. Your functional health and functional fitness depend on it. Once you achieve the goals, try to maintain or improve your levels of cardiorespiratory fitness.

Alternative Evaluations

Some people may have difficulty performing the tests described above. Among these are people with physical disabilities or injuries that prevent them from running, jogging, or walking. Two alternative tests for such individuals are as follows:

- **Steady-state cycle test.** This is *a test that requires you to pace yourself steadily as you pedal for 20 minutes on a stationary cycle.*
- **Steady-state swim test.** This is *a test that requires you to pace yourself steadily as you swim for 20 minutes.*

Others who may experience difficulty are individuals who are sedentary and/or obese. In this case, cardiorespiratory fitness is assessed by means of an **exercise stress test.** This is *an evaluation in which you walk on a treadmill or ride a stationary bicycle under medical supervision.* This method is also used when a medical screening suggests the possibility of a health problem.

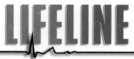

LIFELINE

Becoming a Fitness Mentor

Do you have younger brothers or sisters? Maybe there are younger children in your neighborhood that you know. If so, there is no time like the present to get them involved in their personal fitness.

Becoming a *mentor* (a teacher or adviser) is a way of sharing the information you are learning in this program. It is also a great way to reinforce your knowledge and practice the skills you have learned in this course.

Fitness Check

Estimating Percentage of VO$_2$ max

Cardiorespiratory fitness can be evaluated by measuring *VO$_2$ max*. As discussed in Chapter 7, VO$_2$ max is the largest amount of oxygen your body is able to process during strenuous aerobic exercise. Remember, the more aerobically fit you are, the higher your VO$_2$ max will be. Participate in a variety of activities that develop your health-related fitness, including cardiovascular efficiency. VO$_2$ max can be measured directly with the *maximal exercise test*. This test requires specialized equipment and is performed under the supervision of a health care professional, such as a doctor or exercise physiologist.

However, you can assess your cardiorespiratory fitness on your own by performing one of the tests described in this lesson and calculating your *estimated percentage of VO$_2$ max*. In this activity, you will do 20 to 30 minutes of walking or jogging and try to work at between 50 and 85 percent of your VO$_2$ max.

Procedure:

1. Choose one of the following tests: the steady-state jog test or the steady-state walk test.
2. Before doing the test, make sure you are properly prepared. Use the checklist for cardiorespiratory testing (see "Preparing for Cardiorespiratory Fitness Testing" on page **222**).
3. Do the test you have chosen. (See **Figure 8.2,** page **223** or **Figure 8.3,** page **224**.)
4. If a heart rate monitor is available, use this to measure your heart rate during and after the test. Otherwise, take your pulse (as you learned in Chapter 3) immediately after you complete the test.
5. Record your pulse.

6. Use the formula that follows to determine if you were able to work at between 50 and 85 percent of your maximum estimated VO$_{2max}$. (*Note that the value of k in this equation is 61 for a male and 73 for a female.*)
7. Use the Fitness Ratings Chart for Estimated percentage of VO$_2$ max to assess your performance.
   - If your estimated percentage of VO$_2$ max for the steady-state jog test or the steady-state walk test was between 50 and 85 percent, you are at a good-to-better level of cardiorespiratory fitness.
   - If you do not work at least at 50 percent of your VO$_2$ max, you should continue to condition until you can achieve this aerobic fitness goal.

$$\text{Estimated percentage of VO}_2 \text{ max} = \frac{(\text{Heart Rate} - k) \times 100}{(220 - \text{Age} - k)}$$

Fitness Ratings

Predicted %VO$_2$ max		Rating
50–85%		Good
Greater than 85%	Jogged or ran too fast—needs work	
Less than 50%		Needs work

Preparing for Cardiorespiratory Fitness Testing

To ensure an accurate reading on any endurance test, you need to prime your body. You can accomplish this through regular aerobic conditioning for at least five weeks. **Figure 8.2** provides a sample conditioning routine for the steady-state walk test. **Figure 8.3** on page **224** provides a conditioning routine for Cooper's 1.5-mile run and the steady-state jog tests. **Figure 8.4** on page **225** provides routines for the steady-state cycle and swim tests.

The checklist that follows offers other recommendations that will help you further prepare.

- **Verify the distance.** Make sure the distance you cover is accurate. For all tests except cycling or swimming, it is best to use a regulation track. The distance around a regulation track is exactly 400 meters—about 440 yards.
- **Pace yourself.** For example, by slowing down as needed— until you are able to go the whole distance without stopping. Gradually work at improving your rate of speed.
- **Practice.** Try covering the distance once or twice before the day of the actual test.
- **Consider weather.** Test yourself only when the weather is fair. It should not be too hot, too cold, or too windy.
- **Warm-up and cooldown.** Always perform a proper warm-up before each aerobic workout and the test itself. Do a proper cooldown afterward.

Reading Check

Explain What is the minimum amount of weeks needed to condition one's self for a cardiorespiratory fitness test?

Activities to Develop Cardiorespiratory Efficiency

This lesson provides you with the opportunity to participate in any of the several testing programs for cardiorespiratory fitness. It also provides you with information about conditioning before the test, and evaluating your performance after the test. Any one of these tests can be used to evaluate, develop, and maintain your cardiorespiratory fitness.

The 30-Minute Steady-State Walk Test

The six-week conditioning program, test, and ratings for the steady-state walk test are provided in **Figure 8.2.** For example, if Elena completed the 30-minute walk and covered 1.85 miles, she would be at a good level of cardiorespiratory fitness. A distance of 2.0 miles would be even better for her. Elena could then maintain her performance by following the maintenance program also shown in **Figure 8.2.**

FIGURE 8.2

30-MINUTE STEADY-STATE WALK TEST

	Day 1	Day 2	Day 3
	Minutes of Brisk Walking/Minutes of Slow Walking		
Week #1	3 minutes/1 minute—3/1–3/1	3/1–3/1–3/1	4/1–3/1–3/1
Week #2	5/1–5/1–4/1	7/1–4/1–3/1	9/1–9/1, or 15 minutes nonstop brisk walk
Week #3	10/1–10/1, or 17 minutes nonstop brisk walk	11/1–10/1, or 18 minutes nonstop brisk walk	12/1–11/1, or 19 minutes nonstop brisk walk
Week #4	14/1–9/1, or 20 minutes nonstop brisk walk	15/1–10/1, or 22 minutes nonstop brisk walk	18/1–9/1, or 24 minutes nonstop brisk walk
Week #5	**Perform the test and evaluate yourself** (see box below). If your rating is within the good-to-better range, begin the maintenance program found below. If not, continue conditioning for weeks 5 and 6.	22/1–8/1, or 26 minutes nonstop walk test	24/1–8/1, or 25 minutes nonstop walk test

EVALUATE YOURSELF. *The good-to-better ratings for teens ages 13 to 17 are as follows:*

Males: Walking 2.0 to 2.2 miles in 30 minutes.
Females: Walking 1.8 to 2.0 miles in 30 minutes.

| Week #6 | 25/1–6/1, or 26 minutes nonstop walk test | 26/1–4/1, or 28 minutes nonstop walk test | **Retest.** Those who successfully complete the test can move on to the maintenance program. All others restart conditioning on the Week #5 Program and continue for two additional weeks, then retest on day three of the second additional week. |

Maintenance Walking Program

- **For Moderate Fitness:** Walk 2 miles in 30 minutes, 3 times per week, or accumulate 225 minutes of aerobic activity per week.
- **For High Fitness:** Walk 2 miles in 30 minutes, 5 or more times per week, or accumulate up to 300+ minutes of aerobic activity per week.

Source: Medicine and Science in Sports and Exercise, *1999.*[1,2]

Cooper's 1.5-Mile Run/20-Minute Steady-State Jog

Figure 8.3 on page **224** provides a six-week conditioning program for Cooper's 1.5-mile run and the steady-state jog tests. It also provides a way to rate test performance at week 5. For example, if Joe finished between 9:41 and 10:48 minutes for the 1.5-mile distance, he would be at a good level of cardiorespiratory fitness. A time of 9:40 or faster would place him at a better—or higher—level of fitness.

FIGURE 8.3

COOPER'S 1.5-MILE RUN AND 20-MINUTE STEADY-STATE JOG TESTS

	Day 1	Day 2	Day 3
	Minutes of Jogging or Running/Minutes of Walking		
Week #1	2 minutes/1 minute—2/1—2/1	2/1—2/1—2/1	3/1—2/1—2/1
Week #2	3/1—3/1—3/1	4/1—4/1—2/1	5/1—4/1—4/1
Week #3	7/1—6/2, or 11 minutes steady jog or run	8/1—5/1, or 11 minutes steady jog or run	8/1—6/1, or 13 minutes steady jog or run
Week #4	9/1—6/1, or 13 minutes steady jog or run	10/1—4/1—3/1, or 15 minutes steady jog or run	10/1—8/1, or 16 minutes steady jog or run
Week #5	**Perform the test and evaluate yourself** (see box below). If your rating is within the good-to-better range, begin the maintenance program found below. If not, continue conditioning for weeks 5 and 6.	12/1—7/1, or 15 minutes steady jog or run	13/1—7/1, or 16 minutes steady jog or run

EVALUATE YOURSELF. *The good-to-better ratings for teens ages 13 to 17 are as follows:*

Cooper's 1.5-Mile Run
Males: Jogging or running 1.5 miles in 10:48–9:41.
Females: Jogging or running 1.5 miles in 14:30–12:30.

20-Minute Steady-State Jog (Ages 14–17)
Males: Jogging 1.8 to 2.0 miles in 20 minutes.
Females: Jogging 1.6 to 1.8 miles in 20 minutes.

Week #6	14/1—6/1, or 17 minutes steady jog or run	16/1—4/1, or 18 minutes steady jog or run	**Retest.** Those who successfully complete the test can move on to the maintenance program. All others restart conditioning on the Week #5 Program and continue for two additional weeks, then retest on day three of the second additional week.

Maintenance Walk/Jog/Run Program
- **For Moderate Fitness:** Walk/jog/run 2 miles in 30 minutes, 3 times per week, or accumulate 225 minutes of aerobic activity per week.
- **For High Fitness:** Walk/jog/run 2 miles in 20–24 minutes, 5 or more times per week, or accumulate up to 300+ minutes of aerobic activity per week.

Source: The Aerobics Program for Total Well-Being: Exercise, Diet, Emotional Balance, *1985.*[3] Medicine and Science in Sports and Exercise, *1999.*[1,4]

Similarly, if Lisa covered 1.6 miles in the 20-minute jog, she would be at a good level of cardiorespiratory fitness. A distance of 1.8 miles would place her at a high level. If she was unable to cover at least 1.6 miles, she would need to continue conditioning for two weeks and retest. Once Joe and Lisa are ready, they can begin a maintenance program, provided in **Figure 8.3.**

FIGURE 8.4

20-MINUTE STEADY-STATE STATIONARY CYCLE/ 20-MINUTE STEADY-STATE SWIM TESTS

	Day 1	Day 2	Day 3
	2 minutes of cycling at moderate level of resistance/1 minute of cycling at 0 resistance *or* 2 minutes of moderate forward crawl lap swimming /1 minute of slow swimming		
Week #1	2 minutes/1 minute—2/1—2/1	2/1—2/1—2/1	3/1—2/1—2/1
Week #2	3/1—3/1—3/1	4/1—4/1—3/1	6/1—6/1, or 10 minutes steady cycling with moderate resistance/ moderate forward crawl lap swimming
Week #3	7/1—6/2, or 11 minutes steady cycling with moderate resistance/ moderate forward crawl lap swimming	8/1—5/1, or 11 minutes steady cycling with moderate resistance/moderate forward crawl lap swimming	8/1—6/1, or 13 minutes steady cycling with moderate resistance/ moderate forward crawl lap swimming
Week #4	9/1—6/1, or 13 minutes steady cycling with moderate resistance moderate forward crawl lap swimming	10/1—4/1—3/1, or 15 minutes steady cycling with moderate resistance/moderate forward crawl lap swimming	10/1—8/1, or 16 minutes steady cycling with moderate resistance/ moderate forward crawl lap swimming
Week #5	**Perform the test and evaluate yourself** (see box below). If your rating is within the good-to-better range, begin the maintenance program found below. If not, continue conditioning for weeks 5 and 6.	12/1—7/1, or 15 minutes steady cycling with moderate resistance/moderate forward crawl lap swimming	13/1—7/1, or 16 minutes steady cycling with moderate resistance/ moderate forward crawl lap swimming

EVALUATE YOURSELF. *The good-to-better ratings for teens ages 13 to 17 are as follows:*

Males: Cycling 5 miles or more in 20 minutes.
Females: Cycling 4.5 miles or more in 20 minutes.

Males and Females: Swimming 3/8 mile or more in 20 minutes.

| **Week #6** | 14/1—6/1, or 17 minutes steady cycling with moderate resistance/ moderate forward crawl lap swimming | 16/1—4/1, or 18 minutes steady cycling with moderate resistance/moderate forward crawl lap swimming | **Retest.** Those who successfully complete the test can move on to the maintenance program. All others restart conditioning on the Week #5 Program and continue for two additional weeks, then retest on day three of the second additional week. |

Maintenance Cycling Program

- **For Moderate Fitness:** Cycle 6–7 miles in 30 minutes, 3 times per week, or accumulate 225 minutes of aerobic activity per week.
- **For High Fitness:** Cycle 6–7 miles in 30 minutes, 5 or more times per week, or accumulate up to 300+ minutes of aerobic activity per week.

Maintenance Swimming Program

- **For Moderate Fitness:** Swim 1/2 to 3/4 miles in 30 minutes, 3 times per week, or accumulate 150 minutes of aerobic activity per week.
- **For High Fitness:** Swim 1/2 to 3/4 miles in 30 minutes, 5 or more times per week, or accumulate 200 to 300+ minutes of aerobic activity per week.

Source: Medicine and Science in Sports and Exercise, *1999.*[5]

Steady-State Cycle and Swim Tests

For people who are unable to walk, jog, or run, due to disability or injury, they may perform either the cycle test or swim test as described in **Figure 8.4** on page **225,** which provides appropriate conditioning, testing, ratings, and maintenance for both tests.

The cycle test should be performed on a stationary cycle, alternating periods of cycling at moderate resistance, with periods of cycling using no resistance. As in the steady-state jog test, fitness levels are determined by the distance covered in 20 minutes. For example, if Greg, who is unable to jog, completed the cycle test and covered 5.0 miles in 20 minutes, he would be at a good level of cardiorespiratory fitness. A distance of 6.0 miles would place him at a higher level.

The swim test alternates periods of swimming a forward crawl at moderate intensity with periods of slow swimming. As in the cycle and jog tests, fitness levels are also evaluated based on the distance covered in 20 minutes. For example, if Jamie completed the swim test and covered 0.5 miles in 20 minutes, she would be at a good level of cardiorespiratory fitness. Covering a distance of 0.6 miles in the same time period would put her at a high fitness level. Both Greg and Jamie can maintain their performance by following the appropriate maintenance program shown in **Figure 8.4.**

Lesson 1 Review

Using complete sentences, answer the following questions on a sheet of paper.

Reviewing Facts and Vocabulary

1. **Recall** Describe two alternate evaluations that are used for people who may have difficulty performing the run/walk evaluations.
2. **Recall** Describe the procedure for performing Cooper's 1.5-mile run test.
3. **Vocabulary** Define *steady-state walk test.*

Thinking Critically

4. **Compare and Contrast** Explain the difference between the walking maintenance program for moderate versus high cardiorespiratory fitness.

5. **Evaluate** If a 14-year-old female can walk 2 miles in 30 minutes, how would you rate her cardiorespiratory fitness? Explain your answer.

Personal Fitness Planning

Implementing a Plan Design a maintenance walk/jog/run program to help you maintain a moderate level of cardiorespiratory fitness. Make a walk/jog/run schedule for the next 30 days, and then implement your program by following your schedule. Then evaluate your cardiorespiratory fitness level once more, using one of the tests described in this lesson.

Aerobic Activities

Arthur loves swimming. Beth enjoys jogging. Charlene likes dancing. What do these three teens have in common? All enjoy some form of aerobic activity. Regular aerobic activity promotes moderate-to-high levels of cardiorespiratory fitness. Many aerobic activities require little or no equipment, making them inexpensive to do. Best of all, they are fun.

In this lesson, you'll learn about some popular aerobic activities. These can be done alone, in a group, at home, or at a fitness facility.

Walking

Walking is the simplest and most basic aerobic activity. All you really need for a walking program is a pair of comfortable walking or running shoes and appropriate clothing. You can walk (or jog and run) indoors on a treadmill or outdoors on a track or measured course. You can also get a variation of walking and jogging movements by working out indoors on an **elliptical motion trainer.** This is *an exercise machine that mimics the natural motions of running but without placing stress on the joints.*

What You Will Do

- Identify common aerobic activities and exercises.
- Investigate the benefits of various aerobic activities and exercises.
- Identify the purpose of cardiorespiratory-fitness equipment and accessories.

Terms to Know

elliptical motion trainer
pedometer
heart rate monitor

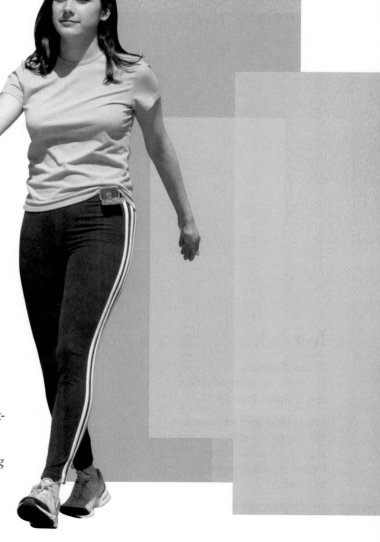

► Walking is a convenient way to improve your cardiorespiratory fitness. It requires little more than a good pair of shoes. *Do you recall the basics of selecting athletic shoes?*

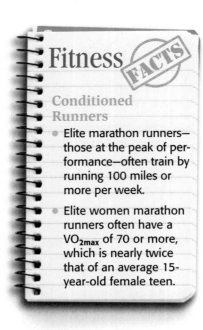
There are several kinds of walking programs that you can participate in. These include:

- **Brisk walking.** At a pace of 3.5 to 4 miles per hour, brisk walking is moderately intense aerobic activity.
- **Power walking.** Power walking is done at a speed of 4 to 5 miles per hour. The intensity level is moderate to vigorous.
- **Race walking.** Race walking is done mainly by competitive athletes. The pace is greater than 5 miles per hour, and the intensity level is vigorous.
- **Water walking.** Water walking is done primarily by people who are injured or in rehabilitation. It is also often prescribed for people who are severely overweight, because it avoids placing excessive stress on the legs and back. Water walking is performed in a pool in chest-deep or deeper water at low, moderate, or vigorous intensity, depending upon the person's needs.

Pedometers

An easy way of monitoring your progress and staying motivated is by using a pedometer (puh-DOM-uh-tuhr). This is *a device that measures the number of steps you take and records the distance you travel on foot.* Pedometers are worn on a belt. They cost about $15 to $20 and can be purchased at sporting-goods stores or department stores. A general cardiorespiratory fitness goal when walking with a pedometer is to try to accumulate 10,000 steps per day, or 4 miles. (Most pedometers require 2,000 steps for each mile for adults and about 2,500 steps for adolescents.)

 Reading Check

Compare Identify the differences between brisk walking and race walking.

Jogging and Running

Two related aerobic activities—jogging and running—are ideal for controlling body weight and maintaining higher levels of cardiorespiratory fitness. The difference between jogging and running is speed. Joggers move at between 4 and 5 miles per hour. Runners move at speeds of 5 to 7 miles per hour or faster. When starting a jogging or running program, progress slowly. (Review **Figure 8.3** in Lesson 1 on page **224** for a sample conditioning program for running or jogging.)

By starting your jogging and running programs slowly and with proper footwear, you can help prevent common injuries. For example, beginning joggers and runners often get shinsplints (pain in the front of the lower leg) due to wearing improper footwear or using improper **biomechanics.** Give your body plenty of time to adjust to the forces of **pronation** and **supination.** This will help you avoid knee and ankle problems that often occur if you begin your program too aggressively.

h⊙t link

biomechanics
For more on biomechanics, see Chapter 2, page **54.**

pronation and supination
For more on pronation and supination and proper footwear, see Chapter 2, page **49.**

Heart Rate Monitors

A good way to monitor the intensity of your jogging or running program is to use a heart rate monitor. This is *a device that records your heart beat by means of a chest transmitter and wrist monitor.* There are many types of heart rate monitors. These can cost between $50 and $100, while more sophisticated models can cost even more. Many heart rate monitors have a function that allows you to set a beeper at a low and higher heart rate zone. You can use this feature to help you jog or run at moderate-to-high intensity without the risk of overtraining.

Bicycling

Bicycling is another way to develop and maintain your cardiorespiratory-fitness levels. It is a low-impact activity and is an excellent activity for overweight individuals because the body weight is supported. There is less of a risk of the types of injuries that can occur from jogging.

It is important to use good biomechanical form while cycling. You will need to make sure the seat is adjusted to a height that gives you good leg extension. (Your leg should remain slightly bent as you push one pedal completely downward.) When bicycling, be sure to wear a safety helmet.

Stationary Cycling

An alternative to conventional bicycling is riding a stationary bicycle. You and your family can purchase a good stationary bicycle for home use. Your school may also have stationary cycles. Some stationary bicycles allow you to monitor your heart rate and the number of calories you are burning.

Many health and fitness clubs offer "spinning" classes. These classes consist of alternating low-intensity stationary cycling with high-intensity cycling. The sessions are often set to music and conducted by a fitness trainer. This type of aerobic activity may be best for those who find that they are getting bored with their personal fitness program. It may help those individuals avoid reaching the relapse stage of the behavioral-change stairway.

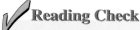

Reading Check

Analyze Why might stationary cycling be a more convenient alternative to cycling outdoors?

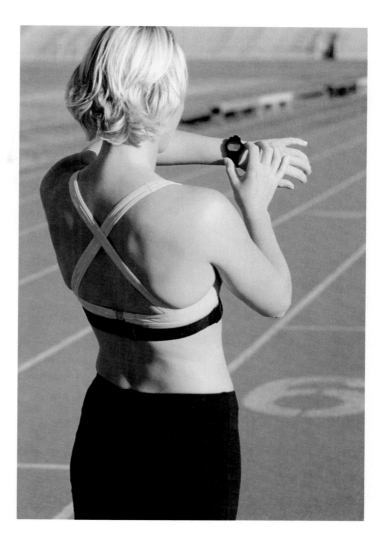

▲ A heart rate monitor is a useful tool in fitness assessments. *Under what other circumstances might you wear a heart rate monitor?*

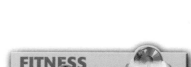

Use online tools to help keep your heart healthy at **fitness.glencoe.com**.

Activity Download information sheets on lifestyle activities and risk reduction. Keep records of your progress to stay fit.

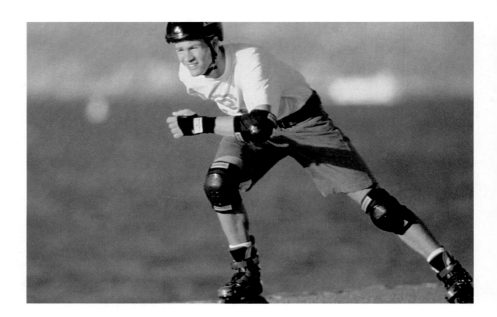

▶ In-line skating is popular in many communities. *What are some safety precautions a person should take when skating?*

hotlink

aerobic dance and stair-stepping
For more on aerobic dance and stair-stepping and how to perform these activities, see Chapter 12, page **366.**

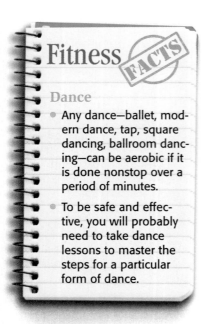

Fitness FACTS

Dance

- Any dance—ballet, modern dance, tap, square dancing, ballroom dancing—can be aerobic if it is done nonstop over a period of minutes.
- To be safe and effective, you will probably need to take dance lessons to master the steps for a particular form of dance.

Other Aerobic Activities on Wheels

Other aerobic activities to increase cardiorespiratory endurance include in-line skating and skateboarding. To perform these activities safely, you need to wear protective equipment, including a helmet, knee pads, elbow pads, and wrist pads.

You will need to practice your balancing and coordination skills to be able to work several minutes at a time at these aerobic activities. When skating or skateboarding, you should avoid hills and congested traffic areas, and always keep your safety and the safety of others a top priority.

Aerobic Dance and Stair-Stepping

Aerobic dance and **stair stepping** are aerobic activities that allow you to exercise and socialize at the same time. Often the two activities are combined, which helps keep participants' interest levels high.

Stair-stepping involves stepping up and down on a single step (usually 6 inches high), or steps stacked on top of one another. This exercise may involve different upper-body movements or routines as well.

Usually aerobic dance is performed in a group and is set to music. The dancing can be done at low, moderate, or high intensities. Most aerobic dance routines last for approximately 45 to 60 minutes. Many beginners find that it takes several weeks before they can complete a full routine. If you participate in aerobic dance, make sure to wear appropriate clothing. Wear supportive footwear to prevent injuries.

Kickboxing

Kickboxing is a popular new aerobic activity. Like aerobic dance, it is usually performed in a group with high-energy or rhythmic music.

In order to begin an aerobic workout program, you need to research and choose an activity that's right for you. This activity will help you find out more about the many activities discussed in this chapter.

What You Will Need

- Pen or pencil
- Paper
- Access to research materials, such as books, periodicals, or catalogues.

What You Will Do

1. Choose one of the aerobic activities discussed in this lesson.
2. Read about the activity.
3. Make a list of equipment, materials, and skills needed to start the activity.
4. Visit a local sporting-goods store, look at a sporting-goods catalogue, or check advertisements to research the price of equipment and supplies.
5. Research the type of lessons necessary to learn appropriate skills for the activity, and check the availability and cost of such lessons in your community.

Apply and Conclude

Share your findings with your classmates. What skills are necessary for your activity? Are there lessons or classes in your area? Compare costs and availability for specific equipment and items needed for your activity. What is the best overall source of supplies and equipment? Share your findings with the class.

It is commonly done with a group in a gym. Kickboxing requires your body to work both aerobically and anaerobically because the routines involve kicks and punches. You may need to practice your program before you can finish the usual 45-to-60 minute class. Make sure you have a knowledgeable instructor and practice appropriate safety measures to avoid injuries.

Cross-Country Skiing

Cross-country skiing is one of the best types of cardiorespiratory-fitness conditioning because it requires the use of both your arms and legs in a continuous activity. Cross-country skiing can be done indoors, on a stationary trainer, or outdoors. For outdoor cross-country skiing, most beginners will need to take lessons. Make sure to wear layers of clothing that can be removed or added as the body heats up or cools down. Cross-country skiing is a low-impact aerobic activity, meaning it puts less stress on your joints than running or jogging.

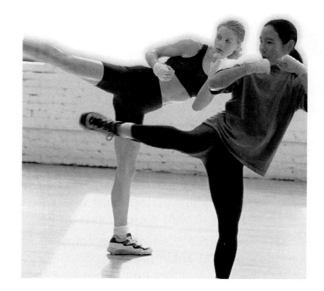

▲ Kickboxing is a popular aerobic activity. *How is kickboxing similar to aerobic dance?*

Water Activities

Exercising in the water is a low-impact activity that improves not only cardiovascular fitness, but also muscular strength and endurance. Aerobic activities in water include lap swimming, aquatic aerobics, aquatic step training, and aquatic line dancing. Swimming laps is a great way to develop and maintain your cardiorespiratory fitness and help control your body composition. It helps to control body fat while improving and maintaining muscle tone. If you choose lap swimming as a regular aerobic activity, you may need to take lessons to master a variety of swim strokes and to improve your efficiency or biomechanics.

Aquatic aerobics and aquatic line dancing incorporate rhythmic movements and dance steps performed in the water. These workouts are often performed to music. Aquatic step training is a cardiovascular workout that involves stepping on weighted steps on the bottom of the pool. Many fitness facilities offer classes in aquatic aerobics for beginner to advanced levels. Because they place less stress on the body than regular aerobics, they are an excellent option for people with arthritis, neck and back problems, and obesity.

Reading Check

Evaluate Of the aerobic activities discussed, which is considered low-impact?

Lesson 2 Review

Using complete sentences, answer the following questions on a sheet of paper.

Reviewing Facts and Vocabulary

1. **Vocabulary** What is a *pedometer*?

2. **Recall** How many steps per day should you try to accumulate if you use a pedometer when you walk for cardiorespiratory fitness?

3. **Recall** How can you prevent shinsplints and knee and ankle problems when beginning a walking/jogging program?

Thinking Critically

4. **Compare and Contrast** Explain the differences between indoor and outdoor cross-country skiing. What are the advantages and disadvantages of each?

5. **Analyze** How might using a pedometer motivate you in your walking/jogging program?

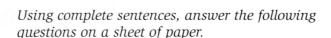

Personal Fitness Planning

Planning for Individual Needs If you became injured or disabled and could not use your legs, how would you design a cardiorespiratory-fitness program for yourself? Design a program that could meet your needs for participation in regular moderate-to-vigorous aerobic activities, using as wide a variety of activities as possible.

Applying FITT to Cardiorespiratory Workouts

What You Will Do

- Apply the physiological principles of overload, progression, and FITT to your cardiorespiratory workout.
- Determine your target heart rate range.
- Evaluate consumer issues and marketing claims promoting fitness products and services.

Terms to Know

target heart rate range
deconditioned

As with any physical activity or exercise, what you get out of an aerobic activity depends on what you put into it. That is, aerobic activities, like other types of exercise, are governed by FITT principles.

Cardiorespiratory FITT and Overload

The physiological principle of *overload* is applied to your cardiorespiratory workout by increasing the amount of aerobic activity that you do. This will overload the main muscle of your cardiovascular system, the heart.

As with any other fitness goal, your cardiorespiratory FITT must be designed to achieve the principle of overload. If the workload is too light, you will not reach your fitness goal. If it is too heavy, you risk serious injury.

Frequency

How frequently should you do aerobic exercise or activity? The answer to that question depends on your current fitness level and age. As a teen, you should try to

- be aerobically active every day.
- accumulate 60 minutes of aerobic activity or exercise per day, or at least 225 minutes per week.

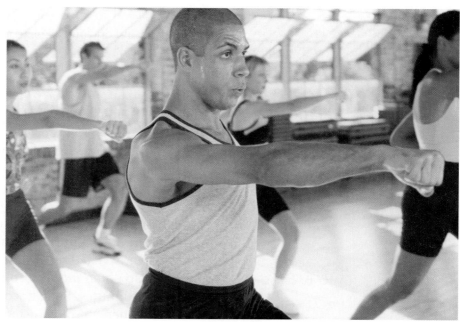

▶ No matter what type of aerobic activities you include in your workout, always apply FITT factors. *What do the letters in FITT stand for?*

FIGURE 8.5

FREQUENCY OF AEROBIC ACTIVITY

Aerobic Fitness Level	Frequency of Conditioning
Beginner	3 to 5 days per week
Moderate-to-High	5 to 7 days per week

hot link

maximum heart rate
For more on maximum heart rate and the formula for computing it, see Chapter 3, page **85.**

FIGURE 8.6

INTENSITY OF AEROBIC ACTIVITY

Aerobic Fitness Level	Intensity (Target Heart Range)
Beginner	120 to 145 beats per minute
Moderate-to-High	145 to 185 beats per minute

If you are just starting out, you can safely begin with three days a week of aerobic activity. Then, as your cardiorespiratory fitness levels increase, gradually add one day at a time. This advice is summed up in **Figure 8.5.**

Intensity

As noted in Chapter 3, the level of intensity in aerobic conditioning can be expressed as a measure of **maximum heart rate.** Most teens are advised to work at between 60 and 90 percent of their target heart rate range. This is *the range your heart rate should be in during aerobic exercise or activity for maximum cardiorespiratory endurance.* Teens that have long been sedentary may need to start out at lower intensities (40 to 50 percent of their target heart rate range). They can then gradually progress to 60 to 90 percent.

To calculate your target heart rate range, first compute your maximum heart rate (220 – *age*). Then determine 60 and 90 percent of that number to get your target heart rate range. Thus, the target heart rate range for a 15-year-old teen would be between 123 and 184 beats per minute.

Note that the lower number in the range represents moderate intensity. If you work at intensity levels lower than this number, you would derive some health benefit. You would not, however, see much change in your physical-fitness levels. If you worked at greater intensity levels than the high-end number (which represents vigorous intensity), you would place yourself at increased risk for overtraining and overuse injuries. **Figure 8.6** shows typical target heart ranges for teens at different levels of cardiorespiratory fitness. For good-to-better cardiorespiratory fitness levels, you do not have to work above the high-end number. However, it is not uncommon to go over the high-end number for short periods when doing anaerobic activities.

 Reading Check

Explain How do you calculate target heart rate range?

Time

Figure 8.7 offers guidelines for how much time you should devote to aerobic activity or exercise sessions. It depends, once again, on your current levels of fitness. If you are just starting cardiorespiratory conditioning, your goal should be 20 to 30 minutes per session. If you are unable to accumulate 20 or 30 minutes continuously, you may have to accumulate 20 or 30 minutes each day in two or three separate aerobic sessions of 10 to 15 minutes each. This may also apply if you are **deconditioned,** meaning *having been out of training for a significant period after achieving at least a moderate level of fitness.* You could also do an *interval workout* at low intensity to accumulate your 20 or 30 minutes. Such a workout might involve jogging for two minutes at 60 percent of your maximum heart rate, then walking for one minute to recover. This routine would be repeated ten times for a total of 30 minutes.

Individuals at good-to-better levels of cardiorespiratory fitness should work at 25 to 40 minutes per session. It should be noted that low intensity for longer durations of time often works best for weight loss and control compared to shorter duration at high intensities.

Type

To maintain or improve your cardiorespiratory endurance, you should choose aerobic activities that elevate your heart rate 60 to 90 percent of its target range, for 20 to 30 minutes at a time whenever possible. Remember, aerobic activities are those that are rhythmic, continuous, and use large muscle groups. Some common examples include, but are not limited to: walking, jogging, running, in-line skating, dance, stair-stepping, kickboxing, cross-country skiing, racquetball, and water activities. Try to think of one you would like to do.

FIGURE 8.7

LENGTH OF AEROBIC ACTIVITY

Aerobic Fitness Level	Time (per Workout)
Beginner	20 to 30 minutes
Moderate-to-High	30 to 60 minutes

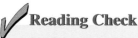

Reading Check

Explain How long should a cardiorespiratory workout last for a person who is just beginning?

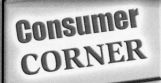

Consumer CORNER

Selling Fitness: Misleading Claims

As with other areas of health and fitness, people look for shortcuts or easy ways out. Although no quick fixes exist, promoters and advertisers suggest that they do. They have come up with a number of products and claims that should be approached with caution. Here are some to watch out for:

- **Promises of quick results.** Unless you already achieved good-to-better levels of fitness, don't expect miracles. A realistic estimate of when you should expect results is between 8 and 30 weeks. The more unhealthy your eating plan and the longer you have been sedentary, the longer it will take to get results.
- **Equipment that does the work for you.** These include motorized exercise machines, belts, and massagers. These do not overload the heart, lungs, or blood vessels. Without

that overload, you cannot improve your cardiorespiratory endurance.

- **Pills and foods.** Contrary to what the ads promise, there are no pills or foods that exercise the heart. Some chemicals may speed up the heart rate, but these do not improve heart and lung function. In fact, some can be dangerous.

Evaluate

Analyze advertisements for fitness products. Then, create your own commercial or written advertisement to encourage people to participate in an aerobic activity discussed in this lesson. Your advertisement should be persuasive and highlight the benefits of the activity you are "selling." Share your ad with the class.

Progression Principle

The rate at which you modify your FITT should be based on your personal fitness goals and your changing levels of cardiorespiratory fitness. To achieve progression, you should adjust FITT factors gradually. Never change your frequency, intensity, time, or the type of activity you are doing all at once or too quickly. Be patient, adjust FITT factors individually, and allow for gradual improvements.

Special Situations

The guidelines for FITT and cardiorespiratory conditioning need to be modified for some people. This includes people with physical disabilities or debilitating injuries. Such people need to consult with a health or fitness professional before participating in a cardiorespiratory program. The same is true for individuals who are obese.

The following are possible activities for people with special needs:

- Water exercises (for individuals unable to walk or jog)
- Arm work (for individuals with lower-body limitations)
- Upper-body cycling (for individuals to reduce weight-bearing exercise)
- Other special modifications that can be made to the aerobic activities described in Lesson 1.

 Reading Check

Identify How should you apply the physiological principle of progression to your cardiorespiratory workout?

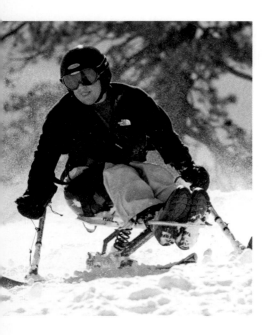

▲ Everyone can improve their levels of cardiorespiratory fitness. *What are some ways in which people with disabilities can achieve levels of cardiorespiratory fitness?*

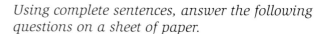

Lesson 3 Review

Using complete sentences, answer the following questions on a sheet of paper.

Reviewing Facts and Vocabulary

1. **Vocabulary** What is *target heart rate range?* How does it apply to the intensity of a workout?

2. **Recall** When applying the physiological principle of overload to a cardiorespiratory workout, what muscle should you target?

3. **Recall** How should you apply frequency to your cardiorespiratory workouts?

Thinking Critically

4. **Analyze** Marla is 16 and has not worked out for several months. Compute Marla's target heart rate range. Review **Figure 8.6** and identify (in beats per minute) the intensity level at which she should work to achieve moderate cardiorespiratory fitness.

Personal Fitness Planning

Researching Activities Do some research in your local community and determine if you can find a health and fitness facility that is offering a new aerobic-fitness activity you would like to try. Find out how much it costs to participate and determine if they have special classes for teens.

Selecting Fitness Equipment

The sale of home exercise equipment has become a big business. Since 1990, the number of people who have bought this type of equipment for the home has tripled. Some people prefer the convenience, while others are more comfortable working out in the privacy of their own homes.

Would you like to have an in-home fitness center? In this lesson you will find out how to go about selecting this equipment. You will also learn the costs involved.

Personal Fitness Equipment

There are a number of factors to consider before setting up a home fitness center and buying equipment. These include the following:

- **Intended use.** How many people will be using the equipment? How flexible is it? What type of exercise is planned? Some machines and devices are designed for cardiorespiratory work, others for resistance, or weight training. It is critical to know which area of fitness will be focused on before making a purchase.
- **Cost.** How much money can you afford to invest in the equipment?

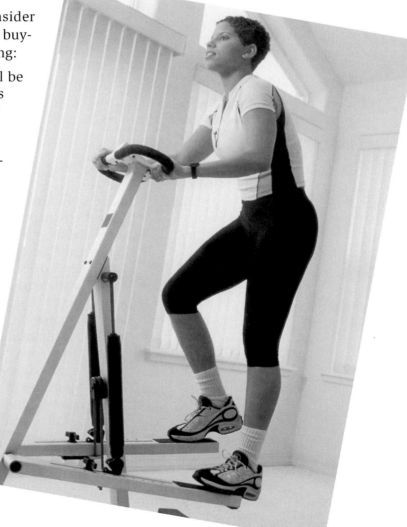

▶ Some people prefer to work out at home. *What are the advantages and disadvantages of having an in-home fitness center?*

Active Mind Active Body

Designing Your Personal Fitness Center

In this activity, you will evaluate your home or apartment setting in terms of a personal fitness center. You will use this information to design a center that will allow your family to maintain its cardiorespiratory-fitness levels.

What You Will Need

- Pen or pencil
- Paper
- Measuring tape

What You Will Do

- Decide where you could set up a fitness center. Consider all possibilities, such as a spare room or den, bedroom, basement area, or garage.
- Review with adults in your family the fitness equipment options described in this lesson. Explain what each piece of equipment does.
- Discuss which type or types would best meet the needs of all members.
- Measure the available space in the areas of your home that you have isolated as possible spots for a fitness center.
- Research the size and cost of the equipment you are considering by visiting local sporting-goods stores, or looking at catalogues. Get size dimensions and costs of the equipment you are considering.
- Rule out items that would not fit the available space or that would be beyond your family's budget.
- Determine which store has the best price for a given item.
- Calculate how much your home fitness center will cost.

Apply and Conclude

What area of your home or apartment seemed to be the most suitable location? Why? Were you able to find equipment that fit this area? What was the cost? Did you include the cost of shipping? How does the cost of this equipment compare with the cost of a year's dues at a health club?

- **Space.** How much space will you need for the equipment? Does such space exist in your home or apartment?
- **Accessibility.** The center must be in a convenient location. At the same time, it must also be out of the way of small children, who could be injured.
- **Safety.** Is the equipment sturdy and built to last? Are there moving parts in which clothing or limbs could accidentally become entangled?
- **Service.** Many brands of fitness equipment are sold. Does the brand under consideration have a warranty? A warranty is *a guarantee on the part of the manufacturer or representative of the manufacturer to repair or replace parts for a predetermined time period.* Also, is the equipment easy to get serviced and repaired? Is the price of labor included in the warranty?

A good starting point for many families is to make a working draft of what the fitness center will look like. This should be based on the dimensions of the home or apartment and the equipment you plan to purchase.

Cardiorespiratory Fitness Equipment

As you learned in Lesson 2, there are many sports, activities, and exercises that develop cardiorespiratory fitness. It should come as no surprise, therefore, that there are many choices for equipment geared to this area. Among these are treadmills, bicycles, stair-steppers, ski machines, elliptical motion trainers, and swimming pools.

Treadmills. Treadmills are the most popular aerobic machines for personal use. You can purchase a good treadmill for as little as $300. The price for state-of-the-art health-club grade models runs as high as $2,000. Most treadmills have basic programming panels for variable speeds, grades (incline), time, and calories expended. If your family can afford one, treadmills are an excellent option for indoor walk/jog/run fitness programs.

Stationary Bicycles. Stationary bicycles are another popular choice for fitness centers. There are two main types of exercise cycles: upright cycles, which function like outdoor bicycles, and recumbent cycles, *bicycles used in a reclining position.* One advantage of the recumbent type is that it offers better lower-back support.

Either type of cycle is easy to use, low-impact, and great for weight control. Most stationary cycles have digital displays that provide you with feedback about the number of calories you are burning. Some also come equipped with levers that you can use to work your upper body at the same time you are cycling.

A less expensive alternative to buying a dedicated stationary bicycle is to attach resistance rollers to a standard bike. These run anywhere from $125 to $250. One downside to rollers is that some models require you to maintain your balance. A solution to this problem is to place the cycle in a doorway. That way, the door frame can be grasped while cycling.

Mind OVER Matter

Exercise Options

Many new types of exercise classes are gaining popularity in health clubs across the country. The emphasis is shifting away from the repetition of traditional exercise and toward motivational routines that help participants enjoy working out.

One example is firefighter training, an advanced cardiorespiratory conditioning class that teaches activities similar to those done by firefighters.

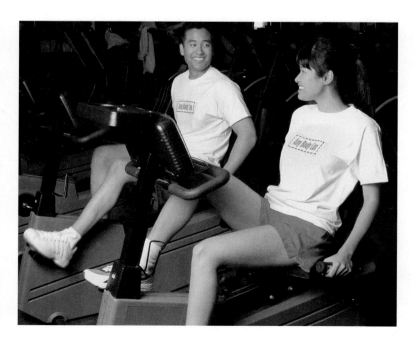

◄ Stationary cycles may be either upright or recumbent. *What are some advantages to using a recumbent stationary exercise bicycle?*

Stair-Steppers. Stair-steppers are machines that simulate the action of walking up a flight of stairs. On some models, you step up and down (usually with a 6-inch stepping action). On others, you walk on escalator-like stairs in a continuous manner, as on an elliptical motion trainer. Stair-steppers do not require much space. Basic steppers cost about $100. More advanced models, which have added features such as calorie counters, can run up to $3,000. Many steppers have levers that you can use to work your upper body at the same time you are stepping.

Cross-Country Ski Machines. Cross-country ski machines provide a low-impact solution to the cardiorespiratory workout. There are two types of ski machines, dependent and independent. On dependent models, the motion of the skis is linked; when you move one ski forward, the other ski moves backward. On independent models, each ski can be moved independently. Independent models are harder to master but can offer a more vigorous workout. They also better simulate the motion of real cross-country skiing.

These machines cost between $200 and $700. It takes some practice to get started on your cross-country ski machine. You will have to learn to adjust the machine to your size and fitness level.

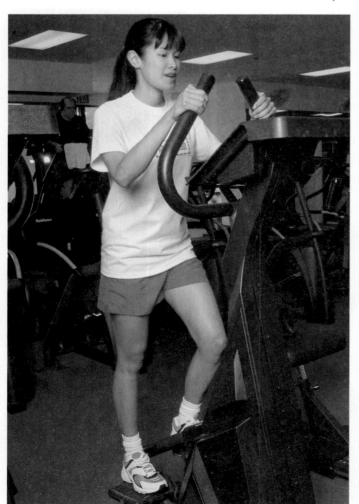

Elliptical Motion Trainer. A recent innovation in cardiorespiratory-exercise equipment is the elliptical motion trainer. Elliptical trainers (like stationary cycles) are easy to use, low-impact, and great for weight control. Many of these machines allow you to train the upper and lower body simultaneously. Reliable elliptical exercisers cost between $100 and $1,200 depending on the features.

Swimming Pool. Some people, especially in hotter parts of the country, have swimming pools at their homes. Others may have access to a swimming pool at school, a local park, or other facility. As discussed in Lesson 2, a swimming pool can provide you with an excellent type of cardiorespiratory training. However, swimming pools will require daily maintenance, and weather conditions may prohibit safe swimming.

◀ Elliptical trainers are easy to use and low-impact. *What's another advantage of these machines?*

Care of Fitness Equipment

If you have home fitness equipment, it is important to maintain this equipment to ensure that it is working safely and effectively. The following tips will help you keep your equipment in top condition.

- Read the operating manual or instructions thoroughly before using the equipment.
- Inspect all equipment regularly.
- Lubricate and repair equipment as advised by the operating manual.
- Use equipment safely and appropriately, as advised by the operating manual.
- Clean equipment, including the benches and work surfaces, before and after each use. Wipe down surfaces with a towel and a disinfectant or 1-percent bleach solution. This will control the spread of germs.
- For safety reasons, pick up and store all loose equipment after use. Keep workout areas free of clutter.
- Know what your warranty covers in the event your machine requires repair.

 Reading Check

Evaluate Which item discussed do you think is the most practical to have in a home? Why?

Lesson 4 Review

Using complete sentences, answer the following questions on a sheet of paper.

Reviewing Facts and Vocabulary

1. **Recall** What are two factors to consider in setting up a home fitness center?
2. **Vocabulary** Explain the difference between a *recumbent* and upright exercise cycle.

Thinking Critically

3. **Compare and Contrast** Compare the costs of the following types of cardiorespiratory home exercise equipment: treadmills and stair-steppers.

4. **Analyze** Explain the sentence "Taking care of your home fitness equipment is like taking out an insurance policy on your investment."

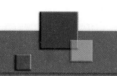 **Personal Fitness Planning**

Investigating Products Visit a local health and fitness club. Learn what the various cardiorespiratory-fitness machines and equipment do. Decide which items you would include in your own dream-home fitness center, and tell why. Finally, investigate whether it would be possible to build your dream fitness center if you had a budget of $2,000.

TRUE/FALSE

On a sheet of paper, write the numbers 1–10. Write True or False for each statement.

1. To achieve a good-to-better score on the Cooper's 1.5-mile run test, a female teen would need to cover the distance in under 1.6 minutes.
2. The exercise stress test is an alternative test for people who are sedentary and/or obese.
3. To achieve accurate results on an endurance test, you should avoid doing any exercise in the weeks leading up to the test.
4. Race walking is done at a pace of 3.5 to 4 miles per hour.
5. A typical kickboxing class lasts between 20 and 30 minutes.
6. Cross-country skiing is a low-impact aerobic sport.
7. Teens who have long been sedentary may need to start out at lower percentages of their target heart rate range than active teens.
8. For moderate-to-high cardiorespiratory fitness levels, you should achieve a time of 30 to 60 minutes per session.
9. Treadmills are the most popular aerobic machines for home exercise use.
10. You can buy a basic fitness stepping bench for $100.

MULTIPLE CHOICE

On a sheet of paper, write the letter of the word or phrase that best completes each statement.

11. The cardiorespiratory evaluation most likely to be done if a medical screening suggests a health problem is
    a. steady-state jog test.
    b. Cooper's 1.5-mile run test.
    c. steady-state swim test.
    d. exercise stress test.

12. To evaluate your cardiorespiratory fitness using estimated $VO_{2\,max}$, you need to do 20 to 30 minutes of aerobic activity at
    a. 30 to 65 percent of your estimated $VO_{2\,max}$.
    b. 40 to 75 percent of your estimated $VO_{2\,max}$.
    c. 60 to 95 percent of your estimated $VO_{2\,max}$.
    d. 50 to 85 percent of your estimated $VO_{2\,max}$.

13. The device used to measure the number of steps you take and estimate the distance you walk is a(n)
    a. heart-rate monitor.
    b. waist/hip pouch.
    c. pedometer.
    d. elliptical motion trainer.

14. Of the following statements about jogging and running, all are true EXCEPT that
    a. the difference between the two is a matter of speed.
    b. a good way to monitor the intensity of either is by using a heart-rate monitor.
    c. both involve the forces of pronation and supination.
    d. neither contributes to cardiorespiratory fitness.

15. Teens who are at least moderately active and in good health are advised to work at
    a. between 60 and 90 percent of their target heart rate range.
    b. 45 percent of their target heart rate range.
    c. between 60 and 90 percent of their estimated $VO_{2\,max}$.
    d. 45 percent of their estimated $VO_{2\,max}$.

16. Of the following, the intensity range recommended for beginners to cardiorespiratory conditioning is
    a. 100 to 110 beats per minute.
    b. 115 to 120 beats per minute.
    c. 120 to 145 beats per minute.
    d. 140 to 170 beats per minute.

17. A person who is deconditioned might BEST be described as
    a. having been kicked off the team for failing to observe training requirements.
    b. having been away from training for a period after achieving at least moderate levels of fitness.
    c. having gained so much weight from years of sedentary living as to be at serious risk.
    d. none of the above.

DISCUSSION

Using complete sentences, answer the following questions on a sheet of paper.

18. **Explain** Describe three ways you can evaluate your cardiorespiratory fitness levels.
19. **Identify** List and describe five different aerobic activities or exercises that will help you improve or maintain your cardiorespiratory-fitness level.
20. **Identify** List and explain four factors to consider when purchasing home exercise equipment.

VOCABULARY

On a sheet of paper, write the letter of the term in Column B that best fits the definition in Column A.

Column A

21. Test that requires you to pace yourself steadily as you walk for a prescribed time.
22. An evaluation in which you walk on a treadmill or ride a stationary bicycle under medical supervision.
23. Numerical range your heart rate should be in during aerobic activity.
24. Test that requires you to pace yourself steadily as you swim for a prescribed time.
25. Device that records your heart beats by means of a chest transmitter and wrist monitor.

Column B

a. exercise stress test
b. steady-state walk
c. heart rate monitor
d. target heart rate range
e. steady-state swim

CRITICAL THINKING

Using complete sentences, answer the following questions on a sheet of paper.

26. **Evaluate** Which method of evaluating cardiorespiratory fitness would you recommend to a friend who was very sedentary and 20 pounds overweight? Describe what is involved in performing the evaluation.

27. **Compare and Contrast** What tips could you give a friend who was considering buying a treadmill for home use? Give the pros and cons of such a purchase.

CASE STUDY

DENISE'S FITNESS PLAN

Denise, who is 16 years old, is physically active and lives in a large city. Her family is going to relocate to a rural community situated several miles from the nearest town. Denise is concerned that she will become less active because she will not have as many resources and opportunities for working out. She has considered asking her parents to convert a room in their new home into a home fitness center. Denise could use some help from a friend who is knowledgeable about setting up a home fitness facility—someone like you.

HERE IS YOUR ASSIGNMENT:

Assume Denise has asked you for help with her plans for designing a personal fitness facility. Organize a list of things Denise should consider and do before purchasing exercise equipment. Use the following keys to help you:

KEYS TO HELP YOU

- Guide Denise in methods to improve her cardiorespiratory fitness.
- Provide her with a list of factors to consider when selecting home fitness equipment.
- Explain the equipment options available.
- Determine a reasonable plan to give Denise that helps her to be successful in developing a fitness facility.

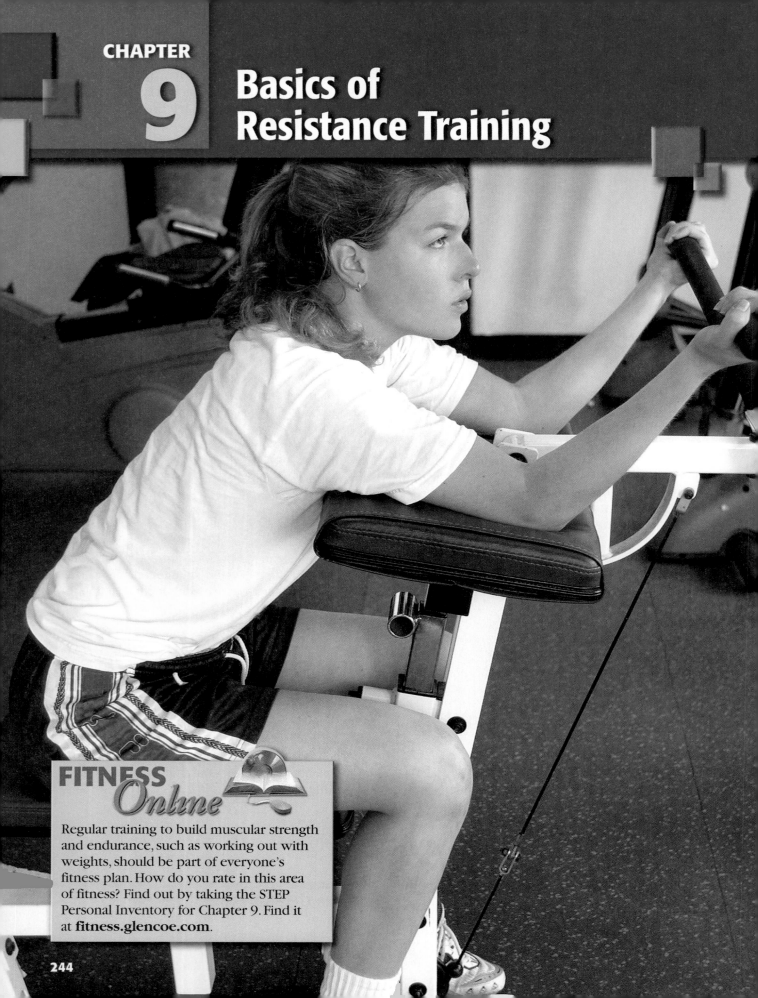

FITNESS Online

Regular training to build muscular strength and endurance, such as working out with weights, should be part of everyone's fitness plan. How do you rate in this area of fitness? Find out by taking the STEP Personal Inventory for Chapter 9. Find it at **fitness.glencoe.com**.

Benefits of Resistance Training

I t was not too long ago that the term *weight lifting* brought to mind an image of body builders with bulging muscles. However, that has changed. Working out with weights is popular among males and females of all ages. In this lesson you will learn more about this trend. You will also discover the many benefits of this form of exercise and of other ways to build muscular strength and endurance.

What is Resistance Training?

The best way to build and tone your muscles is through a program of resistance training. **Resistance training,** or strength training, is *a systematic program of exercises designed to increase an individual's ability to resist or exert force.* Resistance training may involve weights,

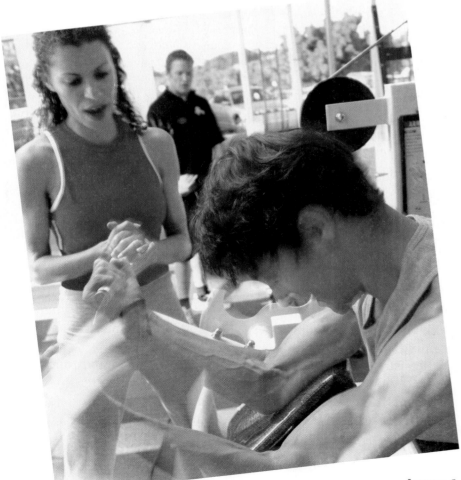

Resistance training builds muscular endurance through use of free weights, weight machines, or elastic bands. *Why do you think it is important to include resistance training in a fitness program?*

FIGURE 9.1

BENEFITS OF RESISTANCE TRAINING

A resistance-training program benefits more than just your muscles. *What other parts of your body can benefit from resistance training?*

Primary Benefits	• Builds and tones muscles • Increases strength and density of bones • Increases strength in ligaments (bone-to-bone connectors) and tendons (bone-to-muscle connectors) • Increases metabolism, which helps control weight (burns more calories) • Reduces body fat and increases lean body mass • Reduces the risk of type 2 diabetes because it improves glucose tolerance and insulin sensitivity • Reduces the risk of osteoporosis

Secondary Benefits	• Increases muscular endurance, which can improve your work capacity (do more work)
	• Helps reduce injury
	  a. serves as shock absorbers for your internal organs when you fall or bump into objects
	  b. protects you from back injuries
	  c. prevents sports injuries
	• Improves personal appearance
	  a. tones, tightens, and shapes muscles
	  b. contributes to good posture
	  c. contributes to positive self-esteem and self-concept
	• Improves flexibility, allowing a full range of motion
	• Enhances sports performance (strength and coordination)
	• Helps reduce stress
	• Can slow down the aging process
	• Helps you perform daily, nonathletic activities with less chance of injury

weight machines, elastic bands, or simply the weight of your own body. Because it often includes weights, it is sometimes called weight training.

Resistance training has many benefits. It builds and tones muscles. It improves metabolism and increases the strength of tendons, ligaments, and bones, which may help to prevent injuries. For other benefits of resistance training, see **Figure 9.1.**

Muscular Strength and Endurance

Building muscular strength and endurance is an integral part of personal fitness for teens and adults of all ages and genders. People with high levels of muscular strength and endurance are able to perform daily tasks more efficiently. This helps them conserve energy and accomplish more in a typical day. They also have better posture and fewer back problems.

Muscular Strength

Muscular strength is *the maximum amount of force a muscle or muscle group can exert against an opposing force.* There are two measures of muscular strength:

- **Absolute muscular strength.** This is *the maximum force you are able to exert regardless of size, age, or weight.* For example, a person able to lift 100 pounds is stronger in an absolute sense than a person able to lift only 80 pounds. The person lifting the 100 pounds generates 20 more pounds of muscular force. Note that females overall have lower percentages of absolute muscular strength than males.
- **Relative muscular strength.** This is *the maximum force you are able to exert in relation to your body weight.* For example, Jim weighs 125 pounds and can lift 130 pounds during a weight training exercise. Tom weighs 160 pounds and can lift 150 pounds on the same exercise. Tom clearly is stronger in an absolute sense, but which of the two teens is the stronger pound for pound? The answer, shown in **Figure 9.2,** can be determined by dividing the amount of weight lifted by the body weight of the individual. The individual with the higher number is exerting more strength per pound of body weight. Thus, in this example, Jim has more relative muscular strength.

From a fitness standpoint, relative muscular strength is more important than absolute muscular strength. In Chapter 10, you will be asked to determine your relative muscular strength for a variety of weight-training exercises.

Mind OVER Matter

Developing Muscular Strength

The strongest person may not be the fittest. Try not to worry about your maximum strength and how it compares to others. Where fitness is concerned, it is your strength in relation to your body weight that matters.

By developing your relative muscular strength, you will have more of the physical energy you need to perform day-to-day physical tasks as well as a more positive outlook.

FIGURE 9.2

RELATIVE MUSCULAR STRENGTH
Below is the formula for calculating relative muscular strength.

	Weight Lifted ÷ Body Weight = Relative Muscular Strength
Jim	130 lbs ÷ 125 lbs = 1.04
Tom	150 lbs ÷ 160 lbs = 0.93

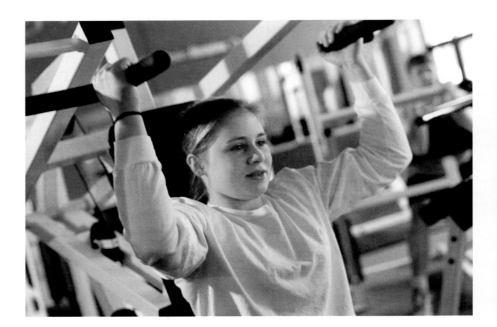

 Improving your muscular strength and endurance can improve the way you look and feel.

repetitions (reps)
For more on repetitions and their role in resistance training, see Chapter 10, page **296**.

Muscular Endurance

Muscular endurance is *the ability of the same muscle or muscle group to contract for an extended period of time without undue fatigue.* Muscle endurance is measured by two numbers: the amount of resistance (or weight) and the number of **repetitions** (or "reps"). A person who can properly lift 75 pounds for 15 reps, for example, has greater muscular endurance than a person (of the same gender) who can only do 10 reps with the same amount of weight.

As with muscular strength, good health and fitness depend more on relative muscular endurance than on absolute endurance. **Relative muscular endurance** is *the maximum number of times you can repeatedly perform a resistance activity in relation to your body weight.*

 Reading Check

Compare How is absolute muscular strength different from relative muscular strength?

Resistance Training and Overload

According to the **overload principle,** to improve a muscle's strength or endurance, you must first overload that muscle. In resistance training, *overloading* means putting more stress, in the form of weight or resistance, on a muscle than it is accustomed to handling. The extra stress load takes the form of weight or some similar force.

Progressive Resistance

As your muscles gradually adjust to the increased stress, you need to increase the workload further. This causes the muscles to become stronger. **Progressive resistance** is *the continued systematic increase of muscle workload by the addition of more weight or resistance.*

overload principle
For more on the overload principle, see Chapter 3, page **83**.

There are many forms of progressive resistance that training can take. Each has its own specific goal. They include:

- **Weight training.** This is a general term that refers to the use of weights to improve general fitness, health, and appearance. Weight training can be done with barbells, dumbbells, and weight machines. It can also be done with a combination of machines and free weights.
- **Weight lifting.** This term refers to a competitive sport done by athletes who follow very specific training programs. Weight lifting is designed to build power and strength.
- **Bodybuilding.** This term refers to a competitive sport in which muscle size and shape are more important than strength. Like weight lifting, bodybuilders follow very specific programs and do many different resistance exercises.
- **Strength training or muscle conditioning.** This term refers to training done by athletes in competitive sports *other than* weight lifting or bodybuilding. Basketball, baseball, and football players all do strength training. Their common goal is to improve performance in their sport and reduce the chance of sports-related injury.
- **Rehabilitation.** This term refers to the use of resistance exercises to recover from a muscle or bone injury. Rehabilitative conditioning usually uses low levels of resistance.

Reading Check

Summarize List the five components of progressive resistance training.

Lesson 1 Review

Using complete sentences, answer the following questions on a sheet of paper.

Reviewing Facts and Vocabulary

1. **Vocabulary** What is *resistance training*?
2. **Recall** Why is relative muscular strength more important to personal fitness than absolute muscular strength?
3. **Recall** What is *muscular endurance*?

Thinking Critically

4. **Compare and Contrast** Explain the difference between weight training and bodybuilding.
5. **Evaluate** Cory and Troy are both 15. Cory weighs 135 pounds and lifts 150 pounds on the bench press exercise. Troy weighs 142 pounds and lifts 165 pounds on the bench press. What is each teen's relative muscular strength? Which teen has the higher absolute strength? Which teen is more fit, generally speaking?

Personal Fitness Planning

Identifying Benefits Review the benefits of resistance training listed in **Figure 9.1.** Consider your personal fitness and choose five benefits that are most important to you. List them in order of importance, and briefly explain why they are important to you.

What You Will Do

- Identify the different types of muscles and explain how muscles work.
- Apply the biomechanical principle of type of contraction to resistance training.
- Identify the role nerves play in muscle function and strength.
- Describe how muscles grow and become stronger.

Terms to Know

cardiac muscle
smooth muscles
skeletal muscles
contraction
extension
dynamic contraction
static contraction
nerves
muscle fiber
muscle hyperplasia
hypertrophy
microtears

Your Muscles and Their Functions

Most of the routine movements you make in a typical day, such as standing and walking, require little conscious thought. Yet, each of these movements involves the complex interaction of many different muscles and muscle groups. Muscles are elastic, stretching to allow a wide range of motion. In this lesson, you will learn about these biomechanical principles and the muscles that make them possible.

Types of Muscles

All body movements depend on muscles. Each muscle is grouped into one of three categories, depending on its function:

- **Cardiac muscle.** This is *a special type of striated tissue that forms the walls of the heart.* Your heart is the most important muscle in your body. Its unique properties enable it to contract rhythmically about 100,000 times a day to pump blood throughout the body. Contraction of cardiac muscle is involuntary.
  - **Smooth muscles.** These are *muscles responsible for the movements of the internal organs, such as the intestines, the bronchi of the lungs, and the bladder.* Also involuntary, they work without a person's conscious control.
  - **Skeletal muscles.** These are *muscles attached to bones that cause body movement.* There are more than 600 such muscles. Unlike the cardiac and smooth muscles, skeletal muscles are voluntary—that is, you consciously control their movement. The major skeletal muscles are shown in **Figure 9.3.**

◀ Resistance training will improve your ability to perform daily tasks. *How can increased muscular strength and endurance reduce your risk of injury when performing daily tasks?*

Resistance training has little effect on involuntary muscles. The remainder of this lesson will focus mainly on skeletal muscles and how resistance training influences them.

Skeletal Muscles

Approximately two-thirds of the muscles in your body are skeletal muscles. They account for 40 percent of your body weight. Skeletal

FIGURE 9.3

THE SKELETAL MUSCLES

Muscles are grouped into three categories: cardiac, smooth, and skeletal. *Which of the three muscle types is most affected by weight training?*

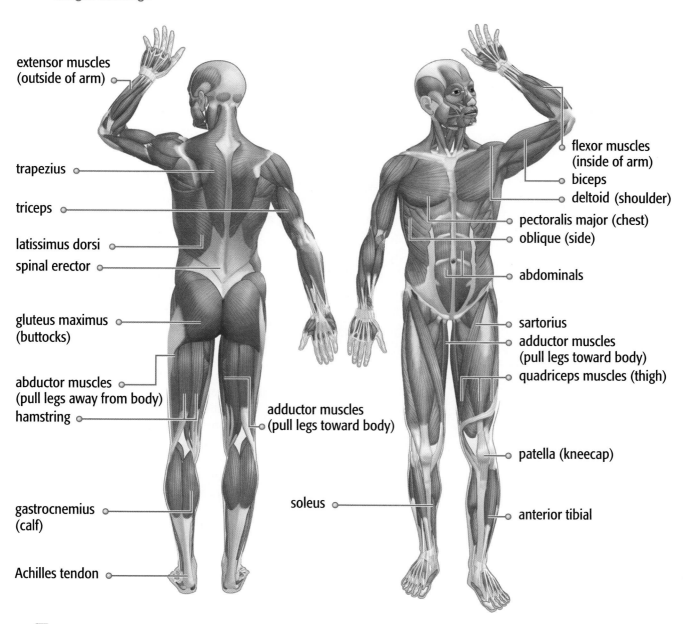

extensor muscles (outside of arm)

trapezius

triceps

latissimus dorsi

spinal erector

gluteus maximus (buttocks)

abductor muscles (pull legs away from body)

hamstring

adductor muscles (pull legs toward body)

gastrocnemius (calf)

soleus

Achilles tendon

flexor muscles (inside of arm)

biceps

deltoid (shoulder)

pectoralis major (chest)

oblique (side)

abdominals

sartorius

adductor muscles (pull legs toward body)

quadriceps muscles (thigh)

patella (kneecap)

anterior tibial

FIGURE 9.4

MUSCLE CONTRACTION

The biceps and triceps are opposing muscles of the arm. Place the fingers of one hand on the triceps of your other arm and flex your biceps. *What do you feel happening to your triceps?*

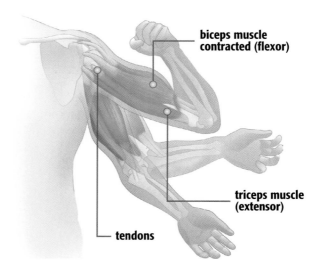

biceps muscle contracted (flexor)

triceps muscle (extensor)

tendons

muscles work together to produce two *complementary*, or opposing, actions. These are contraction, *the shortening of a muscle,* and extension, *the stretching of a muscle.* See this process at work for yourself right now by "making a muscle." When you flex the muscle in your upper arm (your biceps), the bulge you see is caused by the muscle's contraction (see **Figure 9.4**). Notice that as your biceps shortens and compacts, the large muscle on the other side of your arm becomes rigid and stretched tight. This muscle (your triceps) is extending.

Types of Contractions. There are two main types of muscle contractions. These are:

- Dynamic contraction. Also sometimes called *isotonic contraction,* this is *a type of muscle contraction that occurs when the resistance force is movable,* such as a barbell. Dynamic contraction has two phases. In the *concentric phase,* the muscle shortens and exerts force in a direction opposite the pull of gravity. In the *eccentric phase,* the muscle should slowly and smoothly release its contraction and become longer. Arm curls with a dumbbell are an example of an exercise that uses dynamic muscle contraction. If the muscle were simply to relax rather than slowly lengthen, gravity would quickly pull the arm down. This would not allow for any muscle work to be done during the eccentric contraction. Muscle work during the eccentric contractions is necessary for development of muscle strength and growth.

- **Static contraction.** Also sometimes called *isometric contraction,* this is *a type of muscle contraction that occurs absent of any significant movement.* Flexing the muscle in your upper arm is an example of a static contraction. So is pushing against a wall or other immovable object. Pushing your fist with all your might into the palm of your other hand is also a static contraction.

Nerves and Muscle Fibers

For a muscle to contract, it must receive a signal from the brain. This signal is carried by **nerves.** These are *pathways that deliver messages from the brain to other body parts.* The **muscle fiber** is *the specific structure in the muscle that receives this signal.* This is a long, thin strand no wider than a human hair. Bundles of such fibers account for most of a muscle's mass. Blood provides oxygen, energy, and a waste removal system for each muscle fiber.

Connective Tissues

Skeletal muscles are connected to the bones by means of fibrous cords of tissue called tendons. These bind the two together while allowing the muscles to move efficiently. Bones are connected to one another by bands of tissue called *ligaments.*

 Reading Check

Compare What is the difference between a dynamic contraction and a static contraction?

How and Why Muscles Grow

Scientists do not fully understand exactly how and why resistance training builds muscles. However, several theories have emerged.

Muscle Hyperplasia

Some experts believe that muscles get larger during weight training due to **muscle hyperplasia** (hy-per-PLAY-zhuh), *an increase in the number of muscle fibers.* As yet, muscle hyperplasia has been seen only in some animals, such as cats and dogs.

Muscle Hypertrophy

Other researchers contend that a person is born with his or her full number of muscle fibers. According to this view, muscle growth is due to **hypertrophy** (hy-PER-truh-fee), *a thickening of existing muscle fibers,* not to an increase in their number.

During resistance training, chemical and physical changes occur inside the muscle fiber that can cause hypertrophy. If each of the hundreds of thousands of fibers within a muscle slightly increases in size, the entire muscle will become larger.

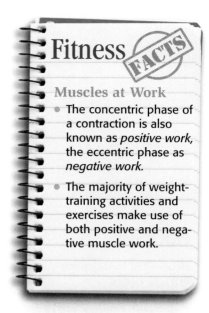

Fitness FACTS

Muscles at Work
- The concentric phase of a contraction is also known as *positive work,* the eccentric phase as *negative work.*
- The majority of weight-training activities and exercises make use of both positive and negative muscle work.

How and Why Muscles Get Stronger

Increased strength is usually the main goal of individuals who begin a resistance-training program. With proper training and good nutrition, weight training can and will improve muscle strength. However, many other factors affect muscle strength. Among these are heredity, muscle size, and nerve function.

Heredity

Heredity is the total of physical and mental traits that you inherit from your biological parents. One inherited trait that directly affects your potential for building muscle strength is your muscle fiber ratio. Specifically, everyone is born with two types of fiber—**slow-twitch** and **fast-twitch.** As noted in Chapter 7, fast-twitch fibers are better suited to anaerobic work than slow-twitch fibers. They also have a greater capacity to increase in size. The greater the proportion of fast-twitch to slow-twitch muscle fibers a person inherits, the greater his or her increase in muscular strength is likely to be. **Figure 9.5** shows the role of slow- and fast-twitch muscle fibers in specific activities.

Muscle Size

The larger the muscle, the greater its potential for strength. Strength, in other words, is directly related to a muscle's size. Researchers have found that muscle fibers are capable of developing

slow- and fast-twitch muscle fibers
For more on the ratio of slow-twitch to fast-twitch muscle fibers, see Chapter 7, page **208.**

FIGURE 9.5

FAST-TWITCH AND SLOW-TWITCH MUSCLE FIBERS

This chart shows the relative involvement of fast-twitch and slow-twitch muscle fibers in sport events. *Which of these activities do you do best? What does this suggest about your ratio of slow-twitch to fast-twitch muscles?*

Event	Involvement of Fast-Twitch Fibers	Involvement of Slow-Twitch Fibers
100-yard dash	High	Low
Marathon	Low	High
Olympic weight lifting	High	Low
Barbell squat	High	High
Soccer	High	High
Basketball	High	Low
Distance cycling	Low	High

a maximal force of 3.5 kg (7.7 lb) per square centimeter (0.4 in^2) of muscle area on average. Supposing, for example, that Kyle increases his muscle size by 50 percent (from 100 to 150 cm^2). Then the maximal force Kyle could exert (his strength) would be increased from 350 kg (770 lb) to 525 kg (1,155 lb).

Nerve Function

Before a muscle can contract, it must receive a message from the brain. That message is carried by nerves. Regular resistance training improves the ability of nerves to carry messages to a muscle. The messages will then arrive faster and cause more muscle fibers to contract. The result is improved strength. A person just beginning weight training can attribute most early gains in strength to improved nerve function.

Other Factors Associated with Muscle Strength

Several other lesser factors can influence the development of muscular strength. These include:

- **Consistent training habits.** People who work out regularly will see more improvement than those who do not.
- **Level of strength.** Beginning lifters will see a more rapid strength improvement than experienced weight trainees.
- **Training intensity.** This includes how hard you work, the kind of program you follow, the number of sets and repetitions, and which muscles you are working. You will learn more about factors associated with weight-training intensity in Chapter 10.
- **Length of your program.** The longer you work, whether it is weeks, months, or years, the more you can improve your strength.

Reading Check

Summarize Name three major factors that influence muscular strength.

Why Muscles Get Sore

Everyone has experienced some muscle soreness at one time or another. This is especially common in the beginning stages of resistance training. This soreness usually occurs within twenty-four to forty-eight hours of the workout.

There are several theories about why muscles get sore. One theory is that **microtears**—*microscopic rips in the muscle fiber and/or surrounding tissues*—occur during greater-than-normal resistance. These tears are most likely to happen during the negative, or eccentric, phase of an activity or exercise. This is especially true when you come down too fast and stop quickly when lowering a heavy weight.

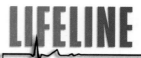

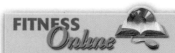

FITNESS *Online*

Learn more about muscles and their function at **fitness.glencoe.com**.

Activity Click on the interactive buttons and test your knowledge of each muscle in the body.

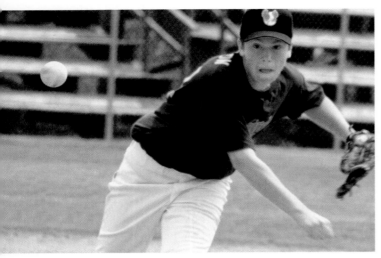

Another theory suggests that during intense exercise, a muscle may not receive all the oxygen it needs. Even though this oxygen shortage is temporary, it may still contribute to soreness.

A third explanation is that waste products build up around the muscles during intense exercise. This accumulation is believed to increase pressure on sensory nerves. The result is muscle pain.

Treating Muscle Soreness

Regardless of the cause of exercise-related muscle soreness, this soreness is not a serious problem. In fact, it is quite normal. With proper training technique and time, the soreness will go away.

In the meantime, there are several steps you can take to help relieve muscle soreness.

- Be sure to perform a proper warm-up and cooldown.
- If the pain is excessive, you are lifting too much. Reduce the amount of weight, and do a lighter workout.
- Drink plenty of water—before, during, and after working out. Eat meals on a regular basis and choose nutritious foods.
- Give the muscles time to repair themselves before reworking them. After two to three days, most soreness is usually gone.

▲ Baseball pitchers often experience soreness in the leg muscles from "braking" too abruptly at the completion of their pitching motion. *What phase of a dynamic muscle contraction is occurring at this point?*

 Reading Check

Explain How can you prevent muscle soreness?

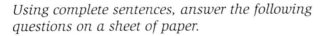

Lesson 2 Review

Using complete sentences, answer the following questions on a sheet of paper.

Reviewing Facts and Vocabulary

1. **Vocabulary** What is *muscle hypertrophy?* What causes it?

2. **Recall** List and explain the two main types of muscle contraction.

3. **Recall** What is one explanation of why and how muscles get stronger?

Thinking Critically

4. **Analyze** Name a sport or activity that you enjoy doing or would like to begin doing. Identify aspects of this sport that involve concentric muscle contractions and aspects that involve eccentric muscle contractions.

5. **Evaluate** What advice would you give a friend who is experiencing muscle soreness after beginning a program of resistance training?

Personal Fitness Planning

Designing a Program Devise a plan for a regular program of resistance training for your upper body, shoulders, arms, and legs. Your plan should not use any additional weights; use only the weight of your body. Start slowly, no more than three days a week. This will allow your muscles time to adapt gradually and begin the strengthening process. Begin your program, and keep a log of your progress.

Resistance-Training Myths

What You Will Do

- Compare differences between the muscles of males and females.
- Identify the age at which a program of resistance training can safely be started.
- Recognize how resistance training can benefit older adults.

Terms to Know

testosterone
osteoporosis
muscle tone

More and more people are recognizing the benefits of resistance training. However, there are several myths about resistance training that may prevent some from making it part of their workout. In this lesson, you will explore some of these myths and understand the reality of resistance training and its benefits.

Resistance-Training Myths Associated with Females

Many of the most widespread and lasting myths about resistance training involve women. The two that follow are among the most commonly repeated.

Myth 1: Bulky Muscles

Females who lift weights will develop big, bulky muscles. The average female has a smaller and lighter skeleton, has narrower shoulders, and is 30 to 40 pounds lighter than the average male. She also has less muscle mass. The total number of muscle fibers tends to be lower in women. Also, there is a difference in testosterone levels between the genders. Testosterone is *a chemical produced by the body that plays an important role in building muscles.* Although

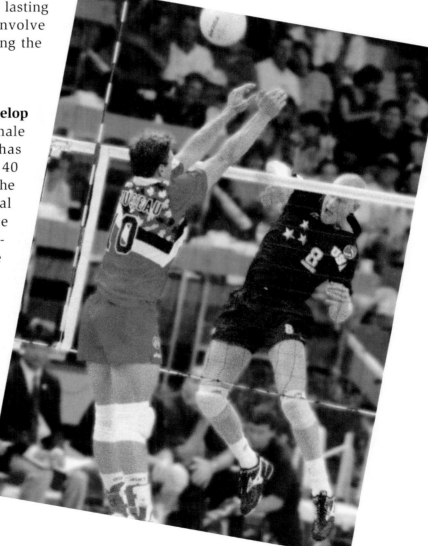

► Contrary to one myth, resistance training can improve athletic performance and skill-related fitness. *What specific advantages does resistance training offer to these volleyball players?*

the female body does produce some testosterone, the level is 1/10 to 1/20 that of males. These factors provide assurance that females who engage in strength training will not develop big, bulky muscles.

Myth 2: Strength

Female muscles will not develop increased strength. Although females typically have less muscular strength than males, this does not mean lesser strength gains. When placed in similar resistance-training programs, females may enjoy *greater* strength improvements than males. This is because of the lower level at which they started. Also, although they may have less muscular strength than males, females who follow regular programs of weight training have a reduced risk of osteoporosis (os-tee-oh-pur-OH-sis). This is *a bone disease that causes decreased bone mass and density,* especially in older women. It is especially important for females during the teen years to build bone mass to reduce the risk of osteoporosis. This can be done through weight-bearing activities and a diet that includes calcium-rich foods.

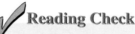 **Reading Check**

Explain Name two benefits of resistance training for females.

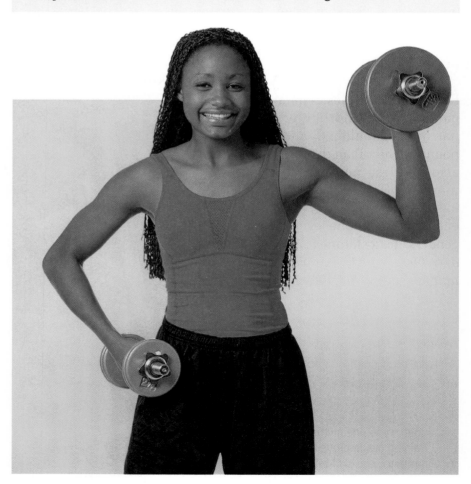

▶ The fear of developing big, bulky muscles has been exposed as a myth. *Can you name another myth about resistance training involving females?*

Other Resistance-Training Myths

Some of the remaining popular myths about resistance training relate to the age of the lifter. Others relate to the lifter's expectations of results.

Myth 3: Children and Teens

Weight training is harmful to the growth and development of children and teens. A recent study by the American Academy of Pediatrics suggests that, with proper supervision, weight training can be done by children as young as age 5. Teens can obtain many of the same benefits as adults through a specially designed program of weight training. Weight training also offers the additional benefit of maximizing bone development during adolescence. This can help reduce your risk of osteoporosis later in life. It also improves glucose tolerance, reducing your risks of obesity and type 2 diabetes.

Serious injury can occur if weight lifting is not done properly. However, if teens observe proper technique and safety precautions when lifting weights, they can avoid injury. Proper supervision and training under a certified fitness trainer or a coach is important. Done correctly, resistance training is not dangerous for teens.

Myth 4: Older Adults

Older adults should avoid weight training. More and more older adults recognize the benefits of resistance training. Medical professionals advise them to participate in a fitness program throughout the life span that includes strength training. The results include improved ability to walk, lift things, climb stairs, and stay active and healthy. Moreover, since older adults rapidly acquire strength gains, they can practice weight training for a lifetime.

Myth 5: Bodybuilders

With enough time and effort, anybody can be a world-class bodybuilder or power weight lifter. Although anyone can expect some strength and size improvements with regular weight training, not everyone will obtain the same results. You are limited by your heredity. This does not mean that you should not work at reaching your maximum potential in the weight room. Resistance training will lead to health and fitness benefits, even if it doesn't make you a world-class bodybuilder.

Myth 6: Muscle and Fat

Muscle can turn to fat if a person stops lifting weights. Muscle and fat are different kinds of tissue. They are not interchangeable. Strength training improves lean body mass and tones muscles. People who stop lifting may see a decrease in muscle size and **muscle tone.** This refers to *a muscle's firmness and definition.* They will not, however, see an increase in body fat unless they discontinue all forms of physical activity while taking in the same number of **calories.**

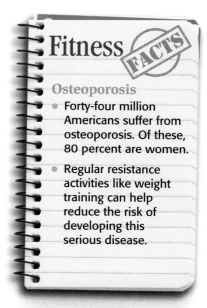

Fitness FACTS

Osteoporosis
- Forty-four million Americans suffer from osteoporosis. Of these, 80 percent are women.
- Regular resistance activities like weight training can help reduce the risk of developing this serious disease.

Source: National Osteoporosis Foundation, 2003.[1]

hot link

calories
For more on the relationship between calories and physical activity, see Chapter 4, page 115.

Myth 7: Muscles and Flexibility

Resistance training will limit my flexibility. Some people believe that increasing muscular strength and endurance means limiting or reducing flexibility. However, weight training will not negatively affect a person's flexibility. Your flexibility is determined primarily by how much you stretch. Proper weight lifting will help you maintain and improve your level of flexibility, as long as your fitness program includes proper stretching. You will learn more about the relationship between muscular strength and flexibility in Chapter 11.

Myth 8: Muscles and Skill-Related Fitness

Larger muscles will hinder athletic performance. Because resistance training increases muscle size, some believe that it decreases certain skills, such as speed and coordination. However, the increased strength those muscles provide allows your body to move *more* quickly. Similarly, because many weight-training exercises involve the coordination of several muscles, resistance training improves coordination and conditions your body to move *more* efficiently.

 Reading Check

Explain Identify and explain a resistance-training myth that is related to physical activity and age. Then give the facts.

Lesson 3 Review

Using complete sentences, answer the following questions on a sheet of paper.

Reviewing Facts and Vocabulary

1. **Recall** Why are females unlikely to develop large, bulky muscles?
2. **Recall** How can weight training help prevent *osteoporosis*?
3. **Vocabulary** What is *muscle tone*?

Thinking Critically

4. **Analyze** What role does weight training play in bone development? In body composition?
5. **Synthesize** Karen is interested in toning and improving the muscular strength of her legs but is afraid bigger muscles will one day turn to fat. What reassurances about weight training could you give her?

Personal Fitness Planning

Identifying Goals List your goals for incorporating resistance activities into your own personal fitness plan. Write them down so they can be used to assist you in the development of your personal fitness program in the future. Keep your goals and review them as you learn more about resistance activities and exercises.

Resistance-Training Equipment and Gear

J orge had read all about the benefits of resistance training. He couldn't wait to put his knowledge to use. After an hour of lifting, he felt a stinging sensation in his right shoulder. By nightfall, the sting had become a searing pain. Jorge could have avoided his misery by learning some key safety facts about weight-training equipment and gear.

What You Will Do

- Evaluate the advantages and disadvantages of various weight-training devices.
- Identify different pieces of equipment in resistance-training areas.
- Evaluate consumer issues related to weight-training equipment.
- Participate in activities to evaluate and develop muscular strength.

Terms to Know

free weights
spotter
weight machines
exercise bands
plyometric exercises
calisthenic exercises
weight-training gloves
weight-training belts

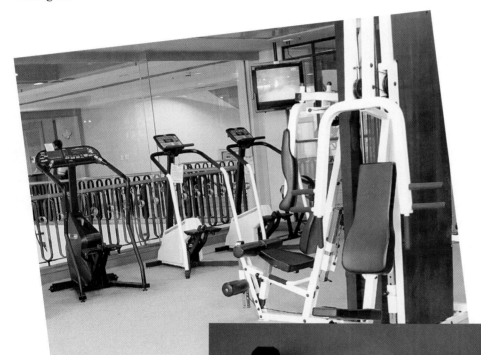

▲ Using equipment correctly is an important aspect of safety in the weight room. *What other precautions can you take to avoid injury and ensure a safe workout?*

Resistance-Training Equipment

Resistance training is performed using a variety of methods with equipment described in **Figure 9.6.** These include free weights, weight machines, exercise bands, plyometric exercise, and calisthenics. Each approach has its pros and cons.

Free Weights

Free weights is *a term applied collectively to dumbbells and barbells, as well as plates and clips.* A *dumbbell* is a short bar with weights at both ends, designed to be held and lifted with one hand. A *barbell* is a long, metal bar with weights at both ends, lifted with both hands at once. The weights placed on a barbell or dumbbell are often referred to as *plates*. They come in a variety of weights and are fastened to the bar using *clips* and *collars*. The reason they are called "free" weights is because of the unlimited direction and movement capabilities of this equipment. Free weights offer the advantage of being more versatile and less expensive than weight machines.

One notable disadvantage of free weights is that their use requires more balance and coordination than machines. The risk of unintentional injury is also greater. When using this equipment, it is vital to have a **spotter.** This is *a partner who can assist with the safe handling of weights and offer encouragement during a training session.*

Active Mind Active Body

What Is in Your Weight Room?

Every weight room is different. Some facilities have mostly machines—others, free weights. Still others have a combination of the two. In this activity, you will get to know the weight-training equipment at your school, a local branch of the YMCA, or another club to which you have access.

What You Will Need

- Pen or pencil
- Paper

What You Will Do

1. Visit the facility you will be using for your resistance training. Refer to the equipment checklist in **Figure 9.6** to identify all the equipment. Place a check mark in the appropriate boxes.
2. If you are unable to identify a particular machine or piece of equipment, speak with a manager or personal trainer. Add categories to your checklist as needed.
3. Complete your inventory by identifying the type(s) of resistance-training equipment available.

Apply and Conclude

Based on your training needs and current level of training (beginning, intermediate, and so on), identify which types of equipment you will work with. State how these will help you achieve your training goals.

FIGURE 9.6

FITNESS FACILITY EQUIPMENT CHECKLIST

Knowing which types of resistance training are available to you is important for planning your workout.

Types of Bars
• Olympic
• Standard
• Cambered/Straight

Types of Plates
• Olympic
• Standard

Types of Dumbbells
• Dumbbell rack
• Hex style
• Pro style
• Adjustable

Types of Benches	
• Flat	• Abdominal
• Incline	• Dipping Bar
• Hyper extension	• Chin-up bar
• Preacher	

Types of Machines	
• Leg press	• Leg abduction
• Back squat	• Leg adduction
• Leg extension	• Seated calf
• Leg curl	• Standing calf
• Lat pull down	

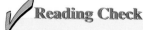

Weight Machines

Weight machines are *mechanical devices that move weights up and down using a system of cables and pulleys.* Some machines have an electronic component that digitally tracks resistance, workout time, and the like. Most machines require little or no balance on the part of the user. Spotters are not required because the weights are connected to the machine and have a predetermined path of movement. Varying the resistance is also easy, in most cases requiring the simple movement of a pin from one weight setting to another.

Anyone planning to buy a weight machine should be mindful of this equipment's expense, which can run into the thousands of dollars. Another problem is that weight machines require large amounts of space. Finally, most machines are targeted at a single muscle area, unlike free weights, which can be used for a multitude of tasks. The chart in **Figure 9.7** on page **264** compares other aspects of weight machines and free weights.

Reading Check

Explain Give one advantage and one disadvantage of using weight machines.

FIGURE 9.7

FREE WEIGHTS VS. WEIGHT MACHINES

Understanding the advantages and disadvantages of both free weights and machines is helpful in planning your program. *Name one advantage and disadvantage of both free weights and machines.*

Factor	Free Weights	Machines	Advantage
Cost	Less expensive, $200 can buy a complete set	Very costly to purchase and maintain, need a variety of machines	Free weights
Space	Take minimal space and may be moved easily	Large, bulky, and heavy; difficult to move	Free weights
Safety	Require a spotter, require balance, greater chance of injury, can cause accidents if not stored in a safe place	Weights are secured, requires no balance or spotters to lift	Machine
Variety	Allow for many different exercises with the same equipment, prevents boredom, works all parts of the body	Usually only one exercise can be done on a machine, many machines are necessary to provide variety	Free weights
Technique/Balance	Difficult to learn, much more complicated technique, balance is a necessity	Much easier to learn, no balance required	Machine
Time	Require a spotter, takes more time to change weight plates	Less total time, can work out alone, easier to change amount of resistance	Machine
Beginning Lifter	Require a spotter, harder technique to learn, balance	Safer, quicker, spotter is unnecessary, easier to learn technique	Machine
Athletic Power and Coordination	Improve coordination and balance of many muscles at the same time	Isolates single muscle and reduces need for balance	Free weights
Motivation	Easier to determine and see strength improvement	More difficult to understand strength improvement	Free weights

Less Expensive Alternatives

Even though free weights are less expensive than weight machines, a complete set can still be quite costly. Certain progressive resistance exercises will call for an adjustable bench, which can cost even more. Fortunately, there are lower-cost and even no-cost alternatives. These include:

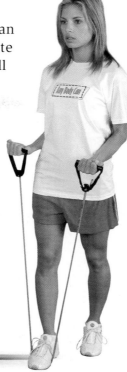

- **Exercise bands.** These are *elastic bands or tubing made of latex that are used to develop muscular strength and endurance.* The bands are color-coded to identify the level of resistance. Although the strips come in set lengths, usually three feet, they may be modified to meet your specific needs.

◀ Using the correct colored exercise band can provide a great strength workout. *What is another advantage of exercise bands?*

Consumer CORNER

Purchasing Weight-Training Equipment

When shopping for weight-training equipment, you need to be a wise consumer. Although equipment may look the same, it may not perform equally well once you get it home. Here are some other points to consider:

- **Quality.** When purchasing free weights, be aware that you get what you pay for. Plastic weights filled with sand, for example, may be less expensive than metal weights. However, they will not last as long.
- **Space.** All weight-training equipment takes up space. Before making a purchase, be sure you have a place where you can work out and, if necessary, store your equipment when you are done.
- **Expense.** Exercising at home with weight machines has become popular. Many different models are available. Before deciding to purchase a weight machine for home use,

you need to consider how much you can afford to spend.
- **Features.** Some weight-training equipment comes with added features that increase the expense of the machine. Determine if the extra features are worth the extra cost.

One last point to consider is whether the equipment lives up to its promise. Many worthless items are sold nowadays. Among these are crude machines that claim to work the abdominal muscles and pills that claim to burn fat.

Evaluate

Find an ad for a weight-training product. Make a list of the features offered, the manufacturer's claims, warranties, and the costs, including hidden costs such as inflated shipping charges. Share your findings in an in-class roundtable discussion of such products.

Proper plyometric technique and adequate strength can provide the athlete with improved muscular force and power. *Who should participate in plyometric training? Explain your answer.*

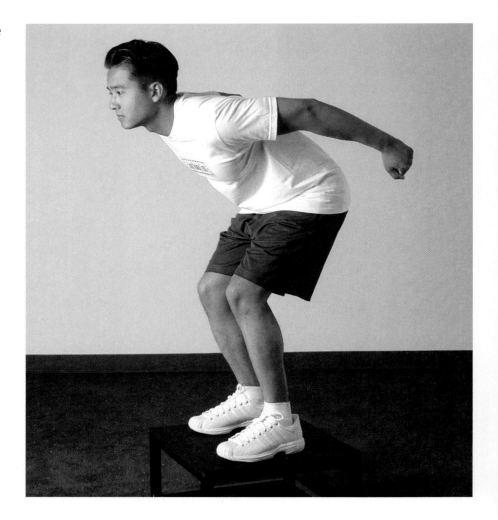

- **Plyometric exercise.** This is *a quick, powerful muscular movement that requires the muscle to be prestretched just before a quick contraction.* Many such exercises require jumping, leaping, and bounding. Common equipment includes boxes of different heights. When used properly, plyometric training can improve muscle force and power. One downside of plyometric exercises is the stress they can place on tendons. This type of training, furthermore, is not recommended for beginners and is most often associated with the improvement of athletic performance.
- **Calisthenic exercises.** These are *exercises that create resistance by using your body weight.* They include such well-known exercises as pull-ups, push-ups, abdominal curl-ups, and jumping jacks. They have been used for many years and were once the main source of fitness training. Calisthenics are low-level resistance activities and provide opportunities for increasing muscular endurance.

 Reading Check

Analyze Which of the less expensive alternatives requires no equipment?

Fitness Check

Evaluating Muscular Endurance

In this activity, you will test two aspects of your muscular strength through resistance exercises. You will test your upper-body endurance by doing push-ups. You will then test your lower-body endurance by doing squats. Remember to warm up before you start. Breathe in a normal pattern and control your speed of movement for each exercise.

Upper-Body Endurance: Push-Ups

- *Primary muscles worked*: chest (pectoralis major), back of upper arm (triceps), shoulder (deltoid)
- *Beginning position*: Begin with your body lying facedown on a mat, legs straight and close together, hands placed palms-down next to your shoulders with fingers facing forward.

Technique:
1. Extend the elbows and push your body up to a fully extended arm position. Keep your back straight at all times.
2. Gradually lower your body to the point where your chest almost touches the ground.
3. Repeat this motion as many times as you can. *Individuals with advanced strength may want to elevate their feet on a box or step at a height of 6 to 24 inches.*
4. Use the Fitness Ratings Chart for Push-ups to assess your performance.

Fitness Ratings: Push-ups

Age/Number of Push-ups	Rating
Males:	
Age 13: 10–25	Acceptable
Age 14: 15–30	Acceptable
Age 15: 15–35	Acceptable
Age 16+: 20–35	Acceptable
Females:	
Age 13–16: 5–15	Acceptable

Lower-Body Endurance: Squats

- *Primary muscles worked*: thighs (quadriceps), buttocks (gluteals), back of upper leg (hamstring).
- *Beginning position*: Begin in a standing position with your feet shoulder width apart. Keep your back straight and your head facing forward with arms at your side.

Technique:
1. Slowly bend your knees, lowering your body to a position where your thighs are parallel to the floor. Avoid bending at the waist as much as possible.
2. Return to the starting position.
3. Repeat this motion as many times as you can.
4. Use the Fitness Ratings Chart for Squats to assess your performance.

Fitness Ratings: Squats

Number of Squats	Rating
Males: 25–50	Acceptable
Females: 20–40	Acceptable

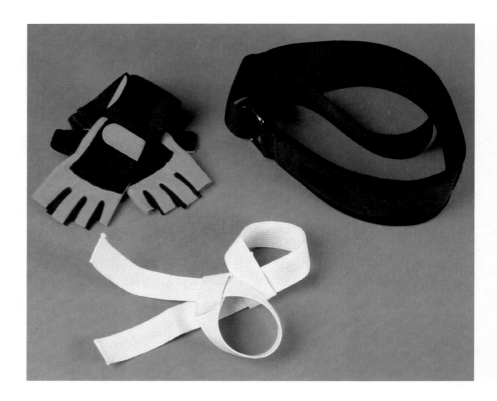

▶ Pictured is an assortment of weight-training gear. *Identify each item and describe its function.*

Resistance-Training Gear

A well-designed program of resistance training begins not just with a decision on which equipment you will use. Careful thought must be given as well to the right clothing and other workout gear. These items, too, will affect the safety, comfort, and cost of your training.

Clothing and Footwear

There are a variety of fabrics to choose from when selecting appropriate clothing for strength training. Everything from nylon to breathable synthetic fabrics to plain old cotton is available. Regardless of which style or color you choose, keep comfort, performance, and safety in mind. Remember these tips.

- Weight-training clothing should be nonbinding to allow full range of motion.
- Your outfit should keep you warm or cool, depending on the temperature of your workout facility. Wearing layers can help you control your body temperature.
- Avoid wearing any item that could easily become tangled or caught on the equipment.

Always wear properly fitted **footwear.** It should be designed to give you good arch support and provide traction. A cross-training shoe is probably the best style because it provides ankle support. Wearing a pair of absorbent socks can also help prevent blisters.

footwear
For more on choosing appropriate footwear, see Chapter 2, page **48.**

Other Gear

The number of accessories available to weight trainees is almost limitless. Many of these are useful and inexpensive, though none are absolutely essential. Here are a few of the more useful items:

- **Weight-training gloves.** Similar to the gloves worn by athletes in some sports, these are designed to *prevent blisters and calluses from forming on your palms.* The most popular styles will have padding on the palms and open fingers. If you have sensitive skin or you want to avoid rough hands, wear gloves. Gloves will also improve your grip.
- **Weight-training belts.** These are used primarily to *protect your lower back and stomach when you lift heavy weights.* The belt is worn tightly around the waist to give the stomach muscles something to push against. As a result, pressure builds up in the abdomen, which in turn pushes against and stabilizes the lower spine. This protects the lower back.
- **Straps and wraps.** These 1½-inch-wide strips of a canvas-like material are wrapped around your wrist and then twisted around a bar. They are used for very heavy lifts when your grip cannot support the weight. Wraps or elastic bandages are used to give additional support to joints. They are most often used during heavy leg exercises. They can provide support, but they also restrict your range of motion.

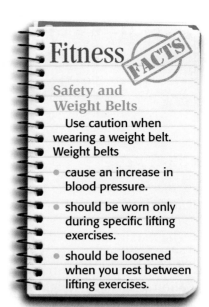

Fitness FACTS

Safety and Weight Belts

Use caution when wearing a weight belt. Weight belts

- cause an increase in blood pressure.
- should be worn only during specific lifting exercises.
- should be loosened when you rest between lifting exercises.

 Reading Check

Explain What is the purpose of a weight-training belt?

Lesson 4 Review

Using complete sentences, answer the following questions on a sheet of paper.

Reviewing Facts and Vocabulary

1. **Vocabulary** What is the collective name by which dumbbells and barbells are known?
2. **Recall** What are *plyometric exercises*? Who should do them?
3. **Recall** What are the advantages of wearing weight-training gloves while lifting?

Thinking Critically

4. **Compare and Contrast** Explain why it is important to consider the advantages and disadvantages of free weights and machines before starting a weight-training program.

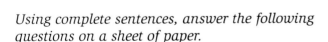

Personal Fitness Planning

Assessing Equipment Make a list of the resistance equipment and gear you might use to meet the goals you stated in Lesson 3. Use the Fitness Check evaluations to better design your resistance goals. Chapter 10 will discuss weight-training exercises and their proper technique as well as programs for the entire body. You may want to consider a variety of exercises that can be used to work on your specific goals.

TRUE/FALSE

On a sheet of paper, write the numbers 1–10. Write True or False for each statement.

1. The maximum amount of force a muscle can exert against a resistance is muscular strength.
2. Relative muscular strength takes into consideration your body weight and your strength.
3. Putting greater stress on a muscle than it is accustomed to is the principle of specificity.
4. Body builders, athletes, and power lifters use the same kind of weight-training programs.
5. A primary benefit of weight training is the prevention of a bone disease called osteoporosis.
6. Tendons and ligaments are forms of connective tissue.
7. Testosterone is a male hormone also found in females that plays a role in building muscles.
8. Isometric contractions start by lengthening and then getting shorter.
9. The term *hypertrophy* is used to describe how muscle fibers get thicker and cause muscles to grow.
10. Most experts believe that weight training and good nutrition will increase the number of a person's muscle fibers.

MULTIPLE CHOICE

On a sheet of paper, write the letter of the word or phrase that best completes each statement.

11. Which of the following is an example of muscular endurance?
    a. Five arm curl reps with 20 pounds
    b. Fifteen bench press reps with 75 pounds
    c. Ten sit-ups
    d. A fifteen-second isometric contraction
12. Which of the following is not a benefit of weight training?
    a. Significant increase in cardiovascular efficiency
    b. Increased bone strength and density
    c. Reduction in stress
    d. Faster metabolism and better self-esteem

13. What term describes the use of barbells, dumbbells, and machines to improve fitness, health, and appearance?
    a. Body building
    b. Strength and conditioning
    c. Weight training
    d. Weight lifting
14. When Bob started weight lifting, he shoulder pressed 50 pounds, eight times. Later, he was able to press the same weight twelve times. He increased the weight to 60 pounds and pressed it eight times. Which of the following exercise principles is Bob using?
    a. Overload
    b. Specificity
    c. Intensity
    d. Progressive resistance
15. Skeletal muscles
    a. move bones and joints.
    b. protect against injury.
    c. burn up calories.
    d. all of the above.
16. Which of the following exercises is done mainly by athletes, involves quick, powerful muscular movements and little equipment?
    a. Plyometric   c. Calisthenics
    b. Isometric   d. Aerobic
17. When the muscle becomes shorter, what kind of a contraction is it?
    a. Eccentric   c. Isometric
    b. Concentric   d. Isotonic
18. Which of the following is a result of steroid use?
    a. violates school rules
    b. is illegal
    c. damages team spirit
    d. all of the above
19. What is the main reason that females do not grow muscles as large as males do?
    a. Females do not lift hard enough.
    b. Females do not have as much testosterone as men.
    c. The female body is not capable of lifting heavy weights.
    d. Females do not spend enough time in the weight room.
20. Which of the following is not an advantage of free weights?
    a. They cost less.
    b. They take up less space.
    c. They are less dangerous.
    d. They require more balance.

DISCUSSION

Using complete sentences, answer the following questions on a sheet of paper.

21. **Explain** Define and give an example of relative muscular endurance.
22. **Describe** What is one method of evaluating upper-body strength and one method of evaluating lower-body strength?
23. **Identify** List and explain five myths associated with weight training.

VOCABULARY

On a sheet of paper, write the letter of the term in Column B that best fits the definition in Column A.

Column A

24. The amount of force a muscle or muscle group can exert in one maximum effort.
25. Applying greater stress to a muscle than it is normally accustomed to.
26. Your strength in relation to your weight.
27. An increase in the size of a muscle.
28. An inherited limitation.

Column B

a. relative muscular strength
b. overload principle
c. hypertrophy
d. genetic potential
e. muscular strength

CRITICAL THINKING

Using complete sentences, answer the following questions on a sheet of paper.

29. **Describe** Explain the difference between weight lifting and strength training.
30. **Evaluate** Respond to the statement, "Resistance training is going to be harmful for me because my body has not finished growing."
31. **Identify** List and explain reasons why females can benefit from weight training.

CASE STUDY

THE TRUTH ABOUT RESISTANCE TRAINING

Terri, who is a softball pitcher, would like to improve her arm strength. A friend recommended resistance training. However, Terri has heard many conflicting claims about this type of training. She isn't sure what to believe. She needs the help of someone knowledgeable to inform her about the benefits and mistruths of resistance training. That someone is you!

HERE IS YOUR ASSIGNMENT

Organize a list of statements that will correct the common misconceptions Terri has about weight training. Then list the recommendations you would make for her to get started in a resistance-training program. Use the following keys to help you prepare your list:

KEYS TO HELP YOU

- Explain the benefits of resistance training.
- Explain the truth behind myths that may be confusing Terri.
- Identify the many different types of equipment and resistance-training exercises.
- Explain the advantages and disadvantages associated with free weights and weight machines.
- Inform Terri of the need for proper gear and how to go about selecting what she may need.

FITNESS *Online*

Do you have resistance-training goals? Are these goals reasonable? Do you know the correct and safe way to use weights and other equipment? Find out by taking the STEP Personal Inventory for Chapter 10. Find it at **fitness.glencoe.com**.

Beginning a Resistance-Training Program

What You Will Do

- Identify the importance of setting resistance-training goals.
- Demonstrate safety procedures, such as spotting.
- Apply rules, procedures, and etiquette to your workout.
- Identify a variety of resistance-training exercises that build muscular strength and endurance.

Terms to Know

clips
overhand grip
underhand grip
alternated grip

Setting goals is essential to the success of any endeavor. It is especially important when improving your muscular strength and endurance. In this lesson, you will learn how to set resistance training goals. You will also learn how to avoid injury when using free weights and resistance-training equipment.

Short- and Long-Term Goals

In Chapter 3, you learned about short- and long-term goals. Improving your muscular strength and endurance requires short-term goals that can be used as stepping stones to achieving long-term goals. Some short-term goals may include:

- Increasing your fluid intake
- Getting adequate rest—at least 8–10 hours of sleep each night

Long-term goals may be more complex and require considerable planning, discipline, and patience to achieve them. These may include:

- Increasing your strength by 10 percent
- Toning selected muscles
- Developing leaner body mass

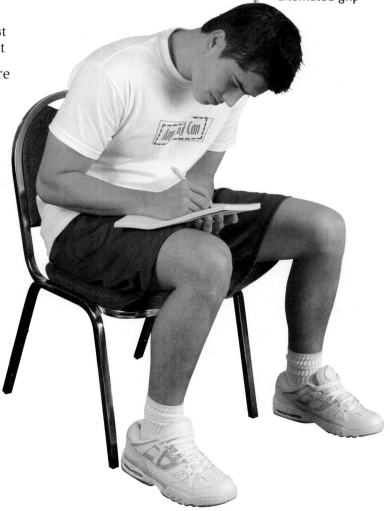

▶ Part of setting a reasonable goal involves setting a reasonable time frame for achieving it. *Why is it important to include this information?*

In Chapter 1, you were introduced to the behavioral-change stairway. This is a step-by-step approach for achieving personal fitness goals. This lesson will provide you with additional tips for planning your resistance-training program.

Setting Your Goals

Plan carefully before you begin your resistance-training program, and write down your goals and how you plan to achieve them. Refer to your plan periodically to stay focused and assess your progress. Consider the following steps as you write your goals.

- **Set reasonable goals.** Your goals should be specific and realistic. They should be goals that are challenging, but that you are capable of attaining.
- **Establish short- and long-term goals.** The short-term goals act as motivators to keep you going and as steps toward reaching your long-term goals. For example, your long-term goal might be to increase your absolute strength from lifting 100 pounds to lifting 135 pounds on the bench press in four months. Your short-term goals could be to lift 110 pounds the first month, then 120 pounds the second month, then 130 pounds the third month, and finally 135 pounds the fourth month.
- **Identify a variety of short-term goals.** Short-term goals enable you to reach your long-term goals. It is important to think of a variety of short-term goals that will help you along the way. Some examples include: strength training three to four hours a week, improving eating habits, drinking plenty of water, and getting adequate rest.
- **Keep written records.** After each workout, record the number of sets and repetitions you performed for each exercise. Periodically, review your progress. This will motivate you to keep going.
- **Revise goals.** Be prepared to accept setbacks. It is not uncommon to have "off" days during resistance training. Learn to accept these days and move on. The same is true of illness or minor injuries, which may cause a delay in training. Don't give up. Revise your goals or end date if necessary. The important thing is to get right back into your workout routine as soon as you can.
- **Think positively.** Believe in yourself and focus on the positive, not the negative. Read your goals aloud each day immediately before and after workouts. Have fun and enjoy the process.

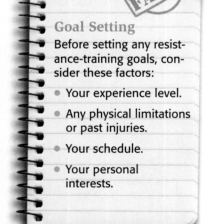

Fitness FACTS

Goal Setting

Before setting any resistance-training goals, consider these factors:

- Your experience level.
- Any physical limitations or past injuries.
- Your schedule.
- Your personal interests.

 Reading Check

Explain Why is it important to set short-term goals as well as long-term goals?

Applying Safety Rules and Procedures

Proper resistance training can improve your fitness, but if done improperly, it can also lead to serious injury. Before beginning your first workout, you need to learn some basic safety guidelines for the proper use of weight machines and free weights.

- **Familiarize yourself with the training facility.** Know where various pieces of equipment can be found.
- **Warm up before each session.** Do a combination of aerobic exercise and stretches of the muscle groups to be worked.
- **Learn and use proper technique on any exercise.** Shortcuts or improper use can minimize your lifting leverage and lead to injury.
- **Use spotters.** When using free weights, have a partner who can support and assist you.
- **Wear a safety belt.** When doing heavy lifting that requires the use of abdominal or back muscles, consider wearing a safety belt.
- **Use clips when adding weights to barbells.** Clips are *clamp-like devices that secure the weights in place.*
- **Practice all lifts.** Practice with very light weights before attempting heavier weight.
- **Control the speed of the resistance movement at all times.** If you find that it is difficult to control the speed, you are probably attempting to lift too much. Reduce the weight.
- **Be alert and act responsibly.** Showing off or behaving irresponsibly can lead to unintentional injury.
- **Return equipment.** Put equipment in its proper place after using it.
- **Allow time for muscles to repair.** Between training sessions, give muscle tissues enough time to repair and renew themselves. For most people, forty-eight hours is enough time.
- **Cool down after each session.** As with the warm-up, combine aerobic exercise and stretches.

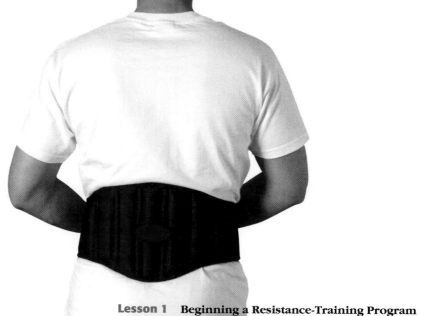

▶ A safe resistance-training workout includes safety belts. *Identify two other ways you can make your workout safe.*

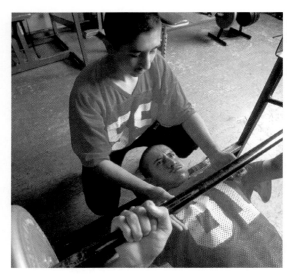

A spotter can help ensure a safe workout. *What else can a spotter provide?*

Spotting

When training with free weights, it is essential to have a spotter. As noted in Chapter 9, a spotter is a partner who can assist with the safe handling of weights and offer encouragement during a session. A spotter has three main jobs:

- Helping the lifter keep the weight moving in a smooth, steady motion
- Observing and pointing out any improper technique being used by the lifter
- Providing motivation and encouragement to the lifter

Spotting is a serious job that demands a high degree of personal responsibility. A good spotter can be the difference between serious injury and a safe, successful workout.

Other Duties of the Spotter. In addition to the three primary jobs just described, a spotter

- keeps the exercise area free of weights or other equipment that could be tripped over.
- puts the proper amount of weight on the bar and spaces it evenly.
- keeps his or her body and hands in a ready position at all times.
- communicates with the lifter. It is important that all verbal and nonverbal commands are understood.
- knows how many repetitions the lifter will be attempting.
- applies assistance without jerking the bar.
- is ready to assume all the weight, if necessary.

 Reading Check

List What are the three main duties of a spotter?

Proper Technique

In resistance training, technique is important. Using proper technique can help you make the most of your training sessions and achieve your goals more quickly. Remember these technique tips.

- Keep your back straight at all times.
- Adjust all weight machines for proper body alignment.
- When performing standing lifts, be sure to have a wide, stable base. Place your feet flat on the floor.
- When lifting objects, use your legs, not your back.
- Keep the weight close to your body to maintain proper leverage.
- All lifts should be done through a full range of motion. Your muscles should be flexed and extended completely.
- Concentrate on the muscles that should be doing the work.
- Make sure you keep your hands on the bar and maintain pressure until all weights are safely put back on the racks.

Breath Control

Learning the proper technique for breathing is critical to the success of your workout. There are three steps involved in breath control.

- Slowly take two or three deep breaths, holding the last breath.
- Begin your lift, exhaling the air slowly.
- Return the weight to its starting position, inhaling as you do.

Getting used to breathing in this manner takes time. Some new lifters practice breath control in front of a mirror.

Proper Grips

One of the most important—and often overlooked—parts of proper lifting technique is gripping the bar correctly. There are three types of grips. The type used depends on the exercise. You will learn more about when to use each grip later in this chapter.

- **Overhand grip.** In the overhand grip, *the bar is grasped with the palms facing downward and the knuckles facing upward* (see **Figure 10.1a**).
- **Underhand grip.** In the underhand grip, *the bar is grasped with the palms facing upward and the knuckles facing downward* (see **Figure 10.1b**).
- **Alternated grip.** In the alternated grip, *the bar is grasped with one palm facing downward and the other palm facing upward* (see **Figure 10.1c**).

Regardless of how you grip the bar, always make sure your fingers are wrapped closely around it so that the thumb meets the index finger. This will ensure that the bar is firmly within your control.

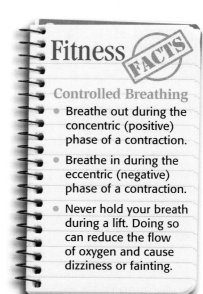

Fitness FACTS

Controlled Breathing

- Breathe out during the concentric (positive) phase of a contraction.
- Breathe in during the eccentric (negative) phase of a contraction.
- Never hold your breath during a lift. Doing so can reduce the flow of oxygen and cause dizziness or fainting.

FIGURE 10.1

PROPER GRIPS

Proper lifting technique involves using one of the three types of grips. *What are the names of each grip?*

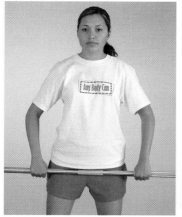

Figure 10.1a

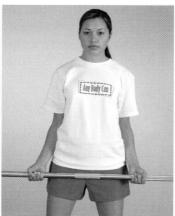

Figure 10.1b

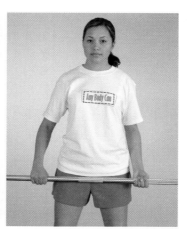

Figure 10.1c

FIGURE 10.2

HAND PLACEMENT

Whether you are using the wide, common, or narrow grip placement, your hands should always be evenly spaced from the ends of the bar. *Why is this important for your safety?*

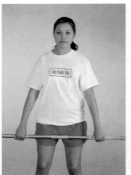

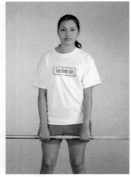

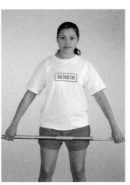

| Figure 10.2a | Figure 10.2b | Figure 10.2c |

Hand Placement

Just as critical as *how* you hold the bar is *where* you hold it. **Figure 10.2** shows the three main grip placements, and the one you choose will depend on the specific exercise. In the common (or standard) grip, your hands are spaced about shoulder width apart (see **Figure 10.2a**). In the narrow grip, your hands are spaced closer together (see **Figure 10.2b**). In the wide grip, your hands are spaced farther apart than your shoulders (see **Figure 10.2c**). No matter which grip you are using, always make sure your hands are evenly spaced from the ends of the bar. This will ensure that the bar remains balanced and reduces the chance of injury. This will also ensure that the muscles on each side of the body receive the same workout.

Weight Room Etiquette

Whether you are working out in the school gym, the YMCA, the YWCA, or some other location, be courteous. Always consider the needs of others.

- Limit your time on a machine or at a work station. This is especially true at peak hours or when others are waiting to use the equipment.
- Use one machine or station at a time. If your training includes alternating between two exercises, choose a time when the facility is less crowded, such as early morning. Even then, be prepared to share.
- Put away free weights and other equipment at the end of your session. In addition to demonstrating courtesy, cleaning up after yourself helps ensure the safety of other users.
- Use a towel. If the facility does not provide towels, bring one from home. Spread the towel on the bench or other surface before your body comes into contact with it. Wipe down the equipment when you have finished using it.

Weight-Training Exercises for the Whole Body

There are many weight-training exercises that may be used to improve strength and fitness. You should choose a variety of exercises that will work all the major muscles and joints of the body.

As you learn and participate in the following exercises, always remember to practice all the resistance-training safety guidelines you have learned. It is especially important for you to strictly follow the lifting procedures described. Have your physical education teacher, trainer, or coach observe your technique to help reduce your chance of injury.

Bench Press

Body area: *middle chest*
Muscles: *pectoralis, deltoid, triceps*
Variation: *dumbbells*
Caution: *Spotter required*

- Lie faceup on a bench. Position your back and buttocks flat on the bench.
- Position your eyes directly under the bar. Keep your head on the bench.
- Position your feet flat on the floor. If the bench is too high, use a chair or the end of the bench to lift your feet. (This prevents injury to your back from arching.) Your legs should remain relaxed.
- Grasp the bar with hands slightly farther apart than shoulder width.
- Your hands should be evenly spaced on each side from the center of the bar; use a wraparound thumb grip, and lock your wrists.
- Move the bar off the rack, and position it over your chest. (Spotter should assist.)
- Keep your elbows out, parallel to the bar.
- Stabilize the bar before lowering it. (Spotter should release the bar.)
- Lower the bar slowly to the middle of your chest. Maintain control and speed; touch, do not bounce the bar off your chest.
- Push upward to the starting position. Go through the full range of motion. (Spotter's hands should be in the ready position.)
- Exhale during the push stage. Do not hold your breath.
- Keep your back, head, and buttocks in contact with the bench at all times.
- When you are done, replace the bar on the rack. Never release your grip until the bar is safely in the rack. (Spotter should assist to replace the bar.)

▼ **Bench Press**

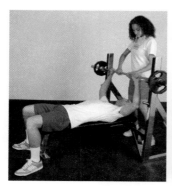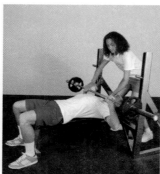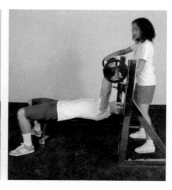

▶ **Variation of Bench Press—Flat Bench Dumbbell Press**

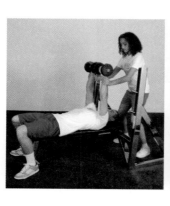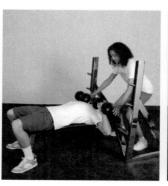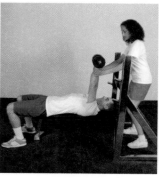

Incline Bench Press

Body area: *upper chest*
Muscles: *upper pectoralis, deltoid, triceps*
Variation: *dumbbells*
Caution: *Spotter required*

- Lie faceup on an incline bench. Position your back and buttocks flat on the bench.
- Position your feet flat on the floor. If the bench is too high, use a chair or the end of the bench to lift your feet. Do not use your feet to lift your body. Your legs should remain relaxed.
- Grasp the bar with hands slightly farther apart than shoulder width.
- Your grip should be evenly spaced. Use a wraparound thumb grip, and lock your wrists.
- Move the bar off the rack, and position it over your chest. (Spotter should assist.)
- Keep your elbows out and parallel to the bar.
- Lower the bar slowly to the top of your chest, near your chin. Maintain control and speed. Touch the bar to your chest. Do not bounce it off your chest.
- Push the bar upward to the starting position. Go through the full range of motion. (Spotter's hands should be in a ready position.)
- Exhale during the push stage. Do not hold your breath.
- Your back, head, and buttocks must remain in contact with the bench at all times.
- At the completion of the reps, replace the bar on the rack. Never release your grip until the bar is safely in the rack. (Spotter should assist in replacing the bar on the rack.)

▼ Incline Bench Press

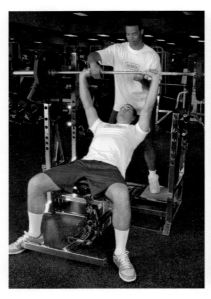
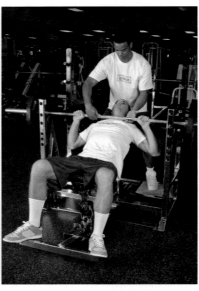
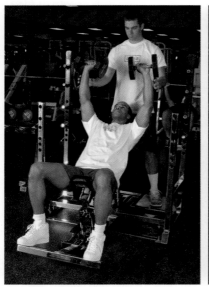
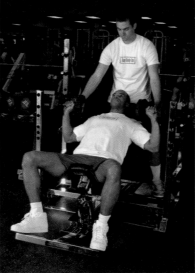

▲ Variation of Incline
Bench Press—Dumbbells

Flat Bench Fly
Body area: *chest*
Muscles: *pectoralis*
Variation: *incline or decline bench*

- Lie faceup on a flat bench. Position your back and buttocks flat on the bench.
- Position your feet flat on the floor. If the bench is too high, use a chair or the end of the bench to lift your feet. Do not use your feet to lift your body. Your legs should remain relaxed.
- Grasp a dumbbell in each hand. Use a wraparound thumb grip.
- Raise your arms and hands to position the dumbbells together over your chest. Your arms should be extended, and your palms should face each other.
- Before you lower the dumbbells, slightly bend both elbows.
- Lower the dumbbells in a wide arc.
- Your elbows should remain slightly bent. Keep your arms in line with your shoulders and chest.
- Lower the dumbbells slowly, controlling their speed until they are level with your shoulders. (Spotter can assist).
- Return the dumbbells to the starting position. Keep your elbows slightly bent until you reach the top of the lift. Continue the reps.
- Exhale during the push stage. Do not hold your breath.

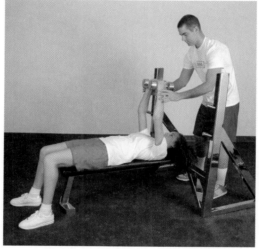

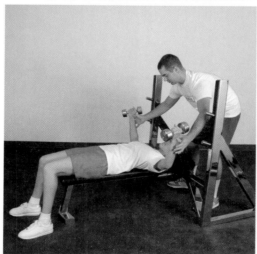

▲ **Flat Bench Fly**

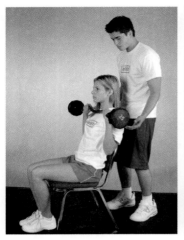
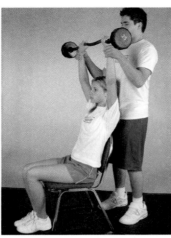

▲ Seated Shoulder
(Military) Press

Seated Shoulder (Military) Press

Body area: *shoulders*
Muscles: *deltoid and triceps*
Variations: *standing dumbbell press, seated dumbbell press, and machine (seated shoulder press, incline shoulder press)*
Caution: *spotter required*

- Sit on a bench or chair. Place your feet flat on the floor.
- Grasp the bar using a standard grip.
- Your grip should be evenly spaced. Use a wraparound thumb grip, and lock your wrists.
- Your elbows should be under the bar and parallel to the bar.
- Your back should be straight (not arched) and your head looking forward.
- The starting position for the bar is at shoulder height and close to the body. (Spotter can assist.)
- The bar is pushed upward to full arm extension.
- Exhale during the push stage. Do not hold your breath.
- Your elbows should remain under, and parallel to, the bar at all times, with your back flat.
- Lower the bar slowly to the top of your chest. Maintain control and speed. Do not let the bar bounce off your chest.
- At the completion of the reps, replace the bar on the rack. (Spotter can assist.)

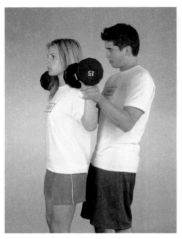
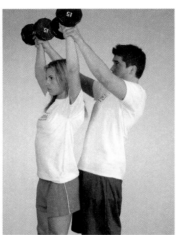

▲ Standing Dumbbell
Overhead (Military) Press

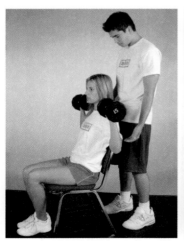
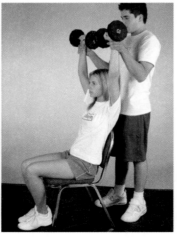

◀ Seated Dumbbell
(Military) Press

Shoulder Shrug

Body area: *shoulders*
Muscles: *trapezius*
Variation: *dumbbell*

- To pick up the bar from the floor, assume a shoulder-width stance, with your feet flat.
- Bend your knees, not your waist. To place your hands on the bar, fully extend your arms.
- Your grip should be slightly wider than your shoulders and outside your knees.
- Your grip should be evenly spaced. Use a wraparound thumb grip.
- The bar should be close to your shins.
- Position your shoulders over the bar.
- Your back must stay flat. Keep your head up. Pull your shoulder blades together. Do not bend at the waist.
- Begin lifting by extending your legs, not your back.
- Move your hips forward, and raise your shoulders.
- Keep the bar close to your body, with your back and feet flat.
- Raise the bar until your knees are slightly bent and your arms are fully extended.
- Exhale during the lifting stage.
- Lift the bar by raising your shoulders toward your ears. Do not bend or pull with your arms.
- Hold this "shrug" position for two counts.
- Exhale during the lifting stage.
- Lower the bar slowly to your waist. Maintain control and speed. Keep your feet flat and your knees slightly bent.
- At the completion of the reps, return the bar to the floor. To protect your back, be sure that you use the same technique you used to pick up the bar to return the bar to the floor.

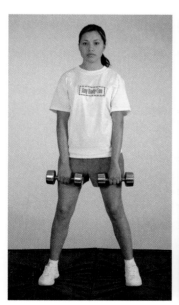
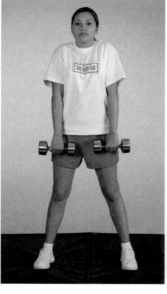
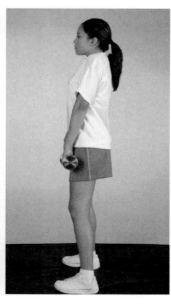

◀ **Variation on Shoulder Shrug (Dumbbell)**

Upright Row

Body area: *shoulders*
Muscles: *deltoids, trapezius, biceps*
Variation: *dumbbells*

- To pick up the bar from the floor, assume shoulder-width stance, with feet flat.
- Bend your knees, not your waist. To place your hands on the bar, fully extend your arms.
- Your hands will grip 8 to 10 inches apart and be placed inside your legs.
- Your hands should be evenly spaced in the grip. Use a wrap-around thumb grip.
- The bar should be close to your shins.
- Position your shoulders over the bar.
- Your back must stay flat. Keep your head up. Pull your shoulder blades together. Do not bend at the waist.
- Begin lifting by extending your legs, not your back.
- Move your hips forward, and raise your shoulders.
- Keep the bar close to your body, with your back and feet flat.

▼ **Upright Row (Barbell)**

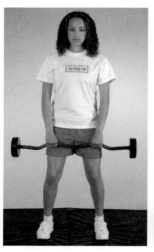 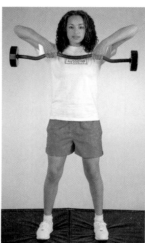 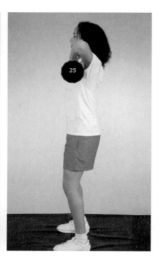

- Raise the bar until your knees are slightly bent and your arms are fully extended.
- Exhale during the lifting stage.
- Pull the bar upward along your stomach and chest toward your chin. Keep the bar close to your body.
- Continue to raise the bar until it is under your chin.
- Your elbows should be higher than your wrist and shoulders.
- Exhale during the lifting stage.
- Lower the bar slowly to your waist. Maintain control and speed. Keep your feet flat, with knees slightly bent.
- At the completion of the reps, return the bar to the floor. To protect your back, be sure to use the same technique you used to pick up the bar to return the bar to the floor.

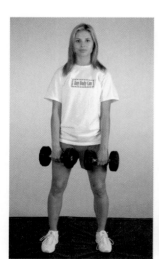 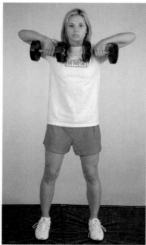 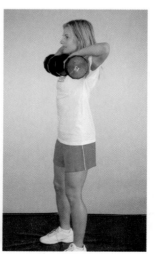

▲ **Upright Row (Dumbbells)**

Front Dumbbell Shoulder Raise

Body area: *shoulders*
Muscles: *front part of deltoids*
Variation: *sitting*

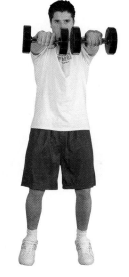
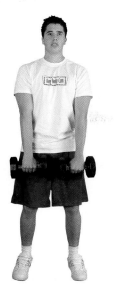
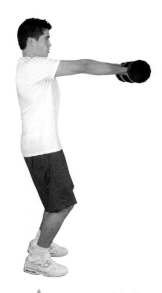

- Start in a standing position with feet shoulder width apart and head up.
- Hold a dumbbell in each hand, with arms hanging on each side of your body and elbows slightly bent.
- Slowly raise your arms in front of your body. Continue to raise your arms until your hands are level with your shoulders. Your arms must stay in front. (The exercise can be done by alternating arms or raising both arms at the same time.)
- Exhale during the lifting stage.
- Hold this position for two counts.
- Lower your arms slowly to the starting position. Maintain control and speed. Continue the reps.

▲ **Front Dumbbell Shoulder Raise**

Side (Lateral) Dumbbell Shoulder Raise

Body area: *shoulders*
Muscles: *middle part of deltoids*
Variation: *sitting*

- Start in a standing position, with feet shoulder width apart and head up.
- Hold a dumbbell in each hand, with arms hanging on each side of your body and elbows slightly bent.
- Slowly raise your arms to the side of your body. Continue to raise your arms until your hands are level with your shoulders. Keep your elbows level with your hands.
- As you raise your arms, rotate your wrists down and elbows up, as if you were pouring water out of a glass. (This exercise may be done by alternating arms or raising both at the same time.)
- Exhale during the lifting stage.
- Hold the position for a count of two.
- Lower your arms slowly to the starting position. Maintain control and speed. Continue the reps.

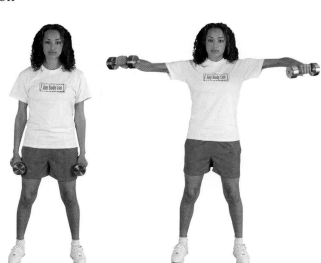

▲ **Side (Lateral) Dumbbell Shoulder Raise**

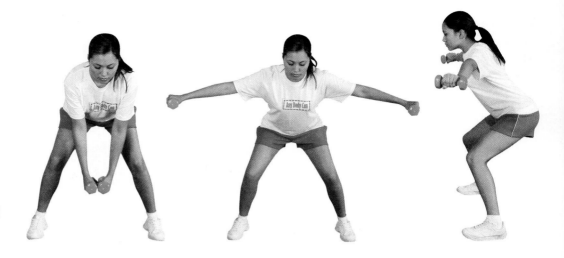

▶ Bent-over Dumbbell Shoulder Raise

Bent-over Dumbbell Shoulder Raise
Body area: *shoulders*
Muscle: *back part of deltoid*
Variation: *sitting*

- Start in a standing position with feet shoulder width apart, knees slightly bent and head up.
- Hold a dumbbell in each hand with arms hanging on each side of your body.
- Bend at the waist. Your arms should be hanging straight down.
- Slowly raise your arms upward. Continue to raise your arms until your hands are almost level with your shoulders.
- Exhale during the lifting stage.
- Hold this position for 2 counts.
- Lower your arms slowly to a starting position. Maintain control and speed. Continue the reps.

Bent-over Row
Body area: *upper back*
Muscles: *latissimus dorsi, trapezius, biceps*
Variation: *one arm dumbbell*
Caution: *Weight belts may be necessary during maximum lifts.*

- To pick up the bar from the floor, assume shoulder-width stance, with feet flat.
- Bend your knees and waist to place your hands on the bar. Fully extend your arms.
- Your grip should be slightly wider than your shoulders.
- Your hands should be evenly spaced in the grip. Use a wrap-around thumb grip.
- The bar should be close to your shins.
- Position your shoulders over the bar.
- Your back must stay flat. Keep your head up, and pull your shoulder blades together.
- Begin lifting by extending your legs until your back is slightly above a parallel position in relation to the floor. Keep your knees flexed and your back flat. Hold this position.

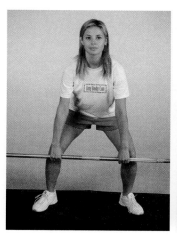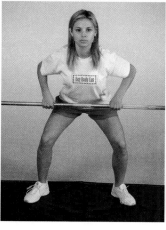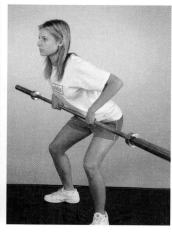

Bent-over Row (Free Weight)

- With arms fully extended, pull the bar up and touch your lower chest or upper abdomen. Keep your elbows out.
- Exhale during the lifting stage.
- Keep your upper body and legs in a set position.
- Lower the bar slowly to the starting position. Maintain control and speed.
- At the completion of the reps, return the bar to the floor. Be sure to use the same technique you used to pick up the bar.

Lat Pulldown

Body area: *midback*
Muscles: *latissimus dorsi, trapezius, biceps*
Variation: *Pull bar to back of neck. (This exercise requires special apparatus.)*

- Grasp the bar with hands 7 to 8 inches wider apart than shoulder width.
- Your hands should be evenly spaced on the grip. Use the wraparound thumb grip, with arms fully extended.
- Pull the bar straight down until you reach a kneeling position, or sit in a chair.
- Your head and torso should remain in an upright position.
- Begin to pull the bar downward toward the top of the chest. Your back muscles, not your arms, should start the motion.
- Continue to pull the bar downward until it touches the top of your chest. Keep your head and torso up. (In an advanced variation, the bar would go to the back of the neck.)
- Exhale during the pulling stage.
- Allow the bar to return slowly to the starting position. Maintain control and speed. Continue the reps.

Lat Pulldown (Machine)

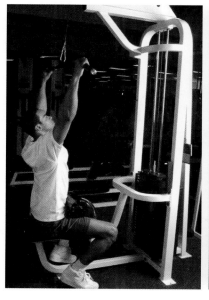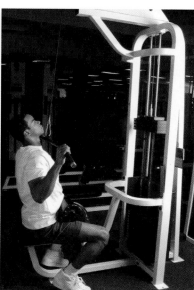

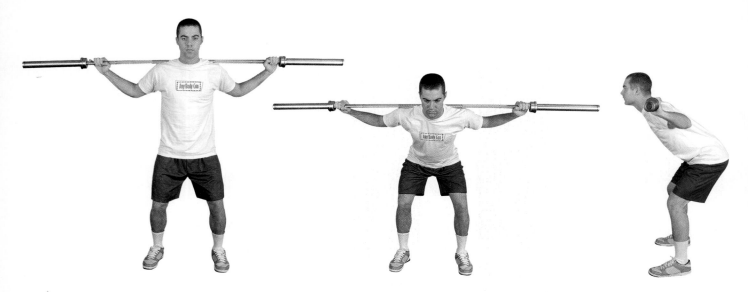

▲ **Straight-back
Good Morning**

Straight-back Good Morning
Body area: *lower back*
Muscles: *spinal erectors*
Caution: *Spotters and light weights recommended*

- Assume shoulder-width stance, with feet flat and head and shoulders up.
- Spotters will lift and place the bar across the back of your shoulders, not your neck. (The lifter could use a weight rack to position the bar.)
- Grasp the bar with hands slightly farther apart than shoulder width.
- Your hands should be evenly spaced in the grip. Use a wrap-around thumb grip.
- Slightly bend your knees. Lean forward by bending at the waist.
- Continue downward. Bend until your back is parallel to the floor. Keep your back and feet flat.
- Slowly return to the starting position. Maintain control and speed.
- Continue the reps. Have spotters remove the bar at the completion of the reps.

Back Squat
Body area: *front upper leg*
Muscles: *quadriceps, gluteals, hamstrings*
Variation: *leg press (machine)*
Caution: *Spotters and squat rack recommended; weight belt required*

- The bar should be positioned on the rack about shoulder high.
- Your hands should be slightly farther apart than your shoulders.
- Your hands should be evenly spaced. Use a wraparound thumb grip.

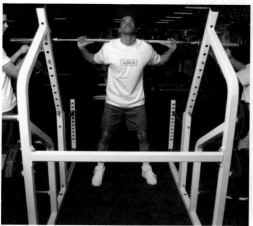
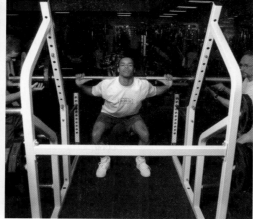
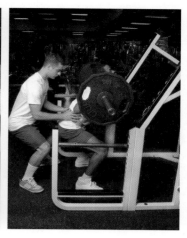

▲ Back Squat

- Position your shoulders, hips, and feet under the bar.
- Place the bar across your shoulders (not on your neck).
- Pull your shoulders back. Straighten your back and raise your chest, with your head up.
- Begin the lift by straightening your legs. (Spotters assist in removing the weight.)
- Take one step away from the rack, and assume shoulder-width stance.
- Your feet should be lined up evenly. Your weight should be evenly distributed on your feet.
- Stabilize the bar before starting the downward motion. (Spotters should release the bar.)
- Slowly bend your knees and lower your hips. Keep your back flat. Do not lean forward.
- Continue to lower the bar until your thighs (quadriceps) are parallel to the floor. Do not bounce or hesitate at the bottom.
- Your knees must stay lined up with your feet. Do not let them point in or out.
- Your heels must stay on the floor. Do not lean forward on your toes.
- Lift the bar by straightening your legs and hips.
- Your head and eyes are up, your knees are aligned with your toes, and your back is flat.
- Your feet are flat, with weight slightly more on the heels.
- Exhale during the lifting stage near the top of the lift.
- Slowly return to the starting position. Maintain control and speed.
- Continue the reps. Replace the bar on the rack. Never release your grip until the bar is safely in the rack. (Spotters should assist in replacing the bar.)

▼ Leg Press (Machine)

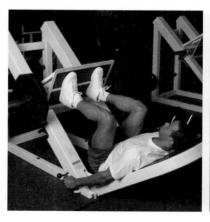
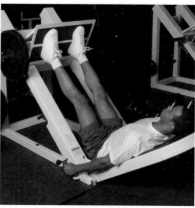

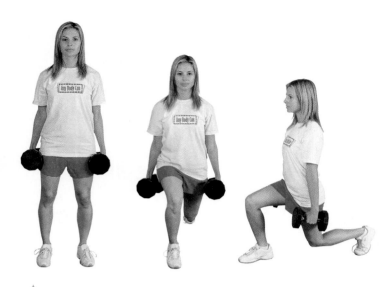

Lunge (Free Weight)

Lunge

Body area: *leg*
Muscles: *quadriceps, gluteals, hamstrings*
Variation: *straight bar*
Caution: *spotters recommended*

- Assume shoulder-width stance, with feet flat on the floor and back straight.
- Bend your knees and waist to place your hands on the dumbbells. Fully extend your arms and grasp the dumbbells with a wraparound grip.
- Your hands should be slightly farther apart than your shoulders.
- Return to a standing position.
- Take one big step directly forward with your right leg.
- Your right foot should hit heel first and go to a flat position.
- Bend your right knee slowly so your thigh is parallel to the floor. Your right knee should not go beyond your toes.
- Your left knee should bend slightly, but not touch the floor.
- Your back should remain straight. Do not lean forward or bend at the waist.
- Return to the starting position by pushing back with your right leg.
- Exhale during the push stage. Do not hold your breath.
- Hesitate at the starting position. Then repeat the same task with your left leg.
- At the completion of the reps, return the dumbbells to the rack.

Leg Curl (Machine)

Body area: *upper back leg*
Muscles: *hamstring*

- Lie facedown on the bench (machine).
- Keep your hips, legs, and chest flat on the bench.
- Your kneecaps should be past the end of the bench.
- Your hands should grasp the bench handles.
- Position the backs of your ankles on the roller pad.
- Begin the lift by flexing your knees. Raise the pad to your buttocks.
- Your hips must remain in contact with the bench.
- Exhale during the pull stage. Do not hold your breath.
- Slowly lower the roller pad to the starting position and continue the reps.

▶ **Leg Curl (Machine)**

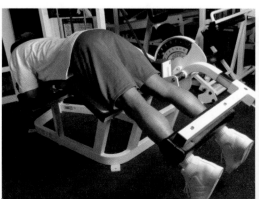
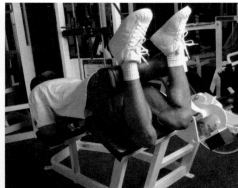

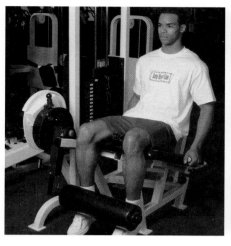
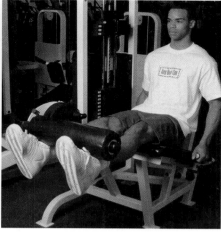

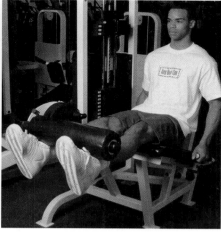
Leg Extension (Machine)

Leg Extension (Machine)
Body area: *front upper leg*
Muscles: *quadriceps*

- Sit in an upright position on the bench with your head up.
- Your back is flat, and your grip is on the handles.
- Place your upper ankles under the roller pad.
- Raise the roller pad by extending your legs at the knee.
- Extend your legs completely, and hold for 2 counts.
- Exhale during the push stage. Do not hold your breath.
- Slowly lower the pad to the starting position.
- Your back and buttocks must stay in contact with the bench.
- Continue the reps.

Standing Heel Raise
Body area: *lower leg*
Muscles: *gastrocnemius*

- The bar should be positioned on the rack about shoulder height.
- Your grip width should be slightly wider than your shoulder width.
- Your hands should be evenly spaced in the grip. Use a wraparound thumb grip.
- Place the bar across your shoulders (not on your neck).
- Your feet should be 8 to 10 inches apart. Place the balls of your feet on a raised surface 1½ to 2 inches high.
- Lock out your knees (straight not flexed).
- Push up on your toes to raise your heels to their highest position.
- Exhale during the push stage. Do not hold your breath.
- Slowly lower your heels until they touch the floor, and continue the reps.
- Replace the bar in the rack.

▼ Standing Heel Raise

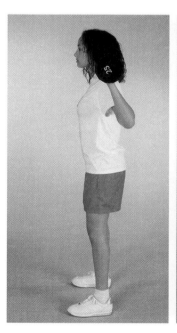
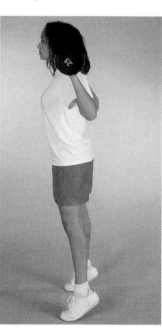

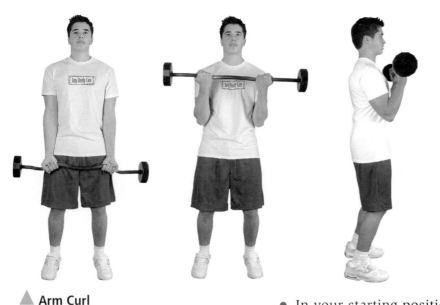

Arm Curl

Body area: *front of upper arm*
Muscles: *biceps*
Variation: *dumbbells*

- Assume shoulder-width stance, with feet flat on the floor.
- Bend your knees, not your waist, to place your hands on the bar.
- Your grip should be the width of your hips.
- Your grip should be evenly spaced. Use a wraparound thumb grip, with palms up.
- Keep your back flat, and straighten your legs to stand up.
- In your starting position, your knees should be slightly bent and your arms fully extended in front.
- Keep your elbows in a stationary position at your side.
- Raise the bar by flexing your arms at the elbows. Raise the bar until your upper and lower arms are squeezed together.
- Keep your back flat and straight. Do not swing your body.
- Exhale during the lifting stage. Do not hold your breath.
- Slowly lower the bar to the starting position. Continue the reps.

▲ Arm Curl

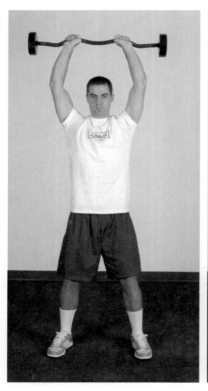
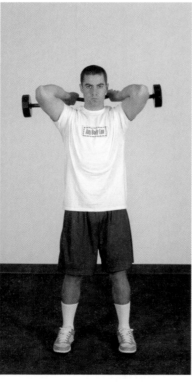

Triceps Extension

Body area: *back of upper arm*
Muscles: *triceps*
Variation: *dumbbells*

- Assume shoulder-width stance, with feet flat on the floor.
- Bend your knees, not your waist, to place your hands on the bar.
- Your grip should be 6 inches apart in the middle of the bar. Use a wraparound thumb grip.
- Keep your back flat, and straighten your legs to stand up.
- Raise the bar over your head, with arms fully extended and knees slightly bent.
- The area from the shoulder to the elbow should stay in this position throughout the exercise.

▲ Triceps Extension

- Slowly lower the bar to the back of your neck by bending your arms at the elbows.
- Keep your elbows close to your head and near your ears.
- When the bar touches the back of your neck, return the bar to the overhead position by straightening your arms.
- Do not allow your elbows to move away from your ears.
- Exhale during the pushing stage. Do not hold your breath.
- Continue the reps.

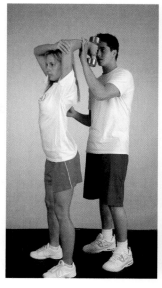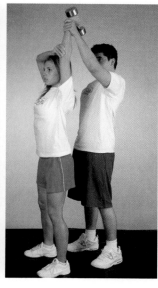

▲ **Variation of Triceps Extension (Dumbbells)**

Dumbbell Kickback
Body area: *back of upper arm*
Muscles: *triceps*

- Assume shoulder-width stance, with feet flat on the floor and knees slightly bent.
- Bend over at the waist until your upper body is parallel to the floor.
- Extend one arm, and place your hand on a bench or chair for balance.
- Place the dumbbell in your other hand. Use a wraparound thumb grip, with your palm facing your leg.
- Raise the dumbbell to your waist. Bend your arm at the elbow so that your upper arm is parallel to the floor and your lower arm is perpendicular to the floor.
- Straighten your elbow until your arm is straight. Do not move the position of your elbow in relation to your waist.
- Exhale during the lifting stage. Do not hold your breath.
- Slowly lower the dumbbell to the starting position. Do not swing your arm.
- Continue the reps, and then switch arms.

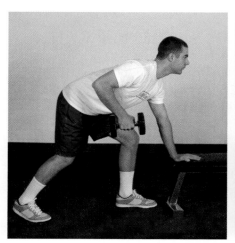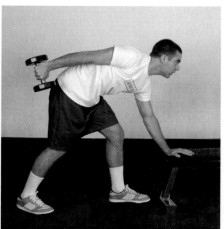

▲ **Dumbbell Kickback**

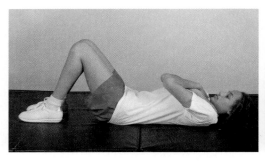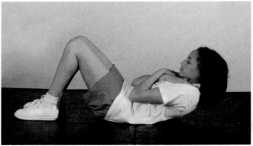

◢ **Abdominal Crunch**

Abdominal Crunch
Body area: *stomach*
Muscles: *abdominals*
Variations: *incline bench, raised feet, machines*

- Lie faceup on a mat or carpeted floor. Your back and buttocks should be flat on the surface.
- Your knees should be bent. Position your feet flat on the floor with your heels 12 to 18 inches from your buttocks.
- Place your hands and arms across your chest. Your hands should be placed near the opposite shoulders.
- Position your chin in a tucked position, allowing your chin to touch your chest.
- Contract your abdominal muscles and raise your torso until your elbows contact your upper thighs.
- Exhale when your elbows contact your thighs.
- Slowly return to the starting position. Do not let your chin lose contact with your chest. Your head should not touch the floor.
- Repeat the process until the reps are completed.

Twisting Abdominal Crunch
Body area: *stomach*
Muscles: *abdominals, obliques*
Variations: *incline bench, raised feet*

- Lie faceup on a mat or carpeted floor. Your back and buttocks should be flat on the surface.
- Your knees should be bent. Position your feet flat on the floor with your heels 12 to 18 inches from your buttocks.
- Place your hands and arms across your chest. Your hands should be placed near the opposite shoulders.
- Keep your chin in a tucked position, which allows your chin to touch your chest.
- Contract your abdominal muscles and raise your torso from the floor. Continue to raise your torso until your elbows are near your thighs.

- Twist your torso to the left and touch your right elbow to your left thigh. If possible, extend your right elbow past the left thigh.
- Exhale when your elbow contacts your thigh.
- Slowly return to the starting position. Do not let your chin lose contact with your chest. Your head should not touch the floor.
- Start the process again, but twist the torso to the right side, touching your left elbow to your right thigh.
- Slowly return to the starting position.
- Repeat the process until the reps are completed.

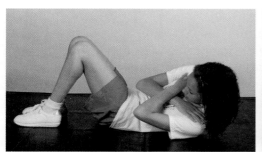
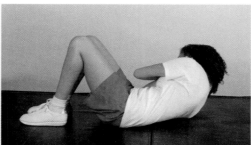

◀ Twisting Abdominal Crunch

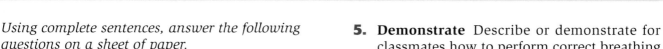

Lesson 1 Review

Using complete sentences, answer the following questions on a sheet of paper.

Reviewing Facts and Vocabulary

1. **Vocabulary** What is the purpose of *clips* in resistance-training safety? Name two other tips that ensure a safe workout.

2. **Recall** Why is proper grip important?

Thinking Critically

3. **Explain** Describe the proper etiquette for using a public weight room.

4. **Apply** Describe or demonstrate the proper procedure for gripping the bar when lifting weights.

5. **Demonstrate** Describe or demonstrate for classmates how to perform correct breathing and spotting techniques when lifting weights.

Personal Fitness Planning

Setting Goals Help a friend or family member determine and set his or her resistance-training goals. Remember to make the goals specific to the person's needs and to write them down. Then make a list of weight-lifting exercises you learned that will help him or her reach these goals. If you do not have access to weights, make a list of other resistance activities you could do together. Discuss how these activities can benefit your mutual health and fitness.

What You Will Do

- Identify components of a resistance-training workout.
- Participate in a variety of exercises that build muscular strength and endurance.
- Describe the exercises that target major muscles.
- Identify various strength-training circuits and explain what each accomplishes.

Terms to Know

repetition (rep)
set
exercise
circuit training
large muscle group
small muscle group

Planning Your Resistance-Training Workout

Imagine going into a weight room and choosing at random the exercises you will do and the equipment you will use. Probably, you would accomplish very little. To be effective, a workout needs to follow a careful plan. In this lesson, you will learn how to create a structured workout.

Components of the Workout

A successful weight-training workout consists of a number of components, or building blocks. These are shown in **Figure 10.3** and described below.

- **Repetition.** More commonly referred to simply as a **rep,** this is *one completion of an activity or exercise.* It is the most basic unit of a workout. A rep consists of lifting a weight and returning it to the starting position. So does doing the negative and positive phases of a push-up. The number of reps done for a particular exercise will vary, depending upon your goals.
- **Set.** A **set** is *a group of consecutive reps for any exercise.* If you do ten push-ups, one right after the other, you have done one set of ten reps. By repeating the process after a short rest of two minutes, you have completed a total of two sets. Like the number of repetitions, the number of sets will be determined by your goals.

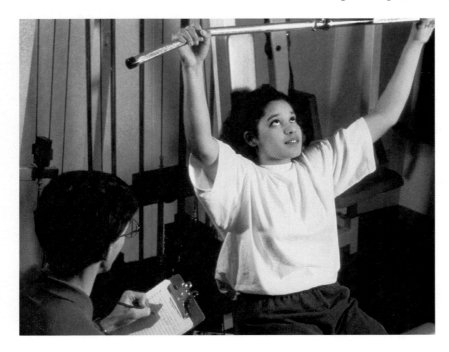

◀ Resistance training exercises target a specific body area. *What body area and muscle group is this teen working?*

- **Exercise.** In a typical workout, you will do several sets of several different exercises. An **exercise,** as the term is used in resistance training, is *a series of repetitive muscle contractions that build strength and endurance.* When the resistance force is movable—the case with free weights and weight machines—the exercise is said to be dynamic. Some of the more common dynamic resistance-training exercises are the bench press, squat, and arm curl. Other examples of resistance-training exercises that do not require free weights or a machine are calisthenic exercises, such as push-ups and pull-ups, in which you apply biomechanical force.
- **Body area.** Every exercise has as its primary target a muscle group within one of the six specific weight-training "body areas," as shown in **Figure 10.4.** The bench press, for example, is targeted primarily at muscles within the chest. Squats work muscles within the leg. The "Active Mind—Active Body" activity on page **298** will give you practice identifying which exercises work which muscle groups.

You cannot expect noticeable results after a single workout. It is only by working out consistently over the course of weeks and months that you will begin to realize a difference.

✔ Reading Check

Identify List and describe the components of a resistance workout.

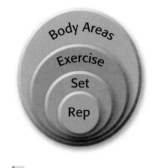

FIGURE 10.3

COMPONENTS OF A WORKOUT

The rep is the most basic component of a resistance-training program. *What is the term given to a series of consecutive reps?*

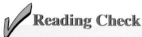

FIGURE 10.4

THE SIX MAJOR BODY AREAS

A workout will include exercises that work one or more of these body muscle areas. *Referring to Figure 9.3 on page 251, name one muscle in each body area.*

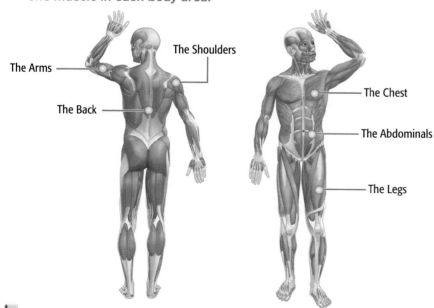

The Arms

The Shoulders

The Back

The Chest

The Abdominals

The Legs

Active Mind Active Body

Participating in Strength-Training Exercises

Can you name an exercise that will strengthen muscles in the upper legs? In the back? After completing this activity, you will be able to identify several exercises and the muscles they work.

What You Will Need

- Pen or pencil
- Paper

What You Will Do

1. Take a moment to identify the major muscle groups shown in **Figure 10.5** on pages **299–300**.
2. Next, copy the following table (which lists some of the more common weight-training exercises) onto a separate sheet of paper.
3. For each exercise, write the muscle group and body area that it targets. You may want to refer to **Figures 10.6** on page **301, 10.7** on page **302,** and **10.8** on page **303** as you complete the table.
4. Finally, attempt each of the exercises so you can feel in your own body

where the work is being done and how biomechanical force is applied. Follow the guidelines for weight-training exercises in Lesson 1 on pages **279–295** to help you prevent injuries.

Apply and Conclude

What similarities did you find among exercises that worked the same muscle groups? How did these activities differ from one another?

Exercise	Muscle Group	Body Area
1. bench press		
2. flat bench fly		
3. military press		
4. shoulder shrug		
5. upright row		
6. front, lateral, and bent-over shoulder raises		
7. bent-over row		
8. Lat pulldown		
9. straight-back good morning		
10. back squat		
11. lunge		
12. leg curl		
13. leg extension		
14. standing heel raise		
15. arm curl		
16. triceps extension		
17. abdominal crunch		

The Strength-Training Circuit

If you are a beginner to weight training, your goal should be to develop a well-designed resistance-training program for all areas of the body. The most efficient way of achieving this goal is through circuit training. Also known as following the strength-training circuit, this is *an approach to resistance training where you rotate from one exercise to the next in a particular sequence.* Training facilities that have a full set of weight machines often arrange these in a training circuit.

FIGURE 10.5

BODY AREAS

Many different types of exercises can be used to develop the same muscle area. *Which will you be including in your workout?*

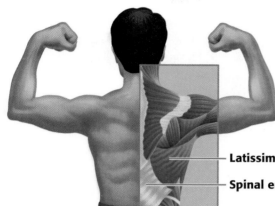

Latissimus dorsi

Spinal erectors

BACK

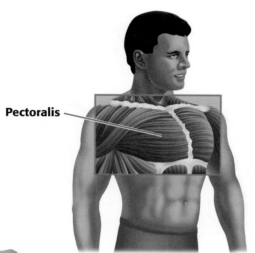

Pectoralis

CHEST

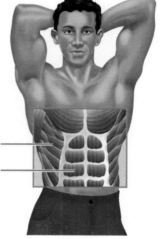

External obliques

Rectus abdominis

ABDOMINALS

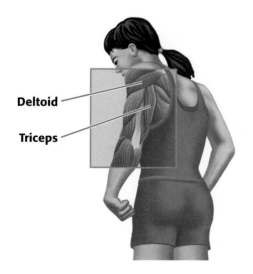

Deltoid

Triceps

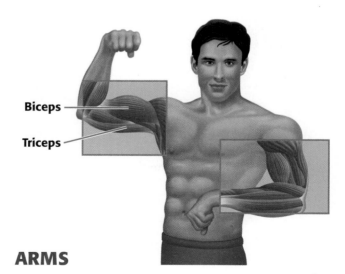

Biceps

Triceps

ARMS

continued on next page

FIGURE 10.5 *continued*

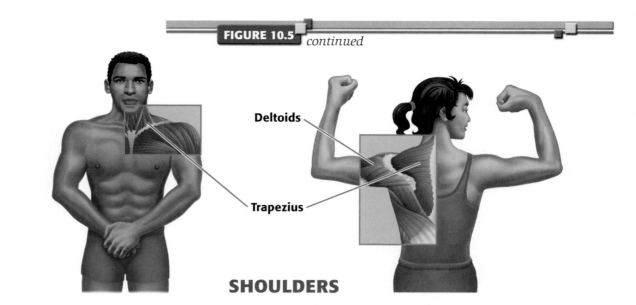

Deltoids

Trapezius

SHOULDERS

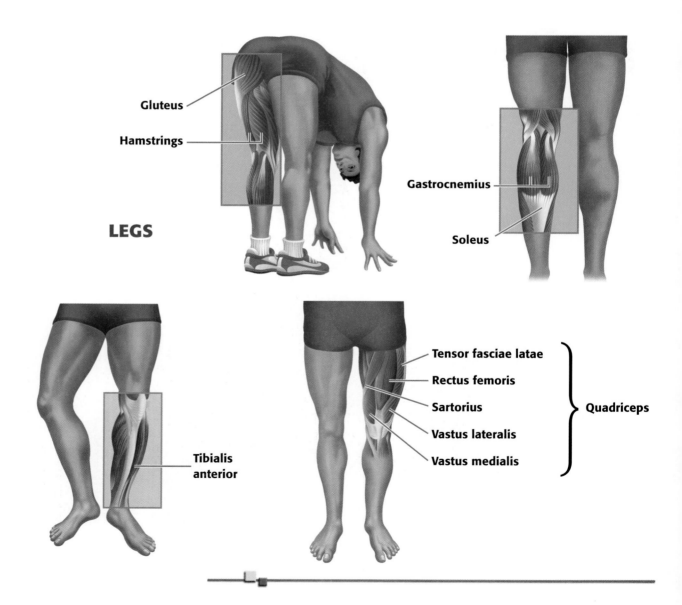

Gluteus

Hamstrings

Gastrocnemius

Soleus

LEGS

Tibialis anterior

Tensor fasciae latae

Rectus femoris

Sartorius

Vastus lateralis

Vastus medialis

Quadriceps

FIGURE 10.6

EXERCISES, MUSCLE GROUPS, EQUIPMENT, AND ACTIVITIES

Exercise	Primary muscle group	Secondary muscle group	Equipment	Sport in which performance is enhanced
Leg extension	Quadriceps		Machine	All activities or sports
Leg curl	Hamstrings	Gastrocnemius	Machine	All activities or sports
Heel raise	Gastrocnemius, soleus		Machine, barbell	All activities or sports
Leg press	Quadriceps, gluteals	Hamstring	Machine	All activities or sports
Lunge	Quadriceps, gluteals	Hamstring	Barbell, dumbbells	All activities or sports
Squat	Quadriceps, gluteals	Hamstring	Barbell	All activities or sports
Sit-ups	Iliopsoas	Abdominals	Floor machine	All activities or sports
Bench press	Pectoralis major, anterior triceps, deltoid	Spinal erectors	Barbell, bench, machine, dumbbells	Football, basketball, wrestling, shot put
Incline press	Anterior pectoralis major, deltoid, triceps		Barbell, dumbbells, incline bench, machine	Football, basketball, wrestling, shot put
Fly (supine)	Pectoralis major	Deltoid	Dumbbells, machine	Football, tennis, discus throw, baseball, softball, wrestling, backstroke
Overhead press	Deltoid, triceps	Trapezius	Barbell, dumbbells, machine	Gymnastics, shot put
Bent-over rowing	Latissimus dorsi, rhomboids	Deltoid, biceps	Barbell, dumbbells, pulley machine	Wrestling, rowing, baseball, basketball
Upright rowing	Trapezius	Deltoid, biceps	Barbell, dumbbells, pulley machine	All activities or sports
Lat pull-down	Latissimus dorsi	Biceps	Pulley machine	Basketball, baseball, swimming, tennis, volleyball, wrestling
Good morning	Spinal erector		Barbell	All activities or sports
Front shoulder raise	Anterior deltoid		Barbell, dumbbells	All activities or sports
Bent-over lateral raise	Posterior deltoid	Rhomboids, latissimus dorsi	Dumbbells, machine	All activities or sports
Lateral shoulder raise	Deltoid	Trapezius	Dumbbells, machine	All activities or sports
Shoulder shrug	Trapezius		Barbell, dumbbells, machine	All activities or sports
Arm curl	Biceps	Forearm muscles	Barbell, dumbbells, pulley machine	All activities or sports
French press	Triceps		Barbell, dumbbells, pulley machine	All activities or sports

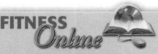
Variations on the Circuit

Today Brian and Jorge both worked on legs. Both used the same equipment during their sessions. However, Brian, who plays soccer, began his workout with squats to develop his thigh muscles. Jorge, who is on the school cross-country team, started with heel raises to build his calf muscles.

As Brian and Jorge's weight room preferences illustrate, circuit training can be customized to meet individual needs. Choosing a variation designed for your personal goals can help you maintain proper intensity for target muscles. It also helps you make the most of your workout time.

The following are three common variations used in circuit training. The remainder of this lesson will explore these approaches.

Training Large Muscle Groups Before Small Muscle Groups. Like Brian, many people who train with weights prefer to work large muscle groups—such as those in the upper leg—before small ones.

- **Large muscle group.** This term designates *any group of muscles of large size as well as any large number of muscles being used at one time.* Examples of large muscle groups are those of the upper legs, chest, and back.
- **Small muscle group.** This term designates *any group of muscles of small size as well as any small number of muscles being used at one time.* Examples of small muscle groups are those of the arms and lower legs.

One advantage of this approach is that large muscle groups require more strength, energy, and mental concentration. You have only limited amounts of each of these resources. Working the large muscles first allows you to make the most of them.

FIGURE 10.7

CIRCUIT TRAINING: LARGE MUSCLES BEFORE SMALL MUSCLES

A bench press, which works the chest muscle (pectoralis), uses the small muscle in the back of the upper arm (triceps). *Which exercise does the chart recommend doing first? Why?*

Exercise Order	Muscle Type	Muscle Groups
1. Squat	Large	Thigh and hips (quadriceps)
2. Heel raise	Small	Calf (gastrocnemius)
3. Bench press	Large	Chest (pectoralis)
4. Triceps extension	Small	Upper arm, back (triceps)
5. Bent-over row	Large	Back (latissimus dorsi)
6. Arm curl	Small	Upper arm, front (biceps)

FIGURE 10.8

CIRCUIT TRAINING: PUSH AND PULL EXERCISES

This chart shows one approach to alternating push- and pull-type exercises. *What is an advantage of following this strategy?*

Exercise Order	Exercise Type	Muscle Groups
1. Leg press	Push	Thigh-front (quadriceps)
2. Leg curl	Pull	Thigh-back (hamstring)
3. Bench press	Push	Chest (pectoralis)
4. Bent-over row	Pull	Back (latissimus dorsi)
5. Military press	Push	Shoulder (deltoid)
6. Arm curl	Pull	Upper arm, front (biceps)
7. Triceps extension	Push	Upper arm, back (triceps)

In addition, small muscle groups often play a supporting role in large muscle group exercises. If these small muscle groups become fatigued, completing the large muscle exercises will be more difficult.

Figure 10.7 shows a sample circuit in which large muscle-group exercises precede those for small muscle groups.

Alternating Push Exercises with Pull Exercises. A second variation on the training circuit is to alternate pulling motions (flexing) with pushing motions (extension). This approach gives the muscles extra time to recover between sets. Another benefit of this approach is that it keeps opposing muscles balanced.

Figure 10.8 shows a method for organizing the strength-training circuit in terms of push and pull exercises. **Figure 10.9** gives an example of how opposite muscles are worked in the push-pull model of the circuit.

Alternating Upper-Body Exercises with Lower-Body Exercises. A third variation of circuit training alternates exercises for the upper body (waist and above) with an exercise for the lower body (hips and below). This method allows muscles more recovery time, but it is more difficult than the other circuit-training options previously discussed.

Workouts alternating upper- and lower-body muscles require an equal number of upper- and lower-body exercises. This means doing two to three more leg exercises than in the two previous types of workouts. These additional leg exercises require more energy, making the workout more difficult. This type of alternating plan is, however, a suitable plan for the individual wanting to perform a higher-intensity leg workout. **Figure 10.10** shows an example of how to organize upper- and lower-body exercises in your workout.

FIGURE 10.9

THE ARM MUSCLES: PUSHING AND PULLING

The triceps create force by pushing and the biceps create force by pulling. *What other pairs of muscles could benefit from a push and pull circuit?*

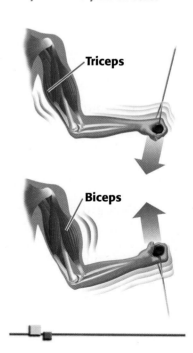

Triceps

Biceps

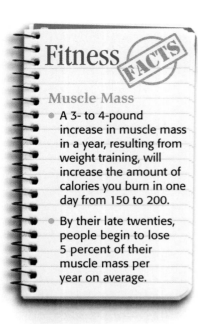

FIGURE 10.10

UPPER-BODY AND LOWER-BODY EXERCISES

Alternating upper-body exercises with lower-body exercises allows muscles more recovery time. *Why is this more difficult than other training circuits?*

Exercise Order	Muscle Type	Muscle Groups
1. Military press	Upper	Shoulder (deltoid)
2. Leg extension	Lower	Thigh (quadriceps)
3. Back lat pull	Upper	Back (latissimus dorsi)
4. Lunge	Lower	Thigh and hip (quadriceps/gluteals)
5. Arm curl	Upper	Upper arm-front (biceps)
6. Leg press	Lower	Thigh-front (quadriceps)

Weakest Muscles Before Strongest Muscles. A final way to order your exercise regimen is to work the weakest muscle first. This approach is adopted commonly by athletes whose muscles have atrophied slightly following an injury. By working a weak muscle when your energy level is at its peak, you can get the muscle back in shape more quickly.

Lesson 2 Review

Using complete sentences, answer the following questions on a sheet of paper.

Reviewing Facts and Vocabulary

1. **Vocabulary** What is a group of *repetitions* called?

2. **Recall** What is *circuit training*?

Thinking Critically

3. **Recognize** Robert is concerned about the lack of muscular development in his legs. What small and large muscle-group exercises should he include in his workout?

4. **Synthesize** Melody, who is a dancer, would like to improve her muscle endurance. List the specific body areas you think she should work and identify the type of circuit you would recommend for her.

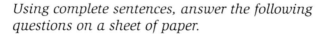

Personal Fitness Planning

Developing Muscular Strength Choose one of the strength-training circuits described in this lesson that best fits your training needs. Extend the circuit by adding at least two more exercises. Under the supervision of your coach or a professional trainer, try this circuit using light weights. Take note of how many sets and reps you did, indicating the weight used.

Applying FITT to Resistance Training

A carefully planned resistance-training program is necessary for building muscular strength and endurance. As you learned in Chapter 3, FITT factors must be properly adjusted in order to achieve your fitness goals. *FITT*, you will recall, stands for *frequency, intensity, time,* and *type.* In order to improve your muscular strength and endurance through a program of resistance training, you must first establish your resistance FITT.

Frequency

Frequency in weight training is how often you work out. For training to succeed, your time between workouts must be measured in days—not weeks. There are no easy shortcuts to muscular fitness. If, for example, you work out only once a week, you will not see any significant gains in your muscular fitness.

What You Will Do

- Apply the physiological principles of frequency, intensity, and time to resistance training.
- Apply intensity to your program by determining your training load.
- Keep accurate records detailing your resistance-training progress.

Terms to Know

total-body workout
split workout
training load
one-rep maximum (1RM)
recovery time
resistance-training cycles

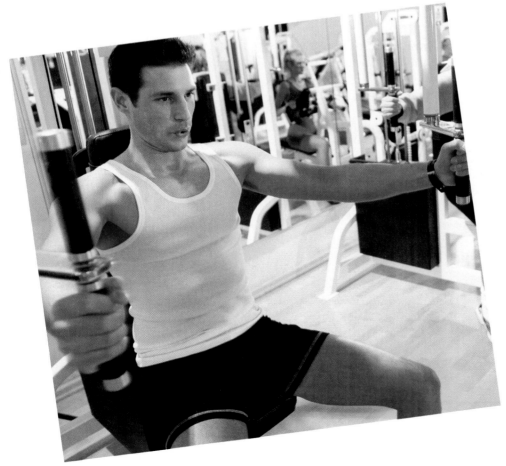

◀ Adjusting FITT factors is necessary to achieve resistance-training goals. *What does FITT stand for?*

As with recovery time, workout frequency requires careful tracking. During an effective workout, your muscles become overloaded. Afterward, they need 48 to 72 hours of rest. Any less, and the muscles won't have a chance to repair themselves. Any more, and the strength training benefits start to diminish.

Most training authorities recommend working out three or four times a week on nonsuccessive days. The following are two popular strategies.

Three-Days-a-Week, Total-Body Workout

A total-body workout is *one in which all major muscle groups are worked three times a week, with at least one day off between workouts.* This is the most popular plan for beginners. It allows for all muscles to receive plenty of work, while at the same time allowing for plenty of rest. **Figure 10.11** shows a three-day, total-body workout.

Four-Days-a-Week, Split Workout

More advanced resistance training requires a split-workout schedule, shown in **Figure 10.12.** A split workout does not work every muscle group at every session. Instead, you *exercise three or four body areas at each session, working at much higher intensities.* You do three or four different exercises per body area and three or four sets for each exercise. Because this places greater demands on your muscles, more recovery time is needed before the same muscle group is worked again.

 Reading Check

Analyze Considering your experience with weights, how frequently should you work out?

FIGURE 10.11

SAMPLE—THREE DAYS, TOTAL BODY

Gill has band practice every Wednesday after school. *How could Gill adjust his workout schedule so that he could get his three sessions in?*

Monday:	Thursday:
Workout	Off
Tuesday:	Friday:
Off	Workout
Wednesday:	Saturday/Sunday:
Workout	Off

FIGURE 10.12

SAMPLE—FOUR DAYS, SPLIT WORKOUT

Examine this schedule. *How much rest time does each group of muscles receive before it is worked again?*

Monday:	**Thursday:**
Chest, Shoulders, Triceps, Abs	Repeat Monday's workout
Tuesday:	**Friday:**
Back, Legs, Biceps, Abs	Repeat Tuesday's workout
Wednesday:	**Saturday/Sunday:**
Rest!	Rest!

Intensity

Intensity, as the term is used in weight training, is the amount of exertion or tension placed on a muscle group. Several factors play a role in determining your training-intensity needs. These are:

- The amount of weight you will lift
- The number of reps and sets you will do
- How many different exercises you will perform per body area

The Amount of Weight

Training load refers to *how much weight you should lift for a given exercise.* This is the single most important factor in your *FITT.* To determine your training load, you must determine your **one-rep maximum (1RM)** for each exercise you plan to do. 1RM is *a measure of a lifter's **absolute muscular strength** for any given exercise.* There are several tests you can do to compute your 1RM. One involves doing one or two reps of the exercise, increasing the weight gradually until you "max out," or cannot complete the lift.

Inexperienced lifters who have not yet mastered proper technique are not advised to do 1RM tests. A safer alternative is finding your *estimated one-rep maximum.* The procedure for this is described in the Fitness Check on pages **308–309.**

Reasons for Testing. First, pretests can be used to determine your training load. Beginners should use 50 to 60 percent of their one-rep maximum, whereas conditioned weight trainers may want to use 75 to 85 percent of their maximum. (See **Figure 10.14** on page **310** to determine your training load). Second, muscular fitness tests help identify strengths and weaknesses, which you can then take into consideration when designing your weight-training program. Finally, these evaluations will help you keep track of your progress—a great motivator for your future workouts.

hot link

absolute muscular strength
For more on absolute muscular strength and what it represents, see Chapter 9, page **247.**

Determining Intensity: One-Repetition Maximum and Relative Muscular Strength

In this activity, you will learn how to compute an estimated one-rep maximum and then use that information to calculate your relative muscular strength.

One-Repetition Maximum

You will determine your estimated 1RM for these exercises: *bench press, squat, military press, biceps curl,* and *bent-over row.* Remember to warm up before you start. Have a spotter assist you with all lifts.

Procedure:

1. Divide a sheet of paper into four columns. In the first column write the name of each of the five exercises listed above. Leave a line or so of space after each exercise.
2. Starting with the bench press, choose a weight with which you can safely perform 6 to 10 repetitions. Write this weight on the appropriate line in the second column.
3. Complete as many full reps of the exercise as you can. Record the number of completed reps in the third column. *Do not count partial reps.*
4. Using **Figure 10.13,** find the column for the amount of reps you completed. Then look down the column to find the amount of weight you lifted. For example, if you completed 7–8 reps, you would use the second column.
5. Read across to the far right column and record the number. This is your estimated 1RM for the bench press. For example, if you lifted 105 pounds 7–8 times, your 1RM is 130.
6. Repeat this procedure for the remaining four exercises.

9-10 Reps Pounds Lifted (70% of Max.)	7–8 Reps Pounds Lifted (80% of Max.)	6 Reps Pounds Lifted (90% of Max.)	1RM Pounds Lifted (100% of Max.)
40	45	50	60
50	55	60	70
55	65	70	80
65	70	75	90
70	80	85	100
75	90	95	110
85	95	100	120
90	105	110	130
100	115	120	140
105	120	130	150
110	130	135	160
120	135	145	170
125	145	155	180
135	150	160	190
140	160	170	200
150	170	180	210
155	175	185	220
160	185	195	230
170	190	205	240
175	200	210	250

Figure 10.13

Calculating Your Relative Muscular Strength

In this activity you will learn how to calculate your relative muscular strength by using your 1RM.

Procedure:

1. Divide a sheet of paper into five columns. In the first column write the name of each of the five exercises listed above.
2. Starting with the bench press, write the weight of your 1RM in the second column.
3. In the third column record your body weight.
4. In the fourth column record the number you get when you divide your body weight into your 1RM.
5. Use the number you got from step 4 and refer to the Fitness Ratings charts at right to determine your relative strength for the bench press. Example: if your number from step 4 was 1.14 and you are a male, your relative strength was average.
6. Repeat this procedure for the remaining four exercises.

Fitness Ratings: Relative Strength (Males)

Relative Strength Rating	Bench Press	Squat	Military Press	Biceps Curl	Bent-over Row
Outstanding	> 1.29	> 1.84	> .99	> .64	> .94
Good	1.15–1.29	1.65–1.84	.90–.99	.55–.64	.85–.94
Average	1.0–1.14	1.30–1.64	.75–.89	.45–.54	.75–.84
Below Average	.85–.99	1.0–1.29	.60–.74	.35–.44	.65–.74
Needs Work	< .85	< 1.0	< .60	< .34	< .64

Fitness Ratings: Relative Strength (Females)

Relative Strength Rating	Bench Press	Squat	Military Press	Biceps Curl	Bent-over Row
Outstanding	> .85	> 1.45	> .50	> .45	> .55
Good	.70–.84	1.30–1.44	.42–.49	.38–.44	.45–.54
Average	.60–.69	1.0–1.29	.32–.41	.32–.37	.35–.44
Below Average	.50–.59	.80–.99	.25–.31	.25–.31	.25–.34
Needs Work	< .50	< .80	< .25	< .25	< .25

Training Load. When you have computed or estimated your 1RM, you can use the results to determine your training load. Training load is expressed as a percentage of your 1RM. Beginners should use 50 to 60 percent of their 1RM. Experienced and conditioned lifters will use a training load that is 75 to 85 percent of their 1RM. **Figure 10.14** shows training loads within this range. The chart covers lifts of up to 350 pounds.

FIGURE 10.14

TRAINING LOADS

Your training load is determined by your 1RM. Beginners should work at 50 to 60 percent of their 1RM. *What would the training load be for a beginning weight trainer with a one-rep maximum of 70?*

1RM	50%	60%	70%	75%	80%	85%	90%
30	15	18	21	23	24	26	27
40	20	24	28	30	32	34	36
50	25	30	35	38	40	43	45
60	30	36	42	45	48	51	54
70	35	42	49	52	56	60	63
80	40	48	56	60	64	68	72
90	45	54	63	68	72	77	81
100	50	60	70	75	80	85	90
110	55	66	77	83	88	94	99
120	60	72	84	90	96	102	108
130	65	78	91	98	104	111	117
140	70	84	98	105	112	119	125
150	75	90	105	113	120	128	135
160	80	96	112	120	128	136	144
170	85	102	119	128	136	145	153
180	90	108	126	135	144	153	162
190	95	114	133	143	152	162	171
200	100	120	140	150	160	170	180
210	105	126	147	158	168	179	189
220	110	132	154	165	176	187	198
230	115	138	161	173	184	196	207
240	120	144	168	180	192	204	216
250	125	150	175	188	200	213	225
260	130	156	182	195	208	221	234
270	135	162	189	203	216	230	243
280	140	168	196	210	224	238	252
290	145	174	203	218	232	247	261
300	150	180	210	225	240	255	270
310	155	186	217	233	248	264	279
320	160	192	224	240	256	272	288
330	165	198	231	248	264	281	297
340	170	204	238	255	272	289	306
350	175	210	245	263	280	298	316

FIGURE 10.15

RECOMMENDATIONS FOR TRAINING GOALS: SETS AND REPS

Some fitness goals are more challenging than others. *Which of the goals shown do you think would be the most challenging?*

Training Goal	Number of Sets and Reps
➤ Fitness and Toning	1–3 Sets of 8–12 Reps
➤ Endurance	2–3 Sets of 12–20+ Reps
➤ Strength	3–5 Sets of 2–6 Reps
➤ Muscle Mass	3–5 Sets of 6–12 Reps

The Number of Reps and Sets

How many reps and sets you do is mainly a function of your fitness goals. Begin by asking yourself what you want to accomplish. Is your goal simply to develop basic muscle fitness? Is it to increase endurance? To add bulk? Maybe it is some combination of these. The chart in **Figure 10.15** shows different training goals and the recommended number of sets and reps for each.

The Variety of Exercises

The more exercises you do to work a body area, the greater the intensity of a workout. Again, your training goals should be the guiding factor. If your goal, for example, is maintaining muscle fitness and overall health, one or two different exercises per body area are enough. Athletes, power lifters, and body builders, by contrast, will do three or four different exercises per body area.

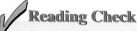 **Reading Check**

Summarize Identify the three factors that shape your resistance-training intensity.

Time

The most important aspect of *time,* as a component of resistance training, is **recovery time.** This is *the duration of the rest periods taken between workout components.* In general, the greater the amount of resistance, the more time your muscles need to recover.

No rest should be taken between reps, which are done in a controlled, continuous fashion. The following are guidelines for recovery time between sets and exercises.

STRESS BREAK
Varying Your Training

A regular resistance-training program can help to reduce feelings of stress in your daily life. However, this benefit will be lost if you become bored with your routine. Varying your exercises, sets, and workout days can help you avoid boredom.

You can also make your program more interesting by adding other types of resistance exercises, such as push-ups, bar dips, chin-ups, or isometrics. Keep your workouts fresh. Don't be afraid to throw in some variety.

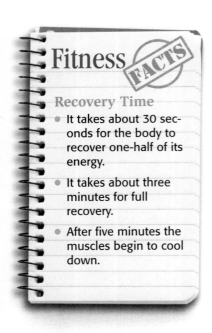

- **Recovery time between reps.** There should be no time between reps. They should be continuous and controlled.
- **Recovery time between sets.** This depends on your weight-training goals. The chart in **Figure 10.16** will give you some specifics.
- **Recovery time between exercises.** This depends on the type of training circuit you are following. The alternating push-pull variation and upper-lower body variation requires $1\frac{1}{2}$ to 2 minutes of recovery time. The large muscle/small muscle variation requires 2 to $2\frac{1}{2}$ minutes.
- **Recovery time between cycles.** Athletes or competitive lifters do not train the same way year-round. Instead, they follow resistance-training cycles. These are *modified programs, designed to meet the needs of off-season, pre-season, and in-season.* Your personal health and fitness resistance-training routine will also require modifications (cycles) throughout the year. You should change your exercises, sets, and workout days to prevent boredom.

Always time your rest periods carefully. Never exceed five minutes. If you do, your muscles will begin to cool down. Allowing too little time will overtax your muscles. Either way you increase your risk of injury.

 Reading Check

Explain Which types of training require the longest rests between exercises? Which require the shortest rests?

FIGURE 10.16

RECOMMENDATIONS FOR TRAINING GOALS: RECOVERY TIME

Find your training goals in the chart. *How much recovery time should you allow between sets?*

Training Goal	Recovery Time
➤ Fitness and Toning	$1\frac{1}{2}$ to 2 minutes
➤ Endurance	30 seconds to 1 minute
➤ Strength	2 to 5 minutes
➤ Muscle Mass	30 seconds to $1\frac{1}{2}$ minutes
➤ Power	3 to 5 minutes

Arnold Schwarzenegger

A Fitness Role Model

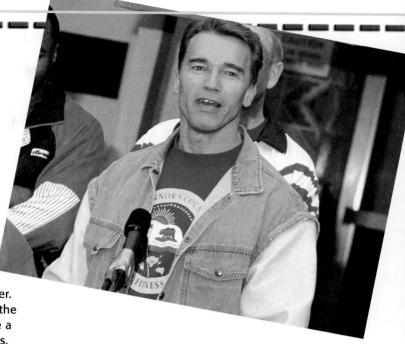

In 1997 at age 49, Arnold Schwarzenegger's peers proclaimed him the greatest bodybuilder of the twentieth century. Schwarzenegger was pleased. Yet, as Arnold will be the first to tell you, there is more to being a big person than having big muscles.

Arnold was born in Austria in 1947. At age 15, he began weight training to strengthen his legs for soccer. He saw results quickly and spent even more time in the weight room. Arnold soon gave up soccer to become a bodybuilder. By 17, he had won his first of many titles.

In the early 1970s, Arnold entered a second career—movie actor. One of his first films, *Pumping Iron,* was the story of a bodybuilder. Audiences loved Arnold. His image began to have a profound impact on how people viewed the benefits of a healthy, fit body.

Off-screen, Arnold has followed up his actions with his words. He has been an outspoken advocate on the benefits of staying fit *and* staying in school. As Chairperson of the President's Council on Physical Fitness, he has delivered his message in all 50 states. He has also assisted in programs to encourage urban youth to stay off the street and to choose athletics as a positive alternative to drugs and violence.

Not everybody can be an award-winning bodybuilder or movie star like Arnold Schwarzenegger. However, Any Body Can learn to be a confident and goal-oriented advocate of physical activity and fitness.

Research

As Arnold Schwarzenegger's example shows, he believes in giving something back to the community. Using print or online resources, learn about the Special Olympics and its goals as well as Arnold's role in this important organization.

Type

Type or mode of resistance training, as it is often referred to, is the specific activities and equipment you might choose to use for your resistance program. This chapter has referred mainly to the use of free weights or weight machines. There are alternative resistance-training programs discussed in Chapter 9, Lesson 4.

Keeping a Workout Record

Today, Jared knows he is supposed to work out but can't remember which body area he should be exercising. Pitfalls like Jared's are easy to avoid. All it takes is keeping accurate records.

FIGURE 10.17

SAMPLE WORKOUT RECORD

In this sample record, *S* stands for sets, *R* for reps, and *Wt* for weight.
What exercises would you include if this were your workout record?

	Date: 10/10			Date: 10/12			Date: 10/14			Date:		
	S	R	Wt	S	R	Wt	S	R	Wt	S	R	Wt
Bench Press	2	10	110	3	10	110	2	11	112			
Incline Press	1	10	90	1	10	90	2	11	90			
Military Press	2	10	40	2	10	40	2	8	50			

Your workout record might resemble the one shown in **Figure 10.17.** Regardless of how you organize your record, be sure to include the date and all the exercises you completed, including the sets and reps.

Other items to consider might include:

- Rest between sets and exercise
- Order of exercises
- Illness and days missed
- Body weight changes
- Nutrition habits

Keeping a record of your workouts helps you avoid forgetting what you did earlier, but it also helps you determine which exercises and training methods work best for you. Also, noting the progress you have made is a great motivator.

Lesson 3 Review

Using complete sentences, answer the following questions on a sheet of paper.

Reviewing Facts and Vocabulary

1. **Vocabulary** What does *1RM* measure?
2. **Recall** What is *recovery time?*
3. **Recall** How does a split workout differ from a total-body workout?

Thinking Critically

4. **Evaluate** Eve's training goal is to improve her fitness and toning. Devise a program that will help her meet her goals. Include details about frequency, intensity, and time of workouts.
5. **Synthesize** Roberto has just begun lifting weights and wants to increase his intensity.

Describe the method he should use for evaluating his relative muscular strength and determining his training load.

Personal Fitness Planning

Keeping Records Design a personalized record-keeping chart. You may either use the model in **Figure 10.17** or create one of your own. If you have already begun a program of resistance training, complete the first entry of your chart for your most recent workout. If you have not begun training, set your chart aside so that you can begin completing it once you start.

Achieving Muscular Fitness

What You Will Do

- Identify the basic eight free-weight routine.
- Identify various programs designed for building strength and power.
- Design and implement resistance programs for strength, power, and muscle mass.

Terms to Know

pyramid training
multiple sets
negative reps
supersets
compound sets
multiple hypertrophy sets

So far, you have learned how to set resistance-training goals. You have also learned how to structure your workouts in a way that achieves your goals. Now it is time to put what you have learned into practice.

The remainder of this lesson will focus on specific training goals. It will also detail exercise programs that can be used to achieve each.

The Basic Resistance Fitness Program

If you have no previous resistance-training experience, your goals should be improving muscle tone and general fitness. Basic resistance-training goals are shown in **Figure 10.18.** A program, known as the "basic eight," can help you reach these goals. The eight exercises in the program work the entire body. They also take relatively little time and a minimum of equipment.

The most popular version of the basic eight is done three times a week, using free weights, one to three sets per exercise. However, variations of these exercises are acceptable as you progress. These are shown in **Figure 10.19,** page **316.**

FIGURE 10.18

TRAINING GOALS AT A GLANCE
This chart shows four main training goals, along with requirements in each category. *Which of these goals is closest to your own?*

Goals	Training Load	Reps	Sets	Recovery Time
Strength	85%–95%	2–6	3–5	2–4 minutes
Hypertrophy	70%–80%	6–12	3–6	30–90 seconds
Endurance	50%–70%	12–20+	2–3	30–60 seconds
Fitness and Toning	60%–80%	8–12	1–3	30–60 seconds

FIGURE 10.19

BASIC EIGHT PROGRAM WITH FREE WEIGHTS

Note that these exercises can also be done with weight machines or exercise bands. *How would you go about determining the number of sets and reps of each exercise you would do?*

Body Area	Exercise/ Technique	Variation/ Technique	Equipment
Chest	Bench Press	Incline Press	Barbell/ Dumbbell
Back	One-arm Dumbbell Row	Bent-over Row	Barbell/ Dumbbell
Shoulder	Military Press	Seated or Standing	Barbell/ Dumbbell
Biceps	Arm Curl	Seated or Standing	Barbell/ Dumbbell
Triceps	Triceps Extension	Triceps Kickbacks	Barbell/ Dumbbell
Thighs	Squats	Lunges	Barbell/ Dumbbell
Calves	Heel Raises	One-leg or Two-leg	Barbell/ Dumbbell
Abdominals	Crunch	Twisting Crunch	None

Programs Designed for Strength and Power

There are several different programs that can be used to increase strength and power. All involve training loads that exceed 80 percent of the lifter's 1RM. These programs are not recommended for beginners. If you do not have adequate training experience, your risk of injury is high.

Pyramid Training

Pyramid training is *an approach to training that uses progressively heavier weights and fewer reps through successive sets of an exercise.* The first set uses relatively light weight. The amount of weight added for each following set is determined by increasing the percentage of the lifter's 1RM for that exercise. Note that each set is followed by a two- to three-minute rest.

Pyramid training is best suited for larger muscle groups, such as those in the chest, back, legs, and shoulders. Athletes frequently use this approach to improve their **skill-related fitness. Figure 10.20** shows a typical pyramid progression for the bench press done by a lifter with an 1RM of 130 pounds.

hot link

skill-related fitness
For more on skill-related fitness, see Chapter 3, page **71**.

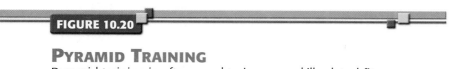

FIGURE 10.20

PYRAMID TRAINING
Pyramid training is often used to improve skill-related fitness.
For which muscle group is pyramid training best suited?

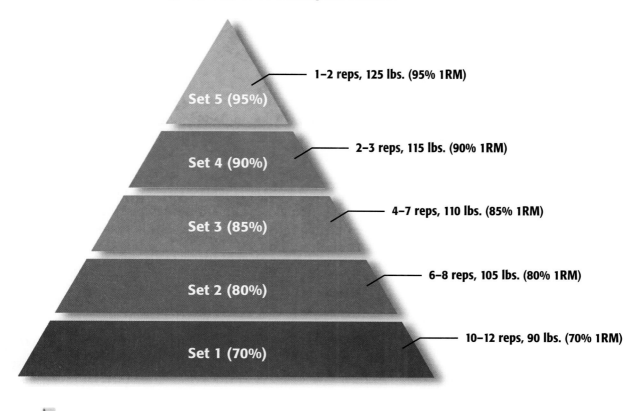

Set 5 (95%) — 1–2 reps, 125 lbs. (95% 1RM)

Set 4 (90%) — 2–3 reps, 115 lbs. (90% 1RM)

Set 3 (85%) — 4–7 reps, 110 lbs. (85% 1RM)

Set 2 (80%) — 6–8 reps, 105 lbs. (80% 1RM)

Set 1 (70%) — 10–12 reps, 90 lbs. (70% 1RM)

FIGURE 10.21

MULTIPLE SETS

This chart shows an example of a multiple-set training program for a lifter with a 1RM of 130 pounds. *How much weight should a person with a 1RM of 200 lift, using this same approach?*

Set	Reps	Weight (% of 1RM)
First	10–12	110 lbs (85% of 130 lbs.)
Second	6–8	110 lbs (85% of 130 lbs.)
Third	4–7	110 lbs (85% of 130 lbs.)

eccentric and concentric
For more on eccentric and concentric muscle work and what occurs during each phase of a contraction, see Chapter 9, page **252.**

Multiple Sets

In the multiple-set approach, *the lifter uses the same amount of weight for three to five sets at a training load of 80 to 95 percent of his or her 1RM.* The number of reps will range from two to six and should be done to the point of fatigue. A recovery time of two to three minutes is allowed between sets. **Figure 10.21** shows multiple sets for the bench press done by a lifter with a 1RM of 130 pounds. A variation on the multiple-set approach, as you will see on page **321,** can be used to gain muscle mass. Unless you have been lifting for at least six to eight weeks, you should not use the higher maximum percentages.

Negative Reps

When doing negative reps, *you do the **eccentric,** or negative, phase of an exercise only, using a weight 10 to 15 percent greater than your 1RM.* The **concentric** phase is handled by one or more spotters. Spotters will raise the bar back to the starting position after you have slowly lowered the bar. Three to four reps per set is the recommended maximum for this exercise.

Negative reps are usually done at the end of a prescribed number of exercises for a particular muscle group. Athletes use these primarily for performance enhancement. Because this system uses eccentric movement, there will be a greater amount of soreness in your workout. Negative reps are an advanced exercise. They should not be done by beginners.

Reading Check

List What three programs are used for building strength and power?

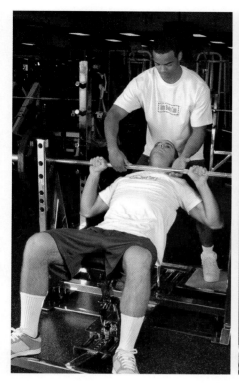
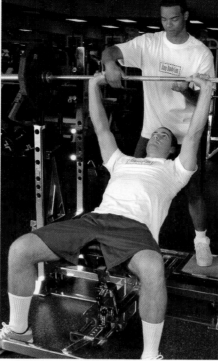

This teen is doing negative reps of the bench press. After he lowers the bar to his chest, the spotter raises it back to the starting position for one rep. *Describe the advantage of this type of workout.*

Programs Designed for Building Muscle Mass

Several programs are available to lifters whose primary training goal is to increase muscle mass, also called hypertrophy. These approaches use training loads of approximately 70 percent of the lifter's 1RM. Again, these should not be attempted by individuals with little or no lifting experience.

Supersets

Doing supersets requires the lifter to *alternately perform sets of exercises that train opposing muscles, without resting between sets.* An example of this approach would be to do ten biceps curls followed immediately by ten triceps extensions to develop the arm muscles.

The main opposing muscle groups are biceps and triceps, quadriceps and hamstrings, chest and back, shoulders and back (latissimus dorsi). Examples of exercise combinations used for supersets include:

- Bench press and seated row for chest and back
- Squats and leg curls for quadriceps and hamstrings
- Shoulder press and lat pulldowns for shoulders and back (latissimus dorsi)
- Biceps and triceps for arms

Supersets are an effective way to keep opposite muscles balanced in strength. They are also extremely efficient, since they allow you to work two muscles at the same time.

Mind OVER Matter

Positive Training Procedures

One of your goals while training should be to make sure that your sessions are safe and injury-free. Be sure to apply rules, procedures, and etiquette while in the weight room. For example, check all equipment before use, take turns at workout stations, wipe down machines, and replace free weights after each use. Explain how these steps can help prevent injury to yourself and others.

Compound Sets

Like supersets, **compound sets** require *doing alternate sets of exercises without allowing for rest between the sets.* Unlike supersets, compound sets train the same muscle group. An example of compound sets would be doing ten bench presses followed by ten flat bench flys.

The major muscle groups involved in compound sets are the chest, back, legs, and shoulders. Examples of common compound exercise combinations include:

- Bench press and flat bench fly for the chest
- Seated rows and lat pulldowns for the back
- Squats and leg press for the legs
- Military and side (lateral) dumbbell shoulder raise for the shoulders

Compound sets are most effective with large muscles or muscle groups and should be done once in a while—approximately every third workout—not every time.

Active Mind Active Body

Designing a Weight-Training Program

Weight training is an activity that you can do for the rest of your life. The skills and knowledge that you have gained in this chapter and Chapter 9 should provide you with the confidence and ability to establish and revise your own resistance program to fit your changing needs and goals.

Using your resistance goals and the results of your estimated 1RM, design a three-week resistance-training program that includes all of the necessary program components. You may record all of this information on the personalized training charts you developed in Lesson 3.

What You Will Need

- Pen or pencil
- Paper

What You Will Do

On a sheet of paper, note the following information:

1. Your goals (hypertrophy, strength, endurance, and so on).
2. Which days of the week you will work out (total body or split week).
3. Which exercises you will do (upper or lower body; big or small muscles).
4. The order of exercises (push-pull or big-small).
5. The weight arrangement (pyramid or same load).
6. Number of reps (based on intensity, such as 60, 75, or 85 percent of maximum).
7. Number of sets (1 to 3 or 4 to 5).
8. Length of rest periods between sets (20 to 30 seconds, 30 to 90 seconds, or 2 to 3 minutes).
9. How to vary the program from week to week (different systems, exercises).

Apply and Conclude

After you have made your list, implement your program. Take note of any changes you had to make to your plan once you put it into practice. What changes did you make and why?

Multiple Hypertrophy Sets

Like the similarly named multiple sets for power, multiple hypertrophy sets require *using the same amount of weight throughout and to the point of fatigue.* Beyond this similarity, the two have several differences.

- The training load for multiple hypertrophy sets, for example, is significantly lower—between 65 to 80 percent of the lifter's 1RM.
- The number of reps per set is higher—between eight and ten.
- The rest period between sets is shorter—only 30 to 90 seconds.

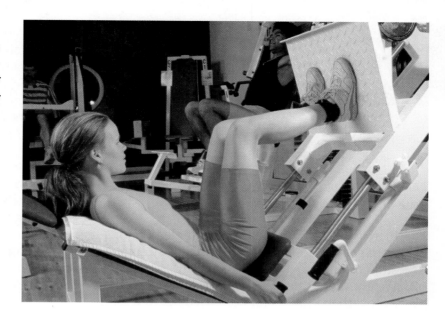

 Reading Check

Compare How are multiple hypertrophy sets the same as multiple sets for power?

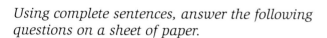

Lesson 4 Review

Using complete sentences, answer the following questions on a sheet of paper.

Reviewing Facts and Vocabulary

1. **Vocabulary** What is a *superset*?
2. **Recall** Explain how *pyramid training* works.
3. **Recall** Which approach to weight training works opposite muscles? Explain.

Thinking Critically

4. **Compare and Contrast** Compare the two different multiple set approaches. Tell how the two are similar and different in terms of their goals and how they are performed.
5. **Evaluate** Read and evaluate each of the following workout plans:
   a. Rudy is interested in adding muscle bulk. He does negative sets twice a week.
   b. Ilana, who is on the volleyball team, wants to develop added power for her serves. Her plan is to do supersets daily, focusing specifically on her triceps and biceps. She has never done resistance training.

Personal Fitness Planning

Designing a Program Your family is planning a skiing vacation this winter. You have two months to get physically fit for the trip. What kind of strength training would be best for downhill skiing? Design the first two weeks of a program that could be used by the members of your family to get them ready for skiing the slopes. This program should provide fitness and injury prevention.

TRUE/FALSE

On a sheet of paper, write the numbers 1–10. Write True or False for each statement.

1. Increasing fluid intake is an example of a long-term goal to improve your muscular strength and endurance.
2. Weight room safety includes having a spotter.
3. An overhand grip should be used on all lifts.
4. Reps are the basic unit of any workout plan.
5. Working larger muscles before smaller muscles allows you to make the most of your strength, energy, and mental concentration.
6. Finding your 1RM can help you determine your training load.
7. Muscle strength can best be developed with heavy weights and low numbers of repetitions.
8. In negative reps, the lifter is responsible only for the concentric phase of the lift.
9. Supersets keep opposite muscles balanced in strength.
10. Compound sets require doing alternate sets of exercises without allowing for rest between the sets.

MULTIPLE CHOICE

On a sheet of paper, write the letter of the word or phrase that best completes each statement.

11. Which of the following exercises does not work the chest?
    a. Bench press
    b. Seated military press
    c. Incline bench press
    d. Flat bench fly
12. Kristin is considering a weight-training program. Which of the following should she consider before developing her goals?
    a. Her current level of strength
    b. Her daily schedule
    c. Past injuries
    d. All of the above
13. Which of the following are not main muscle areas of the body?
    a. Neck and abdominals
    b. Chest and shoulders
    c. Legs and arms
    d. Abdominals and arms
14. Bent-over dumbbell shoulder raises mainly work which muscle?
    a. Trapezius   c. Deltoids
    b. Biceps   d. Latissimus dorsi
15. Weight room safety includes which of the following rules?
    a. Familiarize yourself with the training facility
    b. Control the speed of weights at all times
    c. Practice all lifts before attempting them with heavier weights
    d. All of the above
16. Which of the following is not a responsibility of the spotter?
    a. Stay in a ready position at all times
    b. Motivate your partner
    c. Correct improper technique
    d. Fetching towels for all lifters in the area
17. If you do ten push-ups, one right after the other, you have done which of the following?
    a. One set of ten reps
    b. Ten sets of one rep each
    c. Ten sets of one exercise
    d. None of the above
18. Recovery time for muscles is important at which of the following times?
    a. Between reps   c. Between workouts
    b. Between exercises   d. Both b and c
19. In a total body workout, a person
    a. exercises all major muscle groups, five times a week.
    b. exercises all major muscle groups, three times a week.
    c. alternates the exercising of two major muscle groups, five days a week.
    d. exercises different muscle groups on each day, three days a week.
20. An approach to training that uses progressively heavier weights and fewer reps through successive sets of an exercise is known as which of the following?
    a. Negative reps
    b. Supersets
    c. Pyramid training
    d. All of the above

DISCUSSION

Using complete sentences, answer the following questions on a sheet of paper.

21. Identify List three weight-training exercises that require the use of the common grip and three that require the use of the narrow grip.

22. Identify List and demonstrate six techniques used by spotters. Why are these techniques necessary in the weight room?

23. Design Plan and explain a five-set pyramid workout for the bench press and a three-set superset workout for the arms. Choose your own weight for each workout plan.

VOCABULARY

On a sheet of paper, write the letter of the term in Column B that best fits the definition in Column A.

Column A

24. Exercising three or four body areas at each session, working at much higher intensities.

25. A group of consecutive repetitions for any exercise.

26. The duration of the rest periods taken between workout components.

27. Alternately perform sets of exercises that train opposing muscles, without resting between sets.

28. One completion of an activity or exercise.

29. Doing the eccentric phase of an exercise only, using a weight 10 to 15 percent greater than your 1RM.

Column B

a. repetition
b. split workout
c. superset method
d. recovery time
e. negative workout method
f. set

CRITICAL THINKING

Using complete sentences, answer the following questions on a sheet of paper.

30. Analyze Identify five components of record keeping, and explain why keeping records is important to your weight-training program.

31. Evaluate Respond to the following statement: Megan is a 14-year-old who has never lifted weights and wants to start a weight-training program. She has had some instruction and wants to take a 1RM test to determine her workload. Explain why an estimated 1RM would be more beneficial to her at this stage of lifting.

CASE STUDY

BRET AND ALBERT'S SUMMER RESISTANCE-TRAINING PLAN

The school year is ending. Bret, a ninth grader, has decided to do weight training over the summer. His goal is to develop a program that will meet minimum health and fitness needs. His friend Albert also plans to train with weights. Albert, however, wants to try out for the varsity football team next year. His goal, thus, is to increase his muscle mass and strength.

Neither teen knows how to design a program to meet their specific needs. They need the help of someone knowledgeable about resistance programs. That someone could be you.

HERE IS YOUR ASSIGNMENT:

Organize a list of specific weight-training components for each teen. Then design a two-week sample weight-training program for each.

KEYS TO HELP YOU

- Consider each teen's specific needs and goals (for example, strength, power, or general fitness).
- Determine how to evaluate each teen's current strength.
- Which specific circuit should each teen use?
- Determine the number of reps, sets, and exercises.
- Determine training load.
- Determine frequency and recovery time.

Basics of Flexibility

FITNESS Online

Flexibility offers many benefits to your overall health and fitness. Regular flexibility training should be part of everyone's fitness plan. How do you rate in this area of fitness? Find out by taking the STEP Personal Inventory for Chapter 11. Find it at **fitness.glencoe.com**.

Influences on Flexibility

Bending to tie your shoe or swinging a tennis racquet requires some degree of flexibility. So does twisting around to see who is calling your name. What exactly is flexibility? In this lesson, you will learn about flexibility and its role in functional health.

What Is Flexibility?

Flexibility refers to *a joint's ability to move through its full range of motion.* **Range of motion (ROM)** refers to *the degrees of motion allowed around a joint* (see **Figure 11.1**). ROM varies from joint to joint. Some joints allow a wide ROM. These include ball-and-socket joints, like those in the shoulders and hips. Other joints, such as the

What You Will Do

- Identify factors that can positively or negatively influence your flexibility.
- Apply the biomechanically correct use of leverage to lift objects.
- Explain how good posture may contribute to the prevention of lower-back problems.

Terms to Know

flexibility
range of motion (ROM)
elasticity
posture
static posture
dynamic posture

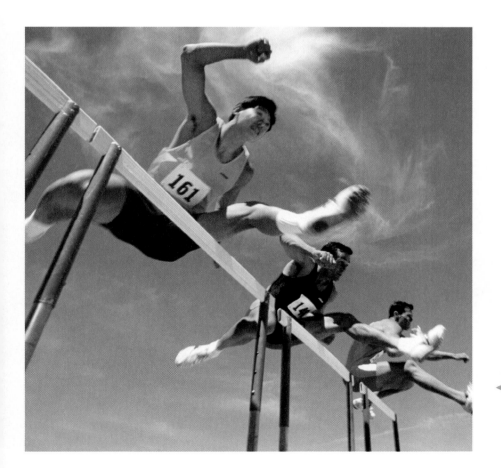

◀ Flexibility is an important part of health-related fitness. *What sports or activities require a high level of flexibility?*

FIGURE 11.1

FULL RANGE OF MOTION

Range of motion refers to the degrees of motion allowed around a joint. *How high can you lift your leg?*

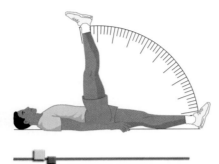

hinge-like joints in your knees, allow only forward and backward movement. Still others, such as those in the neck, allow pivoting and rotation. Yet a fourth type, the joints found in the wrists and ankles, allow bones to glide over one another. These joints and the type of movement allowed by each are shown in **Figure 11.2.**

Factors Affecting Flexibility

How flexible are you? Your answer to this question will be determined by one or more factors. These include:

- **Heredity.** Some people have more flexible joints, tendons, and ligaments than others because of their genetic makeup.
- **Gender.** In general, females are slightly more flexible than males, at least in some movements. For example, females usually have a greater ROM in their hip region. This allows them to touch their toes with greater ease.
- **Age.** Younger people are usually more flexible than older people, mainly because of a loss of elasticity that comes with aging. **Elasticity** is *the ability of the muscles and connective tissues to stretch and give.* You can maintain higher levels of elasticity as you age if you stretch regularly.
- **Body temperature.** Flexibility can change by as much as 20 percent with increases or decreases in muscular temperature. This is one reason why warming up before exercise or physical activity is especially important.

FIGURE 11.2

JOINTS OF THE BODY

Free and smooth range of motion is necessary for a healthy functional life. *What daily activities depend upon these joints?*

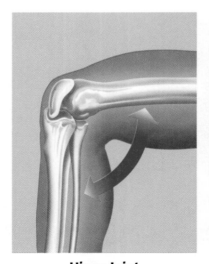

Hinge Joint

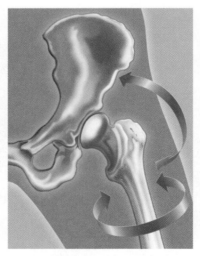

Ball-and-Socket Joint

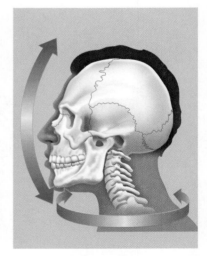

Pivot Joint

- **Injuries.** Injuries to your muscles, skin, bones, or connective tissues may result in the loss of some flexibility. Scar tissue that forms when your body heals itself can limit your ROM. Flexibility exercises can help you regain normal ROM after many types of injury.
- **Percentage of body fat.** Excessive body fat can limit ROM. The excess fat restricts movement around the joints. Losing excess body fat can improve flexibility.
- **Activity level.** The most significant negative influence on your flexibility level is an inactive lifestyle. As you decrease your physical activity or exercise levels, your muscles and connective tissues lose elasticity. If you remain inactive, you will also add body fat, which further limits flexibility.

Reading Check

Explain How does warming up affect your flexibility?

Staying Active, Staying Flexible

To prevent muscles and connective tissue from losing elasticity, you need to stretch your muscles regularly. By doing so, you move your joints through their full ROM. Remember the following guidelines.

- Participate in aerobic activities that do not strain your back to improve strength, endurance, and flexibility function. Options include swimming, walking, jogging, water activities, stationary biking, and hiking.
- Participate in resistance-training activities to condition abdominal and back muscles. These muscles work together to support the back.
- Do simple exercises on a regular basis to help support and align your back.
- Maintain proper body weight.
- Stay active.

Lower-Back Pain

Lower-back pain is often associated with inflexible and weak muscles that support the spine and pelvic girdle. This specific type of pain has become a major health problem in the United States. People with lower-back pain often end up with more serious chronic problems, such as lower-back injuries. The leading cause of back injury is lifting.

Even though back pain is common, simple measures can be taken to prevent it. By maintaining an appropriate amount of flexibility and muscular strength through a basic fitness program, you can condition your muscles to prevent injury. Learning proper lifting techniques and posture also reduces your chance of developing back pain or becoming injured. Later in the chapter, you will learn about exercises that can help prevent lower-back pain.

FIGURE 11.3

PROPER AND IMPROPER LIFTING

Improper lifting is a major cause of lower-back injury. *Do you practice proper lifting?*

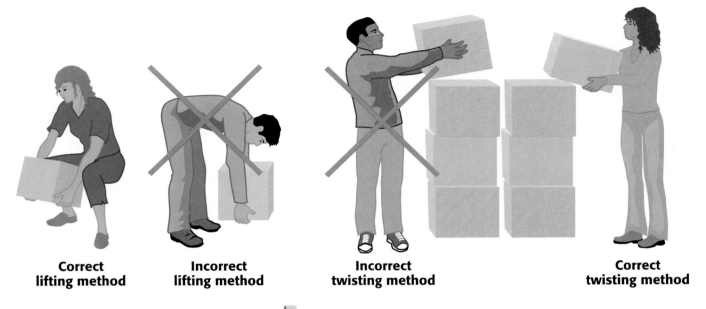

Correct lifting method   **Incorrect lifting method**   **Incorrect twisting method**   **Correct twisting method**

biomechanics
For more on biomechanics, see Chapter 2, page **54.**

Rules for Biomechanically Correct Lifting

As noted in Chapter 2, **biomechanics** is the application of principles of physics to human motion. By applying these principles to the lifting and carrying of heavy objects, you can help prevent lower-back injuries. Imagine you had to lift a heavy box the size of the one in **Figure 11.3.** Would you lean over at the waist and lift upward? If you did, you might hurt your back. When carrying heavy objects, balance the load so that there is equal stress on each of the joints involved. For example, when carrying two sacks of groceries, carry one in each hand, not both in one hand. Avoid excessive twisting, pulling, or pushing movements, which can strain your lower back.

The following are tips on lifting and moving objects of any weight and should be practiced regularly.

- When lifting bulky or heavy items, try to plan ahead. Get a partner to help with the lifting.
- Always position your body close to the object.
- Place your feet shoulder width apart to give yourself a solid base of support.
- Bend your knees when possible and tighten your stomach muscles.
- Use your legs to lift most of the load, keeping it close to your body to apply the correct leverage and prevent injury.

- If only one hand is necessary to pick up the object, use the other hand to support your body weight.
- When walking with the object, try to keep knees slightly bent. Point your toes in the direction you want to move and pivot in that direction. Do not twist at the waist.
- Avoid side bending.
- Lift in a slow, controlled fashion.

 Reading Check

Summarize When lifting, which part of the body should be used to lift most of the load?

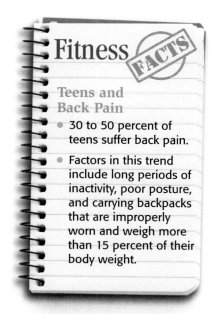
Posture and Lower-Back Pain

Has someone ever said to you, "Sit up straight" or "Don't slouch"? This is advice worth listening to. Good posture habits can reduce stress and strain on your spine and help prevent back injuries. **Posture** refers to *the alignment of the body's muscles and skeleton as they provide support for the total body.* Gravitational forces are at work on your joints, ligaments, and muscles at all times. This is true whether you are standing, sitting, moving, or lying. Good posture helps to distribute the force of gravity through your body. That way, no one structure is overstressed.

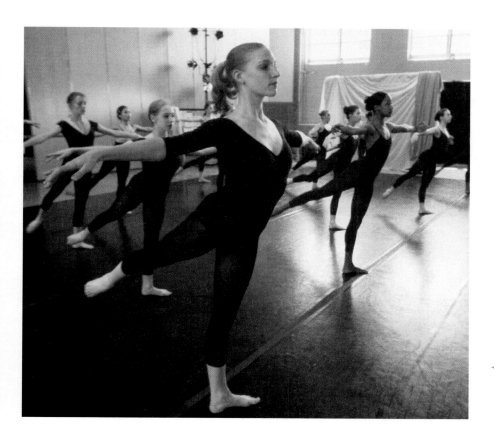

◀ Dynamic posture refers to how you position your body to perform movements. *What is static posture?*

FIGURE 11.4

PROPER AND IMPROPER POSTURE

Improper posture can cause unnecessary stress to your body. *Which of these static posture habits do you practice? Which of the dynamic posture habits do you practice?*

Sleeping

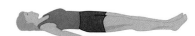

Do not lie flat on your back; this arches the spine too much.

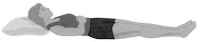

Do not use a high pillow.

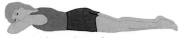

Do not sleep face down.

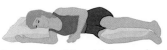

Lie on your back and support your knees.

Lie on your side with knees bent and pillow just high enough to keep your neck straight.

Sitting

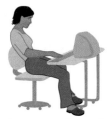

Do not leave your lower back unsupported.

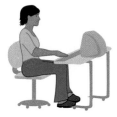

Sit straight with back support, knees higher than hips.

Standing

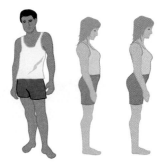

Do not let your back bend out of its natural curve.

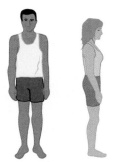

Stand upright, hips tucked, knees slightly bent.

Walking

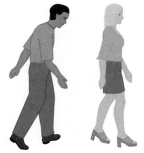

Do not lean forward or wear high heels.

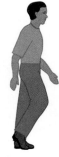

Lead with chest, toes forward.

Most poor posture habits relate to static posture. This refers to *the posture your body exhibits while in a resting position.* Your body is in a state of static posture when you sit at a computer or stand in place. Good dynamic posture, however, is also important. Also known as "posture in motion," dynamic posture refers to *the posture your body exhibits while in motion or preparing to move.* This includes how you position your body to perform movements such as pushing, lifting, carrying, twisting, and swinging. The following tips can also help prevent lower-back pain and injury.

- When sitting, try to keep your back straight.
- When working at a computer, use a chair that provides built-in lower-back support.
- When you need to stand for extended periods, place one foot on a low footstool. Occasionally alternate feet. This will take some of the load off your back.
- When sleeping, use a firm mattress.
- When sleeping, use a pillow that provides support for your head.
- When sleeping on your side, place a pillow between your knees.

Figure 11.4 illustrates improper and proper posture habits. Practicing techniques of good posture will allow your body to work more efficiently. They will also ensure that less stress is placed on a single body part.

FITNESS *Online*

Go to **fitness.glencoe. com** for more accurate information about good posture.

Activity Evaluate your own posture with the self-test, then follow suggestions for improving your posture for a lifetime.

Lesson 1 Review

Using complete sentences, answer the following questions on a sheet of paper.

Reviewing Facts and Vocabulary

1. **Vocabulary** Define *flexibility.*
2. **Recall** What is the meaning of *ROM?*
3. **Recall** List and explain the two types of posture.

Thinking Critically

4. **Analyze** Describe an example of an unsafe lifting technique. Why is biomechanically correct lifting and use of leverage important?
5. **Evaluate** Respond to the following statement: "I am a well-conditioned 15-year-old, so I don't need to worry about my posture." What are the potential dangers of this attitude?

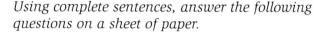

Personal Fitness Planning

Evaluating Fitness Make a list of the activities and chores that you do daily. Evaluate each in terms of your posture and flexibility habits. Which of these could be improved upon? How? How can you apply proper biomechanics to these activities? Is there a pattern regarding when and where you are most likely to exhibit poor posture habits? Attempt to correct any poor habits by becoming more aware of them. Keep a log of your progress.

Evaluating Your Flexibility

What You Will Do

- Identify sports and activities that promote flexibility.
- Explain why too much flexibility can be unsafe.
- Participate in activities to evaluate your flexibility.

Terms to Know

hyperflexibility
muscle imbalance
core stability

How flexible are you? Do you participate in activities and exercises that benefit your flexibility? Can you think of ways your performance in certain activities might improve if you increased your flexibility level? How might flexibility benefit your health in other areas?

In the last lesson, you learned that flexibility is influenced by some factors you cannot control, such as heredity and gender, and several factors you can control, such as your level of activity. In this lesson, you will learn more about the role physical activities and sports play in improving flexibility. You will also learn about the many benefits that improved flexibility offer your overall functional health. In the "Fitness Check" on pages **336–337,** you have a chance to assess your current level of flexibility.

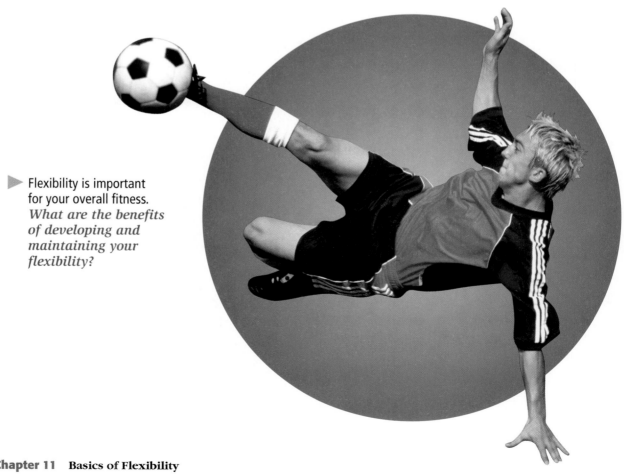

▶ Flexibility is important for your overall fitness. *What are the benefits of developing and maintaining your flexibility?*

FIGURE 11.5

BENEFITS OF FLEXIBILITY CONDITIONING

The chart illustrates the benefits of 8 to 30 weeks of flexibility conditioning in a previously inactive teen. *How can flexibility improve more than just your physical health?*

Healthy Joints	• Increases ROM for the joints conditioned • Promotes more flexible muscles and tendons • Decreases risk of joint injury
Healthy Muscles	• Increases stability for your joints • Increases ROM for strength development
Fewer Health-related Injuries	• Helps control instability • Reduces risk for various chronic muscle/skeletal pain, including lower-back pain
Reduced Stiffness and Soreness	• Increases blood flow • Increases ROM • After physical activities ROM can be regained with stretching, resulting in reduced stiffness and muscular soreness the next day • Stretching after physical activity reduces risk for blood pooling and muscle cramping
Healthy Emotions	• Reduced tension and stress levels
Healthy Image	• Increased functional health and fitness. • Future opportunities to participate in a variety of physical activities and exercises

Benefits of Flexibility

Figure 11.5 reveals how moderate-to-high flexibility contributes to several areas of health. It reduces stiffness and soreness and helps limit the risk of chronic back pain and similar health problems. Flexibility also prevents injury and improves athletic performance.

There are many physical activities that lead to improvements and maintenance of flexibility. There are also many that do not. The list in **Figure 11.6** on page **335** rates sports and activities according to their potential flexibility benefits. Which of these, if any, do you participate in on a regular basis?

Active Mind Active Body

Which Activities Improve Flexibility?

Do you play sports or take part in some other form of regular physical activity? You may be surprised to know that many such activities provide minimal flexibility benefits. In this activity, you will determine how much flexibility conditioning your sports and activities provide.

What You Will Need

- Pen or pencil
- Paper

What You Will Do

1. Make a list of activities you do on a regular basis. Include sports and exercises.
2. Consult **Figure 11.6.** Write down the number of stars indicated next to each activity you identified.
3. Determine which activities are rated at least *Fair* (★★) in terms of the flexibility levels offered.
4. Add activities or sports to your daily activity routine that are rated *Fair, Good,* or *Better.*

Apply and Conclude

Based on your findings, tell whether your activities are providing adequate flexibility benefits. If they are not, what activities can you add to help you meet your flexibility needs? Note specific activities you would like to add to your personal fitness plan.

Hyperflexibility and Muscle Imbalances

You might think that the more flexibility a person has, the better. This is not necessarily true. A joint with too much ROM can become injured easily. This *excessive amount of flexibility* is known as hyperflexibility.

Hyperflexibility can occur when a joint has been stretched beyond its normal ROM or when weak muscles surround a joint (as can happen following a muscle injury). Hyperflexibility can also occur because of hereditary tendencies for "loose joints." A person with a hyperflexible shoulder joint, for example, may have stretched ligaments or tendons. This condition may, in turn, cause the shoulder to dislocate easily. Such a person can improve the stability of his or her shoulder by strengthening the muscles that control its movement. These muscles are the rotator cuff (the muscles that surround the shoulder joint) and the biceps (the muscles in the front of the upper arm).

When you strengthen muscles around a joint, you need to be sure to work the two opposing muscle groups involved. This will help you avoid a muscle imbalance. This is *a condition in which one muscle group becomes too strong in relation to a complementary group.* Muscle imbalances occur when one or more FITT factors are misapplied in the training of opposing muscle groups. The underdeveloped muscles are at increased risk of becoming injured. This, in turn, can reduce your normal ROM and cause pain or injury.

✓ Reading Check

Analyze What is a muscle imbalance? What factors cause muscle imbalances?

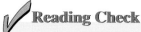
FIGURE 11.6

ACTIVITIES THAT BENEFIT FLEXIBILITY

Not all sports will improve your flexibility. *Which sports or activities provide the most flexibility conditioning? The least?*

Sports or Activity	Flexibility Benefits	Sports or Activity	Flexibility Benefits
Archery	★★	Mountain Climbing	★
Backpacking	★★★	Racquetball	★★
Ballet	★★★★	Rhythmical Exercise	★★★
Badminton	★★		
Baseball	★★★	Rope Jumping	★★
Basketball	★★★	Rowing	★★
Bicycling	★★	Skating: Ice, Roller, or In-line	★★
Bowling	★		
Canoeing	★★		
Circuit Training	★★★	Skiing: Cross-Country or Downhill	★★★
Dance, aerobic	★★★		
Dance, line	★★	Soccer	★★
Dance, social	★★	Softball	★★
Fencing	★★	Surfing	★★★
Fitness: Calisthenics	★★★★	Swimming	★★★
Football	★★	Tennis	★★
Golf (walking)	★★★★	Volleyball	★★
Gymnastics	★★★★	Walking	★
Handball	★★★	Water Polo	★★
Hiking	★★	Waterskiing	★
Jogging	★	Weight Training	★★★
Martial Arts	★★★★	Yoga	★★★★

Better ★★★★ Good ★★★ Fair ★★ Low ★

Evaluating Your Flexibility

Having acceptable levels of flexibility in a variety of joints is an important health and fitness consideration. You may not be aware of your range of motion for various stretches. However, if they are below acceptable levels, you may be at risk for injury.

In this activity, you will work with one or more partners to identify your specific range of motion for three stretches. You may choose to perform any or all of the following evaluations: trunk lift, arm lift, or sit-and-reach test. You will need the following items: paper, pencil, a yardstick, tape, a broomstick (or wooden rod 3 feet long), a mat, and a box that is 12 × 14 × 16 inches. Be sure to do a light warm-up prior to all stretches.

Trunk Lift

Procedure:

1. Lie facedown on the mat with your toes pointed and your hands next to your thighs (see **Figure 11.7a**).
2. While a partner holds your legs, slowly lift your chin as high as possible. Hold this position for about three seconds (see **Figure 11.7b**).
3. A second partner should use a yardstick to measure how many inches above the floor your chin reaches.
4. Repeat twice.
5. Use the Fitness Ratings Chart for Trunk Lift to assess your performance.
6. Reverse roles with each partner and repeat steps 1 through 5.

Fitness Ratings: Trunk Lift	
Inches Lifted	**Rating**
9 to 12 inches	Healthy
Under 9 inches	Low

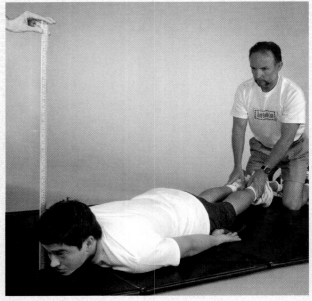

Figure 11.7a

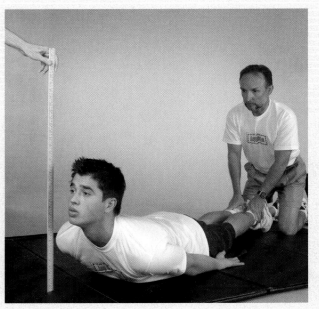

Figure 11.7b

Arm Lift

Procedure:

1. Lie face down on the mat (see **Figure 11.8**).
2. With your arms spread shoulder width apart, hold a broomstick or other light rod out in front of you. Your palms should be face down, with your arms and wrists straight.
3. Keeping your chin on the floor, raise your arms and the rod as high as possible. Hold the position for three seconds.
4. Have a partner use a yardstick to measure how many inches the rod is above the floor. Repeat twice.
5. Use the Fitness Ratings Chart for Arm Lift to assess your performance.
6. Reverse roles with your partner and repeat steps 1 through 5.

Fitness Ratings: Arm Lift	
Inches Lifted	**Rating**
11 to 14 inches	Healthy
Under 11 inches	Low

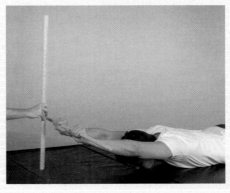

Figure 11.8

Sit-and-Reach Test

Procedure:

1. Tape the yardstick to the top of the box with 9 inches protruding beyond one end.
2. Remove your shoes. Place the box in a stationary position against a wall. Position yourself in a seated position with your legs straight and the protruding end of the yardstick facing you.
3. Place one foot flat against the side of the box nearest you. Bend the other leg.

4. Extend your arms over the yardstick, with your hands placed one on top of the other, palms down. Keep your hands together (see **Figure 11.9**).
5. Reach forward in this manner four times. The fourth time, hold this position for at least one second while a partner records how far you can reach.
6. Repeat with the other leg.
7. Use the Fitness Ratings Chart for the Sit-and-Reach Test to assess your performance.
8. Reverse roles with your partner and repeat steps 1 through 7.

Fitness Ratings: Sit-and-Reach Test	
Inches Stretched	**Rating**
Males:	
8 inches	Healthy
Under 8 inches	Low
Females (Ages 13–14):	
10 inches	Healthy
Under 10 inches	Low
Females (Ages 15 and up):	
12 inches	Healthy
Under 12 inches	Low

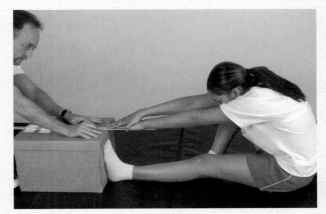

Figure 11.9

Flexibility Training for Core Stability

One way to prevent and treat hyperflexibility and muscle imbalances is by developing core stability, *the stretching and strengthening of muscles around the spine and pelvic muscles.* Increasing core stability involves a combination of strength-training exercises and flexibility training. For example, basic abdominal crunches are a great way to strengthen the necessary muscles for core stability. In addition, many of the free-weight exercises discussed in Chapter 10, such as the incline press, bent-over row, and squats are great ways to increase the strength of one's back and pelvic muscles.

Flexibility training is the other component of developing core stability. You have already performed a few of these stretches in the "Fitness Check" on pages **336–337.** Several more stretches, introduced in Lesson 4, are also effective for this type of training. They include the single knee hug, reverse hurdler, wall slides, and leg raises.

Core stability helps prevent injuries and low back pain. It is also essential for improving and maintaining your performance fitness. Core stability is an important element in developing balance, power, and coordination. When you participate in a variety of physical activities and competitive sports, you will benefit from increasing your core stability.

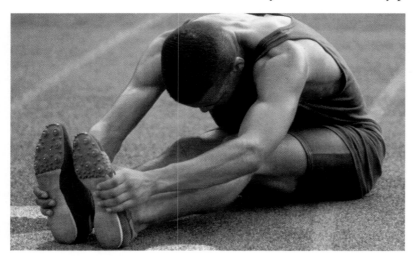

▼ Core stability is developed by stretching and strengthening the back and pelvic muscles. *What aspects of performance fitness benefit from improving core stability?*

Lesson 2 Review

Using complete sentences, answer the following questions on a sheet of paper.

Reviewing Facts and Vocabulary

1. **Vocabulary.** What is *hyperflexibility?*
2. **Recall** Identify two sports that have high ratings for providing flexibility conditioning.

Thinking Critically

3. **Describe** Why might performing too many flexibility exercises or achieving too much flexibility be unsafe?

4. **Analyze** Explain why it is important to maintain adequate strength and flexibility in all the muscles around a joint.

Personal Fitness Planning

Improving Flexibility This activity examines your flexibility scores on the three evaluations you did for the "Fitness Check" activity. Over the next three weeks organize your daily schedule in such a way that allows time for you to practice the three stretches. At the end of the three weeks, retake the evaluations and make note of any improvements.

Lesson 3

Developing Your Flexibility

To develop flexibility, your personal fitness plan needs to include activities and exercises that will maintain or improve your ROM. One easy general approach to achieving this goal is to include stretching exercises in your warm-ups and cooldowns.

This lesson will help you apply physiological principles and develop the particulars of your flexibility program. It will help you determine your flexibility FITT.

FITT and the Principle of Overload

Determining your FITT for any fitness goal, as you have learned, begins with evaluations. For the present purposes, you will use your ratings from the three flexibility evaluations you performed in Lesson 2. If you achieved healthy levels of flexibility, you will design a stretching program that helps you maintain these levels. If your ratings were low, you will need to increase one or more FITT factors to achieve overload.

Remember, never change all four FITT factors at the same time. In addition, do not change any one factor too quickly. Be patient, and allow for gradual improvements.

What You Will Do

- Apply the physiological principles of overload, specificity, and progression to develop your flexibility.
- Apply the FITT formula to your flexibility plan.
- Describe types of stretches and what each type accomplishes.

Terms to Know

static stretching
ballistic stretching
reflexes
reflex-assisted stretching
passive stretching

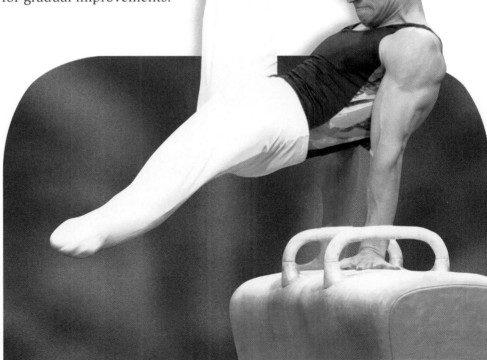

▶ Improving flexibility means increasing FITT factors to achieve overload. *What are the four FITT factors?*

Frequency

How often should you do your stretches? A minimum of three days per week is recommended. However, it is best to do some stretching daily. If you are just starting out, begin with three days per week. Then, during the improvement stage of progression, add more days per week.

Intensity

Because the risk of injury is great, you need to exercise care in establishing your intensity needs when stretching. Your goal should be to reach the point where a muscle or connective tissue is stretched just beyond its normal resting state. You have reached that point during the stretch if you feel slight discomfort but no real pain. Bouncing, jerking, or other sudden movements can increase your risk for injuries.

 Reading Check

Explain How can you achieve overload in your fitness program?

Time

How do you determine the duration of your stretches? For static stretching, begin by holding each stretch for 20 to 30 seconds. Repeat this three times for each static stretch you do. As your ROM increases, try to hold each stretch for 30 to 60 seconds, repeating three times per stretch.

Type and the Principle of Specificity

To improve the flexibility of a particular joint or body area, you need to apply specificity. That is, do stretches that affect the nerves, muscles, and connective tissues that control movement around a specific joint or body part. To maintain or improve your overall flexibility levels, do a variety of stretches that influence all your major body parts. Also, remember to work the two opposing muscle groups involved to avoid a muscle imbalance, as discussed in Lesson 2.

The "Active Mind—Active Body" feature in Chapter 3 (pages **104–105**) provides instruction on twelve basic stretches that could be included in warm-ups and cooldowns. In Lesson 4 of this chapter, you will learn several others.

The Principle of Progression

The rate at which you modify your FITT should be based on your overall fitness goals and changing levels of flexibility. Beginners should progress slowly with regard to time and intensity. It is fine, however, to stretch on a frequent basis.

 Reading Check

Describe How does specificity apply to a flexibility program?

Any Body Can

Tiger Woods

In the Swing of Fitness

Some people claim that sports is in their blood. In the case of Eldrick "Tiger" Woods, this claim is almost fact. As a toddler, Tiger was introduced by his parents to the sport of golf. By the age of 8, he had won his first of six international junior tournaments.

Tiger Woods was born on December 30, 1975, in Orlando, Florida. He grew up in Cypress, California. In 1996, he entered Stanford University on a golf scholarship. There he won the NCAA individual championship.

Since joining the professional golf tour, Tiger Woods has dominated the sport. He was named Player of the Year by the Professional Golf Association (PGA) in 1997, 1999, 2000, and 2001. With a win at the Masters Tournament on April 8, 2001, he became the first player in history to sweep all four major tournaments in a single year.

Tiger is physically active, on and off the golf course. He works out daily and enjoys weight training and flexibility exercises. Both help him maintain his remarkable golf skills.

Not everyone can be as great an athlete as Tiger Woods. However, anyone can learn to develop a

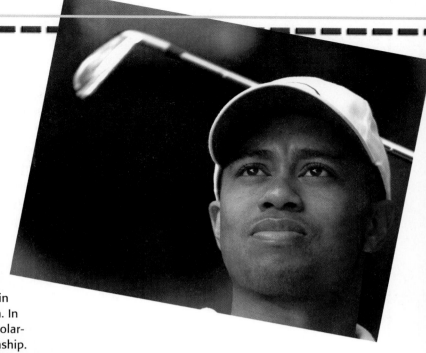

personal-fitness plan and stick with it to improve the quality of his or her life. Yes, Any Body Can!

Research

Although flexibility may not seem important in some sports such as golf, a high level of flexibility has many benefits. Learn more about the role of flexibility in a particular sport by talking to a teacher, coach, or athlete about the type of flexibility exercises that are used in training, and how flexibility can positively impact an athlete's performance.

Types of Stretching and Your Flexibility

Four basic stretching techniques can help improve your flexibility levels. These include static stretching, ballistic stretching, reflex-assisted stretching, and passive stretching.

Static Stretching

Static stretching consists of *doing stretches slowly, smoothly, and in a sustained fashion.* You hold the stretch for 20 to 30 seconds until you feel slight discomfort but no real pain. Static stretching can also be done while sitting (see **Figure 11.10**) to stretch the hamstrings, by making slow circular motions with the arms or by slowly stretching the neck side-to-side. Static stretching, when done regularly, is safe and effective at increasing the ROM of the joints you work. Everyone should do some static stretching to help maintain or improve flexibility.

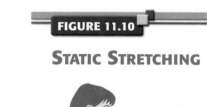

FIGURE 11.10

STATIC STRETCHING

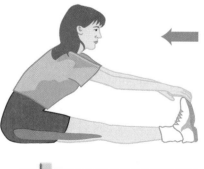

FIGURE 11.11

BALLISTIC STRETCHING

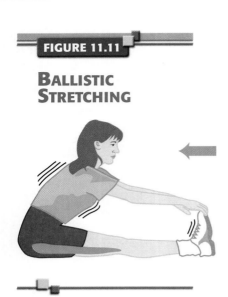

Ballistic Stretching

Ballistic stretching involves *quick up-and-down bobbing movements in which stretches are held very briefly* (see **Figure 11.11**). You may have seen athletes doing ballistic stretches in their warm-ups before a game.

Ballistic stretches are used primarily to build components of performance, or skill-related fitness. They are not necessary, or even recommended, for health-related fitness. The reason is that the short, quick motions involved can increase injury risks, particularly if you are not warmed up before you do them. An athlete doing ballistic stretching might do five to fifteen movements, repeating this three times per stretch. He or she may want to increase the number or sets of stretches over time, based on his or her performance needs.

> ### ✔ Reading Check
>
> **Evaluate** What is the difference between static stretching and ballistic stretching?

Reflex-Assisted Stretching

Your muscle reflexes are *the automatic responses that your nerves and muscles provide to various movements.* An example of a reflex is a simple knee jerk. You have probably experienced this type of involuntary reaction as part of a medical checkup.

Your body performs a variety of reflex actions daily. These keep us from falling and help us maintain balance. Some reflex reactions are very sensitive, others dull. Your reflexes can dull as you age if you fail to remain active. Staying active and stretching regularly can help maintain or improve many of the normal reflex actions that dull with aging.

Reflex-assisted stretching includes *stretching movements that challenge the reflexes to adapt.* Such stretches allow your joints to move more quickly and with more explosive power. An example of reflex-assisted stretching is **plyometric** training (see **Figure 11.12**). Plyometric training includes bounding and jumping exercises. Such training is useful in sports such as basketball and some track events, which require jumping at maximal levels. Individuals interested in plyometric training are advised to seek out a certified strength and conditioning coach. A professional can help you develop a safe and effective program.

Like ballistic stretching, reflex-assisted stretching is not recommended for individuals seeking improvements in general fitness. Remember, reflex-assisted stretches are more hazardous than static stretching in regard to injury risk and, therefore, should be done with caution.

Passive Stretching

Passive stretching is *a type of stretching against a counterforce and in which there is little or no movement.* In passive stretching exercises, the counterforce offers resistance. This force may be provided by a partner or an inanimate object, such as a chair or towel.

hotlink

plyometric
For more on plyometric exercise and training, see Chapter 9, page **266.**

If done slowly and safely, passive stretching can yield considerable gains in your ROM. In this activity, you and a partner will take turns practicing this type of stretching. As you proceed, be sure to communicate about the speed of motion and amount of pressure being applied. The pressure should be stopped if there is significant discomfort.

What You Will Need

- Mat or other comfortable surface

What You Will Do

1. Sit on the mat with your legs together and extended.
2. Have your partner place his or her hands on your back near your shoulders.
3. Place your hands one on top of the other and slowly lean forward at the waist, with arms extended. Your partner should apply slight pressure to the point where you can no longer lean forward. The pressure will continue until you instruct the partner to stop.
4. Relax the exercise and repeat once more. Switch positions with your partner.

Note: This same procedure may be repeated with other flexibility exercises. You will learn about additional exercises in Lesson 4.

Apply and Conclude

Were you able to increase ROM as your partner applied pressure? How much additional distance was obtained? Was the second try easier or harder? Do you think this type of stretching will help you reach your goals sooner? Why is it important for your partner to exercise caution when doing this type of stretching? Explain your answer.

FIGURE 11.12

PLYOMETRIC TRAINING

Plyometric training is one type of reflex-assisted training. *In what sports is plyometric training helpful?*

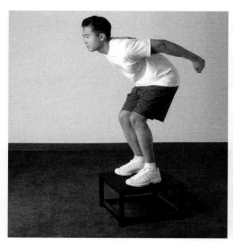
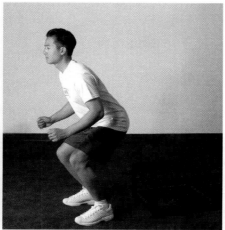

Two examples of passive stretching exercises are illustrated in **Figure 11.13.** In the example below on the right, the person sits on the floor and holds a towel around the heel of one foot. By pulling the towel toward herself while resisting with the foot, she is stretching the hamstring muscles.

Note that passive stretching carries some risks. If you or a partner pulls or pushes too hard, the target muscle or tissue may be overstretched. A muscle or connective tissue pull or tear may result. Passive stretching should thus be done with caution.

FIGURE 11.13

PASSIVE STRETCHING

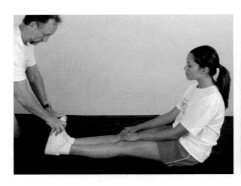 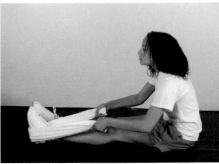

Lesson 3 Review

Using complete sentences, answer the following questions on a sheet of paper.

Reviewing Facts and Vocabulary

1. **Recall** How does frequency apply to your flexibility program?

2. **Vocabulary** What is *static stretching?*

Thinking Critically

3. **Synthesize** Robert has just started a beginner's tennis class and wants to develop some beneficial stretching habits. His level of flexibility is low, but he is eager to improve. How would you advise him to apply progression to his flexibility program, with regard to frequency, intensity, and time?

4. **Compare** What is the difference between ballistic stretching and passive stretching? How might you reduce the risks of these types of stretching?

Personal Fitness Planning

Designing Stretches Design a plan for using a towel as the counterforce in a passive stretching exercise. For example, you might sit on the floor with your legs extended. Place the middle of a towel around your toes, and gently pull the tops of your toes back and hold. Make a list of other ways to incorporate and practice passive stretching on your own.

Flexibility Exercises and Activities

Jo is about to take her daily run in the park. Raul needs to get ready for his team's football game on Friday night. Although these teens have very different interests, they share a common need. Both need to stretch beforehand.

In this lesson, you will learn about many different stretches and the muscles and tissues that benefit from each. The "Active Mind—Active Body" feature on page **349** of this lesson will give you an opportunity to practice many of these stretches and safely introduce them into your flexibility program. You will also learn about some dangerous stretching practices that you should avoid, and alternative modifications of these stretches that are safe and beneficial.

What You Will Do

- Identify flexibility exercises for the whole body.
- Participate in exercises that develop flexibility.
- Identify exercises that are designed specifically to prevent lower-back pain.
- Describe potentially unsafe flexibility exercises.

Terms to Know

adductor muscles

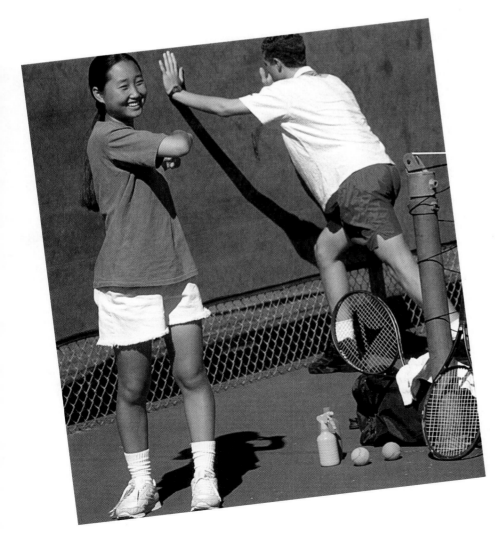

◀ Stretching is an important part of any workout. *What types of stretches do you do as part of your workout routine?*

Stretches for Flexibility

There are many stretches that may be used to improve flexibility. You should choose a variety of stretches and exercises that will work all the major muscles and joints of the body. You may want to review the stretches in Chapter 3, pages **104–105,** for other stretches that are useful for developing flexibility.

As you work through the stretches that follow, remember to
- perform all stretches and exercises slowly.
- always use the technique described.
- review FITT principles on stretching.

Neck

Head Tilts and Turns (neck flexors and extensors and ligaments of spine)

1. Turn your head to the right and hold. Repeat this motion, turning to the left.
2. Tilt your head down to your left shoulder and hold. Repeat this motion, tilting to the right.
3. Tilt your head forward and hold.
   Caution: Do not roll your head in a continuous motion.

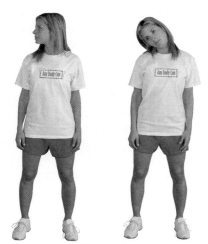

Head Tilts and Turns

Shoulders

Shoulder Shrugs (pectoralis and deltoid)

1. While standing or sitting, raise both shoulders toward your ears without lifting your arms.
2. Relax and repeat.

Shoulder and Triceps Pull (trapezius and triceps)

1. While standing or sitting, place the palm of either hand over the shoulder and on your back.
2. Position the opposite hand on the elbow of other arm. Push toward the back.
3. Repeat the process with the other shoulder.

Shoulder Pulls (trapezius and latissimus dorsi)

1. While standing or sitting, raise your arms to shoulder height.
2. Pull both shoulders toward your spine. Hold and repeat.

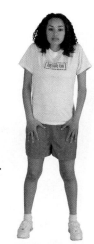

Shoulder Shrugs

Towel Stretch (triceps, shoulder, and chest)

1. Grasp a rolled-up towel with your hands spread shoulder width apart, palms down.
2. Slowly raise the towel from waist height to above your head with your arms extended.
3. Move toward your back as far as possible. Repeat.

Shoulder Pulls

Towel Stretch

Side and Trunk

Trunk Stretches (obliques and latissimus dorsi)

1. While standing or sitting on a chair, place your feet shoulder width apart. If standing, bend your knees slightly.
2. Raise your left arm over your head, and bend to your right side. Do not bend forward. If standing, keep your lower body stationary.
3. Repeat this procedure, this time to the left side.

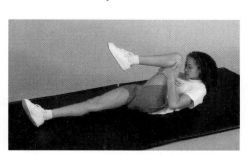

Trunk Stretches

Legs and Back

Single Knee Hug (hamstrings and lower back)

1. Lie flat on your back. Bend one knee toward your chest.
2. Place both hands behind the thigh, and gently pull the leg toward your chest.
3. Switch legs, and repeat. *Modification:* You may bring both knees to the chest at the same time.

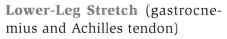

Single Knee Hug

Lower-Leg Stretch (gastrocnemius and Achilles tendon)

1. From a standing position, lean toward a wall with your arms extended.
2. Place one foot in front of the other, and extend the back leg.
3. Keep both feet flat on the ground. Bend your elbows and push toward the wall.

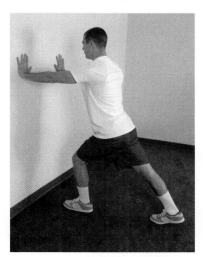

Lower-Leg Stretch

Reverse Hurdler Stretch (hamstring and lower back)

1. Sitting on the floor, extend your left leg forward.
2. Bend your right leg, and place the bottom of the foot on the inside of the left thigh near the knee.
3. Bend at the waist. Extend your body and arms forward toward the toes.
4. Switch legs and repeat.

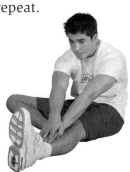

Reverse Hurdler Stretch

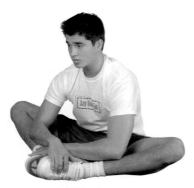

Modified Lotus

Modified Lotus or Adductor Stretch (adductor muscles, lower back) (Your leg adductor muscles are *the muscles on the inside of the leg that pull the legs together.*)

1. Sitting on the floor, bend your knees and place the bottoms of your feet flat against each other.
2. Place your left hand on your right ankle and your right hand on your left ankle.
3. Keep your back straight. Press down on your knees with your elbows.
   Modification: You may grab both feet and pull your upper body toward your feet.

Quadriceps Stretch (quadriceps and knee)

1. From a standing position, bend your left leg toward your back.
2. Lean slightly forward, and balance against a wall or chair.
3. With your right hand, grab your foot and gently pull up and out.
4. Focus on pulling the quadriceps back, instead of compressing the knee. (See **Figure 11.14** on page **353.**)
5. Switch legs and arms and repeat.

Sit-and-Reach Stretch (hamstrings and lower back)

1. Sitting on the floor, extend your legs forward and together.
2. Bend at the waist, and extend your arms and upper body forward. (See **Figure 11.9** on page **337.**)
   Modification: This may be done while sitting in a chair with the knees bent.

Exercises for Prevention of Lower-Back Pain

As noted in Lesson 1, some exercises constitute a kind of insurance against the risk of lower-back pain. Among these are exercises that target the muscles of the back, stomach, hips, and thighs.

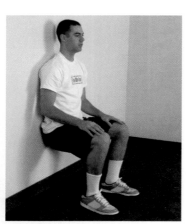

Wall Slides

Wall Slides (hips, back, quadriceps)

1. Position your back against a wall with your feet shoulder width apart.
2. Slide downward into a bent-knee position. Your thighs should be parallel to the ground.
3. Count to 5 or 6. Return to the starting position.
4. Repeat these steps 6 or 7 times.

Rear Leg Raises (lower back and gluteal)

1. Lie facedown with your arms at your sides and your legs straight.
2. With your extended left leg, tighten the muscles of the leg and lift the leg from the floor.
3. Hold this position for 10 seconds, and return to the starting position.
4. Repeat the procedure with the other leg. Continue alternating legs until you have done five repetitions with each leg.

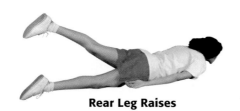

Rear Leg Raises

Front Leg Raises (abdominal and hip adductors)

1. Lie on your back with your legs extended and your arms at your side.
2. Slightly bend the knee and raise your left leg straight above your waist.
3. Hold the position for 10 seconds, then return to the starting position.
4. Repeat the procedure with the other leg. Continue alternating legs until you have done five repetitions with each leg.

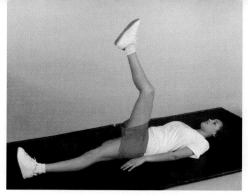

Front Leg Raises

Back Hyperextension Stretch (lower back)

1. Stand with your feet shoulder width apart.
2. Place your hands on your hips.
3. Keep your knees straight, and bend backward at the waist.
4. Hold the position for 2 to 3 seconds. Repeat the exercise 3 times.

Crunches (abdominal)

1. Lie on your back with your knees bent and your feet flat on the floor.
2. Raise your shoulders and head off the floor and extend your arms to your knees.
3. Hold for a 10-second count. Repeat 5 to 10 times.

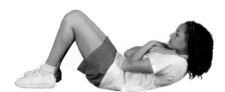

Crunches

Active Mind Active Body

Participating in Flexibility Activities

Choosing the correct stretches for your program is important for your continued success. Equally important is ensuring that these exercises are done correctly. In this activity you will choose a variety of stretches. You will demonstrate how to perform each of them properly and in a safe fashion.

What You Will Need

- Mat or other comfortable surface

What You Will Do

1. Choose at least one stretch for each of the following body parts: neck, shoulders, trunk, lower back, quadriceps, hamstrings, adductors, and lower leg. Three of your choices should be modifications of hazardous stretches found in **Figure 11.14** on pages **350–353.**
2. Demonstrate the safe method for performing each stretch.

Apply and Conclude

Did you find that some stretches were easier to perform correctly than others? Which stretches were you able to demonstrate? Which stretches were you unable to perform correctly? What changes were suggested? Were you able to make the needed corrections? How will these changes improve your flexibility program?

Hazardous Stretches and Their Modification

There are many flexibility stretches that have been practiced for years. A great number of these, including those demonstrated so far in this lesson, are beneficial. Some, however, have been identified by sports-medicine specialists to be high-risk. These hazardous stretches have been linked to a number of sports- and health-related injuries, including:

- **strains**
- sprains
- excess pressure on discs of the back
- overstress of ligaments and muscles

Modifications have been devised for some of these exercises that reduce injury risk. **Figure 11.14** illustrates both the unsafe and safe ways of performing these stretches. If you plan to do any of the following stretches, make sure you are doing the safe, modified version.

 Reading Check

Explain What are the risks of performing hazardous stretches? Describe examples that may be harmful.

hot link

strains
For more on strains, see Chapter 2, page **58**.

FIGURE 11.14

UNSAFE STRETCHES WITH MODIFICATIONS
The stretches shown on the right provide a modified version of the stretch pictured on the left. *Why were these modified stretches developed?*

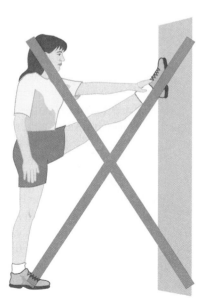

Bar Stretch

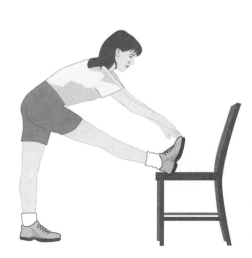

Modified Bar Stretch

FIGURE 11.14 *continued*

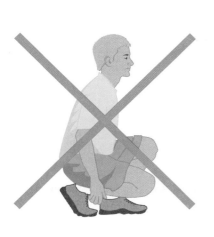

Deep Knee Bend

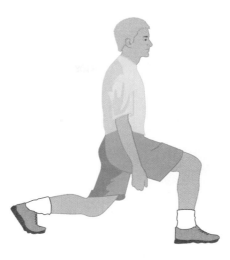

Forward Lunge

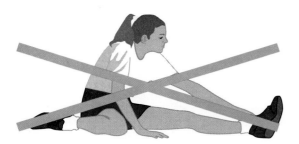

Hurdler Stretch

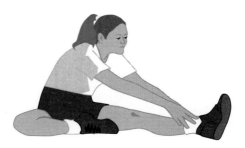

Reverse Hurdler Stretch

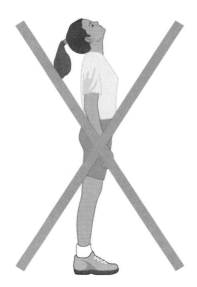

Stretch Neck Roll

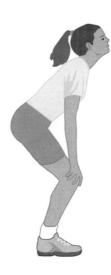

Bent-Knee Neck Stretch

continued on next page

FIGURE 11.14 *continued*

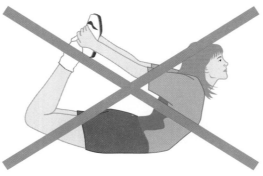

Prone Arch

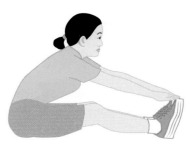

Modified Back Hyperextension

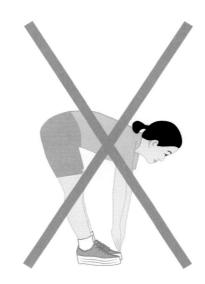

Toe Touch

Sit-and-Reach

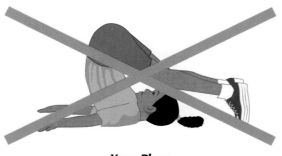

Yoga Plow

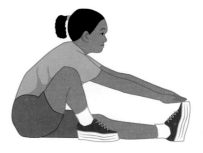

Single-Leg Sit-and-Reach

FIGURE 11.14 *continued*

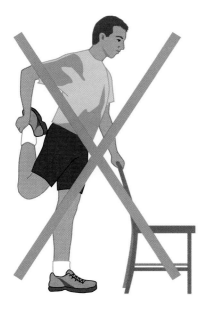

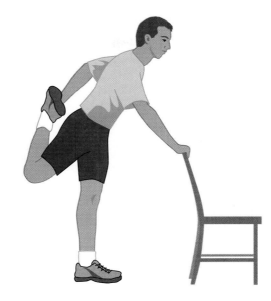

Quadriceps Stretch   **Modified Quadriceps Stretch**

Source: President's Council on Physical Fitness and Sports, 1999.[1]

Lesson 4 Review

Using complete sentences, answer the following questions on a sheet of paper.

Reviewing Facts and Vocabulary

1. **Recall** Name two stretches that benefit the shoulders.

2. **Recall** Describe two of the unsafe stretches illustrated in this lesson. What is the safe method of performing these stretches?

Thinking Critically

3. **Extend** Elma has been studying hard over the last few weeks and has noticed some tightness in her lower back while she sits at her desk. She is concerned that her muscles are not strong enough in the back and hip region. What exercises and stretches would help her solve this problem?

4. **Analyze** Why are head tilts and turns safer than doing the yoga plow stretch?

Personal Fitness Planning

Demonstrating Stretches Work with the adult members of your family to incorporate stretches and lower-back pain prevention exercises into their lifestyles. Caution them against improper stretching by explaining the unsafe versions of the stretches. Demonstrate the safe, modified versions of the exercises. Then observe their technique as family members perform the stretches.

CHAPTER 11 Review

TRUE/FALSE

On a sheet of paper, write the numbers 1–10. Write True *or* False *for each statement below.*

1. ROM is the same for every joint.
2. Hinge-like joints allow you to move forward and backward.
3. Your risk of back injuries is increased if you have inflexible and weak muscles that support your spine and pelvic girdle.
4. Hyperflexibility is a positive trait found only in people with very high levels of flexibility.
5. Muscle imbalances occur when one muscle group is worked and its opposing group is not.
6. The minimum recommended frequency for stretching is three days per week.
7. Static stretches are unsafe and are not recommended.
8. Ballistic stretching is done very slowly without bouncing up and down.
9. Passive stretches require either a partner or a device that offers counterforce.
10. The yoga plow is a safe and effective stretch for hamstrings and lower back.

MULTIPLE CHOICE

On a sheet of paper, write the letter of the word or phrase that best completes each statement.

11. The condition of hyperflexibility is associated with
    a. loose joints.
    b. tight connective tissue.
    c. strong muscles.
    d. strong ligaments.
12. Of the following posture practices, the one that is NOT beneficial is
    a. using a soft mattress.
    b. maintaining a straight back when sitting.
    c. using computer chairs with lower-back support.
    d. using a footstool for one leg if standing for an extended period of time.

13. Your flexibility is influenced by all of the following EXCEPT
    a. heredity.
    b. age.
    c. height.
    d. physical-activity level.
14. The one factor that has the greatest negative influence on your flexibility levels is
    a. lack of physical activity.
    b. excess body fat.
    c. injured joints.
    d. your gender.
15. Biomechanical lifting
    a. includes twisting, pulling, or pushing movements.
    b. should be performed only by athletes.
    c. should be done only with a partner.
    d. can help prevent lower-back injuries.
16. Plyometric training is a type of
    a. static stretching.
    b. ballistic stretching.
    c. reflex-assisted stretching.
    d. passive stretching.
17. The type of stretching that requires a partner or device to help you complete a stretch is
    a. static stretching.
    b. ballistic stretching.
    c. reflex-assisted stretching.
    d. passive stretching.
18. When stretching, your goal should be to reach the point where
    a. a muscle or connective tissue is barely stretched.
    b. a muscle or connective tissue is stretched just beyond its normal resting state.
    c. a muscle or connective tissue is stretched well beyond its normal resting state.
    d. none of the above.
19. The stretch most associated with stretching the lower back is
    a. the knee hug.
    b. the wall slide.
    c. the quadriceps stretch.
    d. the reverse hurdler stretch.
20. Which of the following stretches is hazardous and may cause injury?
    a. the knee hug
    b. the calf stretch
    c. the adductor stretch
    d. the stretch neck roll

DISCUSSION

Using complete sentences, answer the following questions on a sheet of paper.

21. **Identify** Describe five ways you can help reduce your risk for lower-back pain and injuries.
22. **Explain** Give five benefits that typically follow 8 to 30 weeks of flexibility conditioning in a previously inactive teen.
23. **Identify** List five stretches that are safe and effective for increasing or maintaining your flexibility levels.

VOCABULARY

On a sheet of paper, write the letter of the term in Column B that best fits the definition in Column A.

Column A

24. A condition in which one muscle group becomes too strong in relation to a complementary group.
25. Stretching with bobbing movements.
26. The automatic responses that your nerves and muscles provide to various movements.
27. A type of stretching against a counterforce in which there is little or no movement.
28. Range of motion or varying degrees of movement.
29. The ability of the muscles and connective tissues to stretch and give.
30. Stretching movements that challenge the reflexes to adapt.

Column B

a. elasticity
b. passive stretching
c. muscle imbalance
d. ROM
e. reflexes
f. ballistic stretching
g. reflex-assisted stretching

CRITICAL THINKING

Using complete sentences, answer the following questions on a sheet of paper.

31. **Analyze** Respond to this statement: You can never have enough flexibility.

32. **Explain** Explain the relationship between physical fitness and health. How does maintaining an active lifestyle contribute to your flexibility?
33. **Synthesize** Most lower-back pain and injuries are preventable by practicing proper lifting and stretches. Identify enough examples of both to create a total program for the back.

CASE STUDY

CASE STUDY—BOB'S INJURY

Bob is a fifteen-year-old who is very active. He enjoys jogging 3 to 5 miles daily. However, in the past year he has noticed that his muscles feel very tight, his lower back hurts occasionally, and he feels like he has lost some flexibility. Bob does not like to stretch and really sees no benefit in it. However, he is concerned about his loss of flexibility, because he thinks it may increase his risk for injuries during jogging. He would like to improve his flexibility levels, but he is not sure how to do so. Therefore, he needs the help of someone knowledgeable about designing and implementing fitness programs—someone like you!

HERE IS YOUR ASSIGNMENT:

Assume that Bob has asked you for some assistance. Organize a list of factors Bob should consider before beginning flexibility conditioning. Then list the recommendations you would give Bob for his first two weeks of flexibility conditioning. Use these suggestions as a guide:

KEYS TO HELP YOU

- Consider Bob's history of flexibility conditioning.
- Consider how he should evaluate his current flexibility levels.
- Consider his needs and goals. (For example, how will he find time to do flexibility exercises?)
- Determine a reasonable plan for Bob that covers the concepts of overload, frequency, intensity, time, type, and progression.

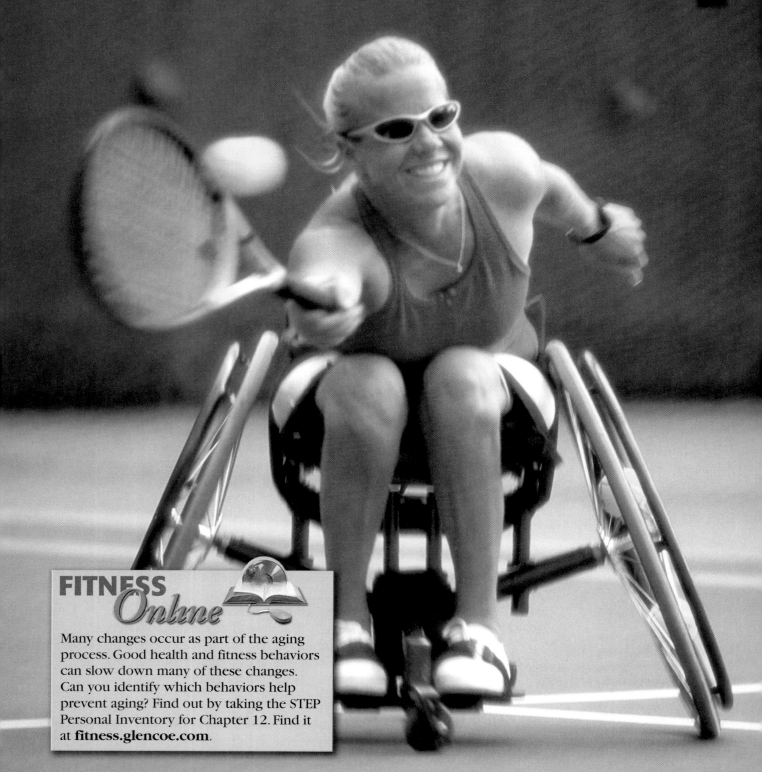

CHAPTER
12
Personal Fitness Throughout Life

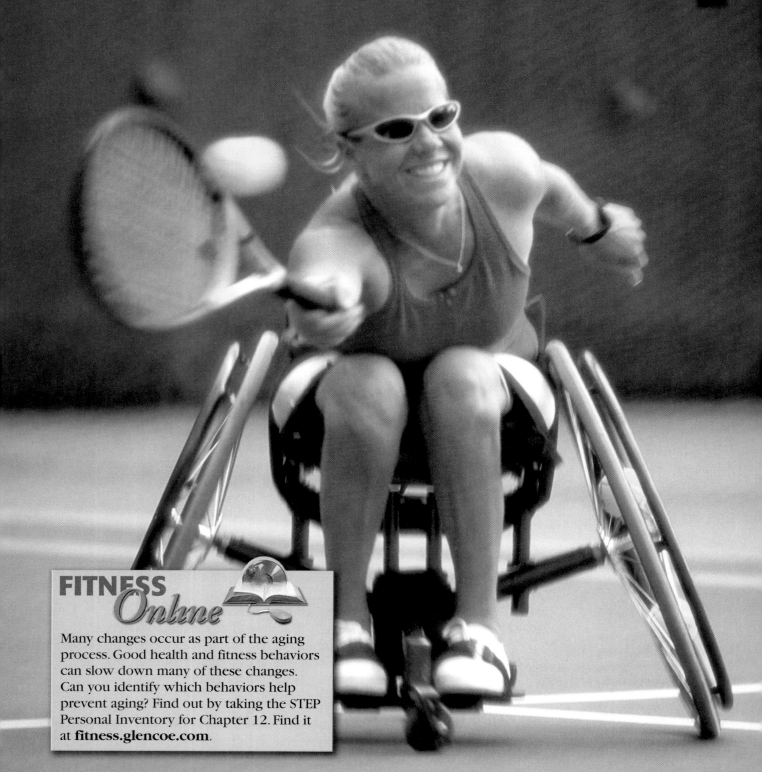

FITNESS
Online

Many changes occur as part of the aging process. Good health and fitness behaviors can slow down many of these changes. Can you identify which behaviors help prevent aging? Find out by taking the STEP Personal Inventory for Chapter 12. Find it at **fitness.glencoe.com**.

Fitness: A Lifetime Goal

Developing personal fitness during your teen years is essential to maintaining good health throughout your life. As an adult, you will benefit from the fitness habits you develop as a teen, and it is important to maintain a high level of fitness as you begin to age. Although you may need to adjust your personal fitness as you get older, personal fitness throughout your life is an achievable goal.

Understanding the Aging Process

The aging process is *the manner in which the body changes as a natural result of growing older.* Some aging-related changes, such as gray hair and wrinkled skin, are outwardly visible. Others are not. The line graph in **Figure 12.1** on page **358** illustrates four internal changes. All are declines in bodily functions of inactive individuals as they get older. Take a moment to examine this graph. Notice that these declines do not occur at the same rate. For example, compare the changes in resting metabolic rate (RMR) and lung capacity from ages 30 to 90. You find that RMR declines only about 10 percent, while lung capacity decreases 25 percent for nonsmokers. While these declines are to some degree inevitable, they do occur more slowly in physically active individuals.

What You Will Do

- Explain the body's natural aging process.
- Identify the physical changes that occur as people age.
- Recognize and explain the relationship between physical fitness and health throughout the lifespan.

Terms to Know

aging process

Personal fitness is a lifetime goal. *Why is it important to remain physically active as an older adult?*

The Aging Process and Health

Although the aging process cannot be reversed or halted, it can be slowed. You probably know some people who look and feel much younger than others their age. You may know people in their fifties, sixties, and seventies who are able to do more physical work than many younger people. For at least some of these people, the key to slowing down the clock is personal fitness. Many of them developed positive attitudes and behaviors early on, when they were your age.

Among these positive behaviors are an active lifestyle and proper nutrition. **Figure 12.2** shows their impact on a number of aging-related changes. As you can see, staying active and eating right will not necessarily keep you from getting gray hair or going bald. You can, however, make a positive impact on health areas such as levels of body fat, blood pressure, resting heart rate, and many other factors that will decrease your risk for diseases later in life.

Preventing or Slowing the Loss of Bone Mass

One physical change that occurs with age is a gradual loss of bone mass. When you are young, your bones are dense. As you progress into young adulthood, this density—or bone mass—will increase. Typically, peak bone mass occurs between the ages of 27 and 32. After this, bone density begins to decline.

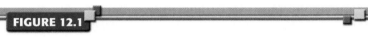

FIGURE 12.1

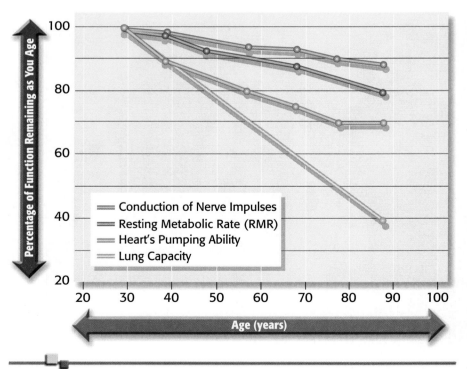

AGING AND PHYSICAL FUNCTIONS

The body's physical functions decline with age. *Which of these body processes declines the most rapidly? The most slowly?*

- Conduction of Nerve Impulses
- Resting Metabolic Rate (RMR)
- Heart's Pumping Ability
- Lung Capacity

Percentage of Function Remaining as You Age

Age (years)

FIGURE 12.2

EFFECT OF EXERCISE AND NUTRITION ON AGING

Staying physically active and eating healthfully will help you maintain your health as you age. *Which of these changes is related to mental/emotional health? To physical health?*

Aging-Related Change	Can (✓) Cannot (X) Make Positive Impact	
Graying of hair		X
Balding		X
Resting energy metabolism	✓	
Increased body fat	✓	
Increased blood pressure	✓	
Increased resting pulse	✓	
Elevated cholesterol levels	✓	
Decreased functional health	✓	
Inherited diseases		X
Hypokinetic diseases	✓	
Loss of elasticity of joints*		X
Loss of flexibility of joints**	✓	
Bone loss	✓	
Mental confusion	✓	
Reduced self-esteem	✓	
Depression	✓	

* elasticity = ability to return immediately to original size and shape

** flexibility = ability to bend without breaking

Source: Adapted with permission from Health: Making Life Choices, *1994.*[1]

Researchers have established a relationship between loss of bone mass and physical activity levels. **Figure 12.3** on page **360** shows this relationship. The graph reveals that more active people have greater bone mass than inactive people. This means that as active people age, they will be at a lower risk for **osteoporosis** than inactive people. Instead of developing brittle bones by age 65, they delay this onset into their seventies or eighties.

Proper nutrition is also important for preventing osteoporosis. Eating foods rich in the mineral calcium offsets some bone loss. Such foods include milk, yogurt, and canned salmon.

osteoporosis
For more on osteoporosis and ways to slow this disease, see Chapter 9, page **258**.

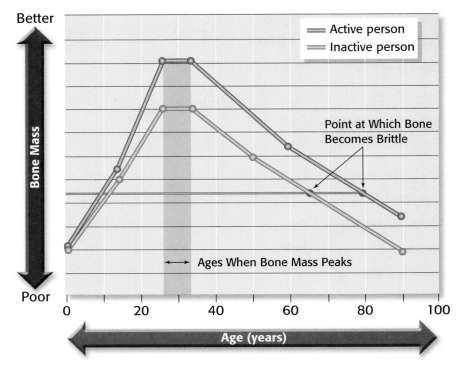

FIGURE 12.3

BONE MASS AND PHYSICAL ACTIVITY

Being physically active can increase peak bone mass and prevent osteoporosis. *At what age does bone become brittle in active people? In inactive people?*

Better

Poor

Bone Mass

— Active person
— Inactive person

Point at Which Bone Becomes Brittle

Ages When Bone Mass Peaks

0   20   40   60   80   100

Age (years)

Source: Adapted with permission from *New Horizons in Pediatric Exercise Science, 1995.*[2]

Modifying Your Activities

As you age, you will need to adjust your personal fitness program to meet your changing needs. For example, you may have to adjust your FITT for selected activities to enable you to recover more completely between workouts. You may find that you need to vary your exercise or activity routine or type to avoid boredom and to help maintain your **adherence.** You will need to understand your mental and physical limitations. Only then will you be able to meet special situations and needs effectively. By staying active throughout your life, you will learn to pay even closer attention to your body, which will help you recognize possible health problems. Then you will be able to maintain a healthy, active, and productive lifestyle throughout your life.

adherence
For more on adherence and strategies for maintaining it, see Chapter 1, page **21.**

 Reading Check

Evaluate What are two behaviors that can slow the aging process? How does physical activity affect bone mass?

The Physical Activity Pyramid: Fitness for Life

In Chapter 1 you learned about the Physical Activity Pyramid. It is a guide for developing and maintaining regular physical-activity patterns that will reduce your risks for chronic diseases as you age. The pyramid illustrates a sensible, step-by-step plan to becoming and staying active. If you currently maintain moderate-to-high levels of fitness, you are off to a good start. As you age, you may need to adjust the types of activities you do, but you can always maintain your overall fitness.

Remember that daily physical activities, such as walking the dog, form the base of the pyramid. The next level up includes aerobic exercise and leisure-time activities. The third level promotes the development and maintenance of strength and flexibility. The top step reminds you to cut down on your sedentary habits.

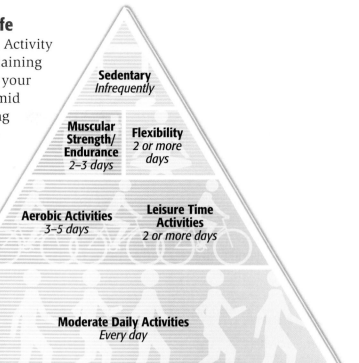

 Reading Check

Explain What type of activities form the base, or first step, of the Physical Activity Pyramid?

▲ The Physical Activity Pyramid can help you plan your physical activities. *What are some examples of each type of activity listed?*

Lesson 1 Review

Using complete sentences, answer the following questions on a sheet of paper.

Reviewing Facts and Vocabulary

1. **Vocabulary** What is the *aging process?*
2. **Recall** List and explain three examples of how your body changes as it ages.

Thinking Critically

3. **Analyze** What effect does physical activity have on health, as one ages?
4. **Evaluate** Explain the saying "Old age is a state of mind."

Personal Fitness Planning

Evaluating Physical Activities Review the Physical Activity Pyramid to determine if you are doing enough of the right activities. You may want to refer to **Figure 1.8** in Chapter 1 on page **10**. Make a list of the things you do daily at each level of the pyramid. Then make a list of the activities you hope to see yourself doing as an older adult. Which activities are the same? Which are different? Explain the relationship between physical fitness and health in your choices.

Your Changing Personal Fitness Goals

Throughout this text you have been encouraged to develop and maintain an active lifestyle. A broad spectrum of physical activities, exercises, and sports can help you achieve that goal. Many of these have appeared in earlier chapters. In this lesson, you will explore several others.

What You Will Do

- Discuss the health benefits of leisure-time activities.
- Identify leisure-time activities that meet your fitness goals.
- Recognize why people should vary their activity selection as they age.
- Design and implement an aerobic-workout routine.

Terms to Know

leisure-time activities
martial arts
t'ai chi

Leisure-Time Activities

Leisure-time activities include *sports and other action-oriented pursuits done for recreation.* Leisure-time activities do not focus on developing health-related or skill-related fitness the way other physical activities might, such as competitive sports. However, done regularly, leisure-time activities can improve some aspects of health-related or skill-related fitness. They also provide other benefits, such as

- reducing stress levels.
- providing an opportunity for social interaction.
- burning calories.
- developing and maintaining self-esteem.

As you continue to develop and refine your personal fitness program, you should experiment with and try a variety of leisure-time activities. Then you can select ones that you find enjoyable and, if possible, help you meet your personal fitness goals.

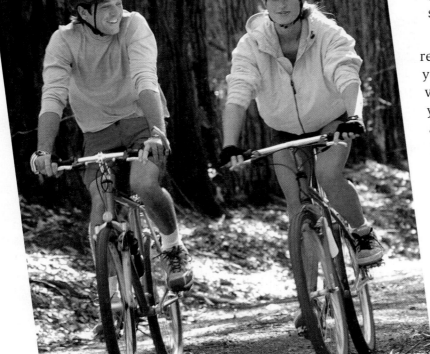

◄ A great way to maintain your personal fitness is by finding leisure-time activities that you enjoy. *What are some benefits of leisure-time activities?*

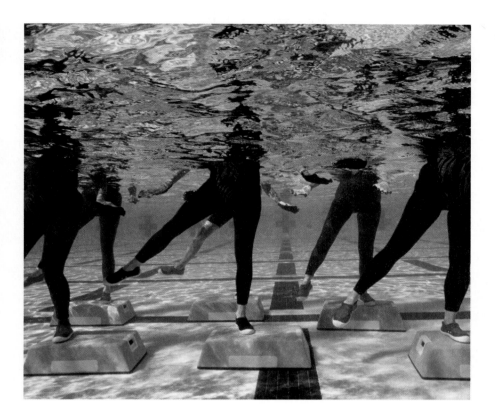

Many people enjoy resistance training as an aquatic activity. *What aspects of fitness do aquatic activities develop?*

Aquatic Activities

Many people enjoy swimming as a leisure-time activity. In Chapter 8, you learned about **lap swimming** as a way to develop and maintain your cardiorespiratory fitness. In addition to swimming laps, many people enjoy working out in the pool by doing exercises against the resistance provided by the water. For example, when you stand in a pool with water at chest level and move your arms back and forth through the water, you can feel the resistance of the water. Aquatic activities reduce the pounding that your body takes in weight-bearing activities (for example, walking or jogging) and can be modified in intensity by working in the shallow or deep ends of the pool. You can use aquatic activities to develop and maintain good to better levels of cardiorespiratory fitness, muscular endurance, and body composition.

Cycling

As noted in Chapter 8, **cycling** is excellent for developing balance and cardiorespiratory fitness and for controlling body composition. It is also a very popular form of exercise with all age groups. Tour cycling is usually done on roads with a light-framed bike that has thin tires. Mountain biking is done on trails with a bike that has a heavier frame and wider tires for better traction. These activities are made more enjoyable and safer when done in groups. Also for safety, always wear a helmet for touring or mountain bike cycling.

LIFELINE

Applying Etiquette
Choose two or three activities from this lesson, or identify some of your favorite activities. Share with the class specific etiquette involved with these activities. For example, you might discuss who has the right of way on trails shared by runners, hikers, and mountain bikers; or how skiers and snowboarders can share the slopes to avoid injury.

hotlink

lap swimming
For more on lap swimming and its benefits, see Chapter 8, page **232.**

cycling
For more on cycling, see Chapter 8, page **229.**

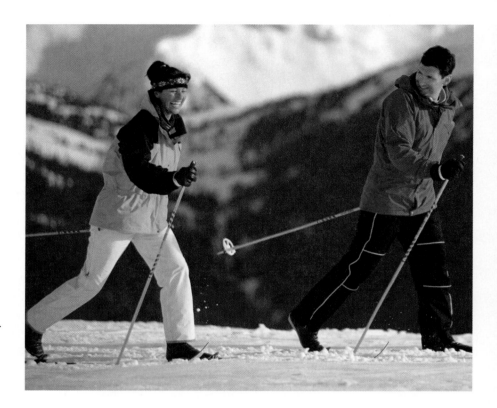

▶ Snow skiing requires excellent coordination and power. *What are the benefits of skiing to your personal fitness?*

h⊙t link

cross-country skiing
For more on cross-country skiing, see Chapter 8, page **231.**

h⊙t link

aerobic dance
For more on aerobic dance, see Chapter 8, page **230.**

Water and Snow Skiing

Whether you're on the water or the snow, skiing allows you to enjoy the great outdoors. The safest way to participate in skiing is to take lessons and purchase or rent quality equipment. Skiing of any type requires excellent coordination and power. As mentioned in Chapter 8, **cross-country skiing** is an excellent way to develop and maintain your cardiorespiratory fitness and body composition.

Dance

As discussed in Chapter 8, participating in **aerobic-dance** classes is an excellent way to improve your cardiorespiratory fitness. However, a fitness center is not the only place to experience the benefits of dance. There are many popular types of dance that are easy to do once you've had a few lessons. Dancing helps develop balance, coordination, and agility. Many forms of dance are also good for aerobic conditioning and weight control, provided they are done regularly and for long enough periods of time. (As you have learned, health-related fitness results depend on your FITT.) Dancing is also an excellent way to interact socially with others while achieving your fitness goals.

 Reading Check

Analyze Does dance improve health-related fitness, skill-related fitness, or both? Explain your answer.

Designing an Aerobic-Exercise Routine

When planning your personal fitness program, you may decide to incorporate aerobic exercise as part of your plan. An aerobic workout is a convenient and enjoyable way to improve and maintain cardiorespiratory endurance.

In this activity, you will apply the physiological principle related to intensity to an aerobic-exercise routine by designing your own routine and evaluating its intensity, using your heart rate. Remember, for any fitness plan to be a success, you need to apply all FITT factors correctly. Once you have verified an appropriate intensity level for your aerobic-exercise routine, you may choose to integrate it as the cardiovascular component of your personal fitness program.

Procedure:

1. If possible, view two or three videotapes of aerobic workout routines. Determine the types of music used, intensities of the exercises done (low, moderate, or high), the types of warm-up and cooldown done, and the types of movements performed.
2. Design your own 12- to 15-minute aerobic-exercise routine.
3. Vary the routine intensity with low-impact and high-impact exercises.
4. Set the routine cadence to a count of 8.
5. Do not repeat any exercises for more than two sets of 8 counts.
6. Use correct exercise technique and develop smooth transitions from one exercise to the next.
7. Make sure your routine includes a warm-up (no longer than 2–3 minutes), aerobic activities that work the arms and shoulders, abdominals, and legs, followed by a cooldown (no longer than 2–3 minutes).
8. After you have practiced your routine, evaluate the intensity of your workout by taking your pulse a total of four times: before you begin, after the warm-up, after the main aerobic activities, and two minutes after the completion of the cooldown.

9. Copy the graph in **Figure 12.4** and chart your results. The shaded areas of the chart indicate an appropriate range of intensity for each phase of your routine. Take note of any areas where your results fall outside the shaded areas.
10. If the intensity was below moderate intensity or above vigorous intensity, plan how you can adjust the intensity level. If the intensity was within an appropriate range, incorporate the aerobic-exercise routine into your personal fitness plan and regularly assess your progress (every four to six weeks) by using one of the Cardiorespiratory Endurance evaluations from Chapter 7 or Chapter 8.

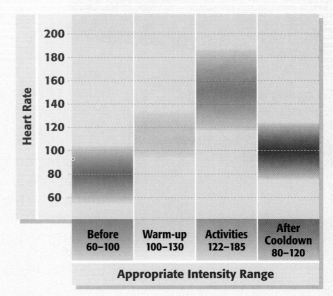

Figure 12.4 INTENSITY OF YOUR AEROBIC WORKOUT

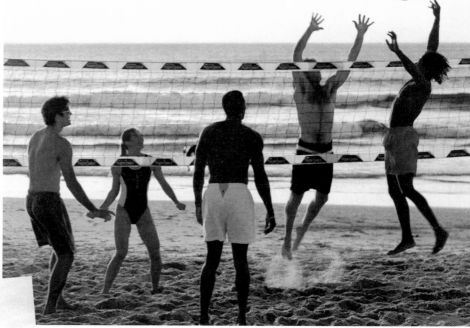

▶ Volleyball is an activity that can be played at the recreational or competitive level. *What other activities mentioned in this lesson can also be competitive?*

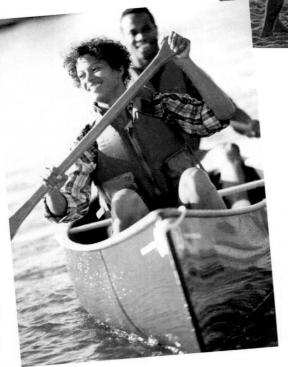

▲ Canoeing is a good way to get outside and enjoy nature. *What are some other health benefits of this activity?*

Volleyball and Basketball

Basketball is excellent for developing coordination, reaction time, and power. They can also provide an excellent cardiovascular- and muscular-endurance workout. Two-person sand volleyball has become very popular. More and more communities are building sand courts to promote participation. Playing half-court or full-court basketball is a challenging activity, but many people are able to participate in it well into middle age by maintaining good-to-better fitness levels.

Racquetball and Tennis

Racquetball and tennis are excellent ways to develop cardiorespiratory endurance and body composition. They require high levels of coordination and agility. Racquetball is one of the most popular indoor leisure-time activities.

If you like to compete, racquetball tournaments are regularly held at many fitness clubs and are designed to challenge players of all ages and abilities. If you prefer tennis, many city parks, recreation departments, and private tennis clubs offer lessons for people of all ages and abilities.

Kayaking and Canoeing

Kayaking and canoeing can be done recreationally or at competitive levels. These activities help develop your power. When done for long periods of time per session, they promote cardiorespiratory fitness, muscular strength, and muscular endurance. You will need to take time to develop the specific skills necessary for these activities to be done safely, but they are great ways to get outside, explore new areas, and help control stress levels.

Rowing

Rowing in all its different forms is an excellent activity to develop your coordination, power, cardiorespiratory fitness, and muscular endurance. It is also a great way to control your body composition. Rowing in a crew can be a great way to meet other people and be part of a team, even if it's just for recreation. Stationary rowing can be fun if you have access to a rowing machine with interactive video feedback to enhance your workout.

 Reading Check

Explain Which activities help to develop coordination? Power?

Martial Arts

The martial arts, which originated in Eastern Asia, are practiced by some 100 million people worldwide. The original purpose of the martial arts was self-defense. Today, martial arts are seen as *activities that combine exercise and relaxation techniques.* Many of these activities teach controlled breathing, which helps reduce stress.

There are approximately 200 separate martial arts. Karate and judo are two of the most well-known. Another popular form of martial arts is t'ai chi (DYE JEE). This is *a martial art that involves fluid, graceful movements, demanding precise muscular control.* Practicing t'ai chi provides excellent muscle tone.

Hiking and Backpacking

Hiking and backpacking are excellent ways to get outside and enjoy nature while developing muscular endurance and cardiorespiratory fitness. Most areas of the country provide numerous opportunities for these activities. For personal safety, you should hike with someone else, using well-marked trails. Carry a water supply to prevent dehydration. If you hike in an area you're not familiar with, make sure you carry a map and compass. These can help you avoid becoming lost. A good pair of hiking shoes or boots is also indispensable. It is a good idea to let someone know where you are going, or, if possible, carry a cellular phone.

Backpacking requires more planning than does a day of hiking. If you will be gone for several days, you will need a tent, food, and fluids. You also need to determine how much weight you are able to carry for extended periods of time.

Hiking and backpacking are useful for maintaining good levels of health-related fitness. However, you need to do some cardiovascular conditioning and muscular-endurance training prior to an extended hiking or backpacking trip.

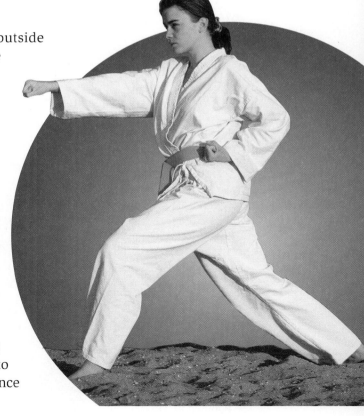
You can increase your self-confidence and self-esteem by participating in the martial arts. *What are the other benefits of the martial arts?*

anaerobic activity
For more on anaerobic activity and how it differs from aerobic activity, see Chapter 7, page **212.**

Rock Climbing

Rock climbing is a challenging activity that requires high levels of muscular strength and endurance. Excellent balance and coordination are also necessary. Though rock climbing is chiefly an **anaerobic activity,** longer climbs will also stress you aerobically. Although typically an outdoor activity, indoor facilities for rock climbing are becoming increasingly popular in many communities. No matter where you climb, you should practice safe climbing skills by always climbing with a partner and using your safety gear.

Calisthenics

Calisthenics are a convenient activity because they can be done in your own home, perhaps with the guidance of a workout video or television show. Doing regular calisthenics (push-ups, abdominal crunches, jumping jacks, and so on) can help you improve your muscular endurance and flexibility. If you do calisthenics in a continuous, rhythmic manner, you can also develop and maintain your cardiorespiratory fitness and control your body composition.

Triathlons, Biathlons, and Marathons

Triathlons are endurance competitions that include swimming, cycling, and running for various distances. Biathlons are endurance events that usually combine two activities—for example, running and cycling, swimming and running, or cross-country skiing and rifle shooting. Marathons are endurance competitions that include running distances of at least 26.2 miles. Triathlons, biathlons, and marathons require high levels of performance fitness, but they do have varied lengths and many participants can find a distance they can complete.

Most people will never try to complete a triathlon, biathlon, or marathon. However, you may want to challenge yourself to compete

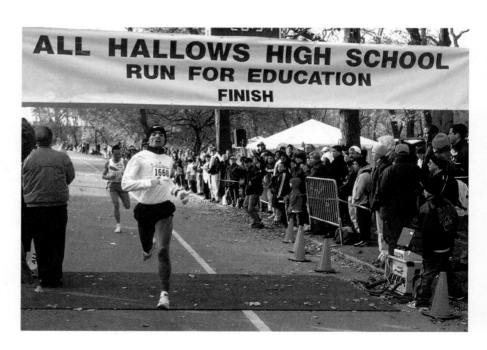

▶ Running in a marathon requires at least several months of preparation.

in one of these events just for your own satisfaction. If you decide to attempt one of these activities, make sure you seek out professional advice beforehand. You will need a sequential training program with periodic checkpoints for at least several months to condition yourself properly before the event.

 Reading Check

Extend What specific types of conditioning does a person need to do in preparation for a marathon?

Activities for a Lifetime

It is only natural that your interests will change as you age. So will your levels of health-related fitness. Your choice of leisure-time activities, thus, should change to reflect your changing needs. Your ultimate goal should be to make physical activity a lifetime habit.

Learn to analyze your lifetime activities to make sure they help you meet your personal needs for health-related fitness, skill-related fitness, stress reduction, and worthwhile leisure pursuits. Also, determine which lifetime activities are realistic for you based on the following:

- **Cost.** Can you afford to participate in the activity?
- **Your personality and attitude.** Does the activity fit your style?
- **Availability of equipment and facilities.** Where can you find equipment or facilities for the activity?
- **Your social needs.** Will you do the activity alone or with friends?
- **Environmental hazards.** Can you engage in the activity safely?

Exercise You Can Enjoy

Working out doesn't have to be work. Leisure-time activities are an enjoyable and effective way of staying physically fit throughout your life.

Whether you enjoy swimming, cycling, dancing, or another action-oriented pursuit, leisure-time activities are a great way of staying physically fit and having fun. Take time to find a leisure-time activity that works for you.

Lesson 2 Review

Using complete sentences, answer the following questions on a sheet of paper.

Reviewing Facts and Vocabulary

1. **Vocabulary** Define *leisure-time activities.*
2. **Recall** Name two activities that promote cardiorespiratory fitness.

Thinking Critically

3. **Compare and Contrast** In what ways are the benefits of hiking and backpacking similar to those of rock climbing? In what ways are they different?

4. **Extend** Jay has been an avid runner for the last five years. He has recently considered the possibility of entering a triathlon. What advice would you give him and why?

Personal Fitness Planning

Assessing Physical Activities Make a list of all the activities named in this lesson that you have personally participated in. Then make a list of those that you have not tried but would like to learn more about. What are the special considerations you need to examine before starting these activities?

Choosing Fitness Professionals

Sheila had been lifting weights for only a short time when she began to experience back pain. She knew she needed to see someone who could tell her what was wrong. She also knew she needed future guidance about lifting techniques.

Would you know who to turn to if you were Sheila? After reading this lesson, you will learn about fitness professionals who are able to help you solve your health and fitness questions.

Finding Qualified Fitness Experts

If you feel you need expert advice in the areas of health and fitness during your teen years, it is always best to first seek the advice of your parents or guardian. As you reach adulthood, however, you will be increasingly responsible for your own health and well-being.

There are a number of professionals who can provide advice and counseling about nutrition, health, exercise, and more. All are required to complete specialized training and have appropriate licensing or certification. To ensure you are choosing a qualified professional, verify that they have the appropriate **credentials.** These are *a summary of the person's professional training and experience in a given field.*

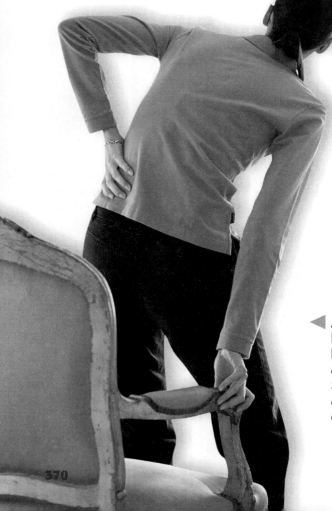

A qualified fitness professional can help with problems such as lower-back pain. *Aside from your parents, who is a good person to talk to if you think you need advice from a health or fitness expert?*

When choosing a fitness or health expert, the following guidelines may be helpful.

- Ask friends or relatives for recommendations.
- Ask other health care professionals you know for a referral.
- Ask a local librarian or consumer protection agency if a directory of such professionals is available. A directory will provide information about their professional credentials and areas of specialization.

Physicians

This grouping includes doctors in general practice who treat day-to-day health problems or injuries. Although a general physician, such as your family doctor, may not specialize in fitness-related problems, he or she can help you determine if you have a fitness-related problem and refer you to the appropriate professional. If you have a specific concern about your health or fitness, a general physician is a great place to start.

Some doctors do have particular specialties. One specialty with particularly strong ties to fitness is orthopedics. This is *a branch of medicine that deals with bone and joint injuries and disorders.* Another physician who often treats fitness-related problems is a podiatrist. A podiatrist is *a physician trained specifically to treat disorders of the feet.* Typically, a family doctor will refer patients to see a specialist if necessary.

 Reading Check

Summarize What do orthopedists do?

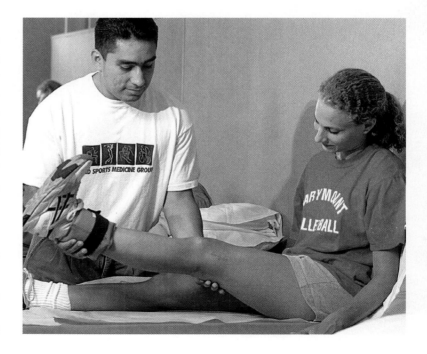

▼ Physical therapists are specially trained to work with people who are rehabilitating from injuries. *What type of personal skills do you think physical therapists need in their line of work?*

Physical Therapists

Physical therapists are *health professionals specially trained to work with people recovering from injuries.* They use a variety of treatments and techniques to help manage their patients' problems. Physical therapists undergo four to six years of academic and clinical training and must be licensed by the state. If you suffer an injury, your physician will most likely refer you to a physical therapist.

Athletic Trainers

Athletic trainers are *professionals who work with athletes undergoing rehabilitation.* Settings may include high schools, colleges, or traveling with professional sports teams. Athletic trainers undergo at least four years of academic and clinical training before they can practice. They work under the supervision of physicians and are often licensed by the state. If you would like advice from an athletic trainer, speak to your physical education instructor, coach, or doctor.

Registered Dietitians

Registered dietitians (RDs) are *professionals who specialize in providing nutritional advice and helping people control their weight.* Registered dietitians undergo at least four years of training and register with the American Dietetic Association before they can practice as a registered dietitian.

Be careful when choosing a professional to advise you about nutrition. Someone may call him- or herself a nutritionist, but they may not have the proper training. When choosing a dietitian, make sure he or she has the initials "RD" after his or her name. This ensures they have the appropriate qualifications.

Exercise Physiologists

Exercise physiologists are *specially trained to understand the body's physical reactions to exercise.* They must earn a college degree with an emphasis in exercise physiology. They are not licensed by the state but must be certified by a national organization. To do so, they must pass written tests and demonstrate their skill as leaders of physical activity.

Exercise physiologists work under the supervision of a doctor to administer medical tests to evaluate a person's fitness. They also develop, implement, and coordinate exercise programs. Often, they work with people who have physical problems, such as diabetes, obesity, or heart disease. Many also work with the general population to provide fitness evaluations and advice about physical activity and exercise.

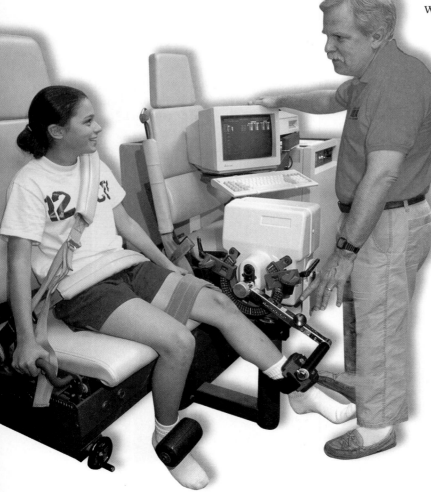

◀ Personal trainers, exercise physiologists, and athletic trainers are just a few of the health and fitness specialists who can advise you about your personal fitness.

Any Body Can

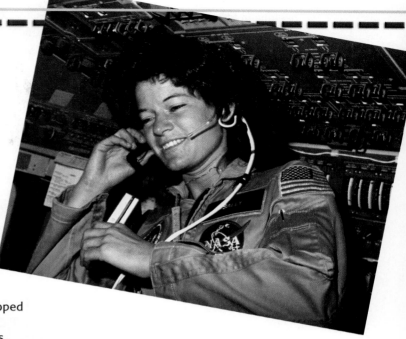

Dr. Sally Ride

When the Sky Is Not *the Limit*

Some people are willing to go far to achieve their goals. Astrophysicist and astronaut Sally Ride has indeed gone far, both scholastically and in physical miles. In 1983, she became the first American woman to go into space.

Sally Kristen Ride was born in Los Angeles, California, on May 26, 1951. She grew up dreaming of being a professional tennis player. She also developed a love for science. She attended Stanford University, where she eventually earned her doctorate in physics.

In 1978, Dr. Ride applied to become an astronaut with the National Aeronautics and Space Administration (NASA). She was one of 35 applicants selected out of a field of 8,000. She was selected partly on the basis of her ability to pass rigorous medical and physical tests. During her training, she mastered the extraordinarily high levels of fitness any person needs to travel in space.

After retiring from NASA, Dr. Ride returned to Stanford University as a professor. Currently she is director of the California Space Institute at the University of California at San Diego. She also continues to be physically active.

Not everyone can be a rocket scientist like Dr. Sally Ride. However, anyone can learn to optimize his or her functional health and fitness with age. Yes, Any Body Can!

Interview

What are other careers that demand high levels of health and fitness? Choose one such career. Interview a person in that field to find out more. Consider asking: What are the physical requirements of the job? How does one train for the tests? What do the physical tests and medical evaluations involve? Does the screening process involve any other types of testing?

Careers in Health and Fitness

Fitness-related professions include personal trainers, aerobic-dance instructors, and fitness specialists. All share a common interest in working with people, alone or in groups, whose goal is to achieve individual personal fitness. These professionals may or may not have formal academic or clinical training. Many organizations sponsor programs that provide professional health and fitness certification in these areas. Individuals must pass written and practical examinations.

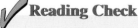 **Reading Check**

Extend Which health professional would you be most likely to see if you wanted to control your body composition? Explain.

▶ If you are interested in health and fitness, there are many careers you may want to consider. *What is required to become a high school physical educator?*

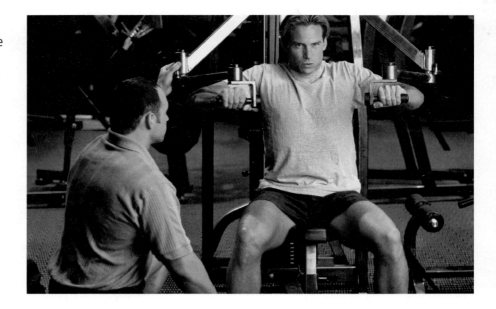

FITNESS
Online

Learn more about careers in health and fitness by visiting **fitness.glencoe.com**.

Activity Visit the online Career Corner. Find careers under Fitness and Nutrition to determine what you can do to prepare for a career in fitness.

Health Educators and Physical Education Teachers

Do you enjoy sharing information with others? Are you interested in wellness, personal fitness, and possibly coaching? If so, a career in physical and/or health education might be right for you. Instructors in these areas must complete four to six years of college, earning degrees in health or physical education specialties. They are certified by the state to teach. The instructor for this class is most likely a health or physical educator or coach. He or she is a valuable resource when you are seeking personal fitness advice.

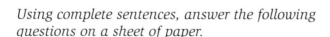

Lesson 3 Review

Using complete sentences, answer the following questions on a sheet of paper.

Reviewing Facts and Vocabulary

1. **Recall** What are two types of doctors who are likely to treat fitness-related problems?
2. **Vocabulary** Define *registered dietitian*.
3. **Vocabulary** Define *athletic trainer*.

Thinking Critically

4. **Compare and Contrast** Explain the differences between a physical therapist and an exercise physiologist.
5. **Synthesize** Imagine you felt a pain in the arch of your foot after playing basketball.

Which fitness professional would you most likely go to? Why would you select this person?

Personal Fitness Planning

Identifying Fitness Professionals How available are fitness experts in your immediate community? Make a list of all the fitness experts in your school. Prepare another list for your local area. Lastly, identify types of fitness experts not available in your immediate area. Contact at least two people on your lists and ask about their credentials and certifications.

Choosing Fitness Products

There are a number of fitness products and facilities available for you to choose from. However, knowing whether a product is safe and effective can be a challenge. So can finding a gym or health club that will help you achieve your fitness goals.

In this lesson, you will learn how to evaluate fitness information related to fitness products and facilities. You will also learn questions to ask when choosing a health and fitness club.

Evaluating Health and Fitness Information

As consumers, we are bombarded by advertisements for health and fitness products. All carry claims that their product will make you fitter, look better, or feel better. While some of these claims are valid, many are false or misleading. The products that they sell are unsafe or ineffective. How can you separate fact from fiction when it comes to media ads, not to mention the countless fitness books and magazines that are available? Here are some guidelines that can help.

- Be suspicious of claims for quick and simple results.
- Beware of miracle breakthroughs that have not been reported by reputable sources.
- Beware of testimonials claiming great results with a product.
- When reading magazine articles or books, examine the writer's credentials. If no credentials are listed, there may be a good reason.
- Beware of mail-order sales or infomercials that promote products or services not endorsed by qualified health and fitness professionals.

In general, never spend money on a health or fitness product until you've had a chance to evaluate it. You'll practice your skills at doing just that in the "Active Mind—Active Body" activity on page **376.**

What You Will Do

- Analyze strategies for becoming a more informed fitness consumer.
- Evaluate consumer issues related to fitness, including health and fitness claims and services.
- Identify the characteristics of a reputable fitness center.

Terms to Know

commercial fitness centers
corporate fitness centers
sports medicine clinic centers

▼ When evaluating a fitness facility, it is a good idea to take notes on the equipment and features. This will enable you to compare options later.

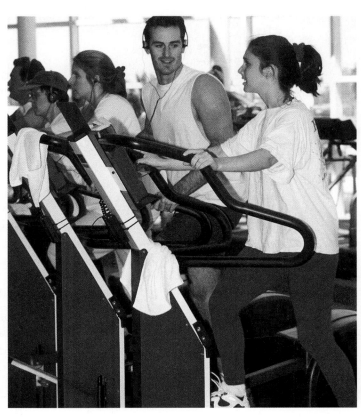

Health and Fitness Facilities

Many people choose health clubs and fitness facilities as a place to develop their personal fitness. As a teen, you will most likely need permission from your parents to join a fitness club. If you have access to a fitness facility, it can be a great place to focus on your fitness. You may not belong to any kind of club now, but you may decide to join one in the future. It is important to choose your fitness facility wisely.

Kinds of Facilities

The first thing you will need to know is that not all health and fitness facilities are alike. Despite some surface similarities, different clubs meet different needs. The services offered and the goals that members can realize also vary. **Figure 12.5** provides a listing of the types of health and fitness facilities described in the following sections. Advantages and disadvantages are also indicated.

Commercial Gyms. These health and fitness facilities are usually small in size and have relatively few members. These centers are geared toward the serious weight trainer or high-performance athlete. The exercise and activity opportunities may thus be limited.

Commercial Fitness Centers. These are *health and fitness facilities that offer a wide variety of resistance- and aerobic-training equipment.*

Active Mind Active Body
Evaluating Health and Fitness Information

This activity will give you and a small group of classmates some practice at evaluating claims for health and fitness products.

What You Will Need

- Pen or pencil
- Paper
- Recent newspapers
- Health and fitness magazines

What You Will Do

1. Each member of the group should select a different medium to investigate. One person should select TV, another magazines, another newspapers, and so on.
2. Look carefully through the examples of the medium you have chosen. Find advertisements for or articles on fitness products.
3. Carefully analyze the claims made in your source. To do this, apply the guidelines from page **375** of your textbook under the heading "Evaluating Health and Fitness Information."
4. Share your findings with your fellow group members.
5. Share these with the class in the form of a report or display (such as a bulletin board with clippings and critiques).

Apply and Conclude

Which of the claims analyzed turned out to be valid? What percentage of the total claims did this number represent? What did this activity teach you about the importance of evaluating health and fitness information?

FIGURE 12.5

VARIOUS TYPES OF HEALTH AND FITNESS FACILITIES

Fitness facilities vary greatly. *What type of fitness facility would be the most convenient choice for you as a teen?*

Health and Fitness Facility	Advantages	Disadvantages
Commercial gym	Is good for high performance	Has limited facilities; members may be too serious for your needs
Commercial fitness center	Has a large variety of activities	May be expensive or too crowded
Commercial dance studio	Usually has certified instructors	Has a limited number of fitness activities
Hospital-based wellness center	Has medical supervision and highly trained personnel	Has a relatively higher cost
Corporate fitness center	Has a variety of recreational and fitness activities	Is limited to employees and family members
Community recreational center	Has a variety of recreational activities and is economical	May have limited health and fitness activities
College- or university-based fitness center	Has a wide variety of programs and trained personnel	To join, you must be associated with the school (student, faculty, or staff); it may be very expensive for others to join
Sports medicine clinic center	Has comprehensive programs and medical supervision; is research based	Is expensive

These centers cater to the general public. YMCAs and YWCAs are examples of facilities that are considered commercial fitness centers.

Commercial Dance Studios. As their name suggests, these are facilities targeted at individuals interested in aerobic dance and jazz forms of exercise. They usually have little in the way of exercise equipment, but offer a variety of dance and aerobic classes that develop cardiovascular fitness and flexibility.

Hospital-Based Wellness Centers. As strides are made in preventive medicine, some hospitals are adding wellness centers. These centers usually offer a variety of exercise and educational programs focusing on personal fitness. They primarily serve "special needs" individuals. These include people who require medical screening before beginning a fitness program and/or medical supervision during physical activity.

Corporate Fitness Centers. The cost of health care in this country has risen dramatically in recent years. Large corporations have borne the burden of these expenses for their employees. Some have developed preventive strategies by featuring *on-site health and fitness facilities available to employees and their families.* At some larger companies, these corporate fitness centers rival local health clubs in the equipment and services offered.

College-Based Fitness Centers. Operated by state or private colleges and universities, these centers are available to students, faculty, and staff. Oftentimes, the centers are housed in the same campus building as the school's physical education department.

Sports Medicine Clinic Centers. Frequently associated with local universities and/or hospitals, sports medicine clinic centers are multipurpose facilities. They *focus on research promoting health and fitness, as well as on the development and operation of health, fitness, recreation, and educational programs.*

Community Recreational Centers. These health and fitness facilities are operated by city park and recreation departments. They offer a variety of recreational activities and programs to community members.

 Reading Check

Explain Which fitness facilities are designed for specific types of exercises? Which are used for developing general fitness?

Choosing a Fitness Facility

Selecting a health and fitness club is a two-step process. First, you need to determine your fitness needs. Then you can explore facilities in your community that best meet those needs. It is also wise to visit several competing facilities to get an idea of what they offer. Here are some questions to ask yourself at each facility you visit:

Cost and Convenience.

- What are the prices? Does the club offer package deals or seasonal specials?
- Is it conveniently located?
- What time does it open and close? Is it open on holidays?
- Does it tend to be crowded at the time you plan to use it?
- Can you fit in and socialize easily with the other members?

Equipment and Facilities.

- Is the equipment well cared for and in top working condition?
- Does the facility have a variety of machines and free weights?
- Does the facility have a variety of aerobic conditioning activities (swimming, cycles, treadmills, stair-steppers, and so on)?
- Are aerobic-exercise classes offered?
- Are racquetball, basketball, or tennis courts available?
- Are there indoor and outdoor hiking and jogging tracks or trails?

- Does the facility have a locker room? If so, are there towels and laundry service?
- Does it have enough showers, hot tubs, saunas, and steam rooms?
- Is there a system in place for evaluating your progress?
- Does the facility have computers to log or chart your progress?

Programs and Staff.

- Are the instructors or personal trainers certified and knowledgeable about resistance training?
- Are individual exercise programs available?
- Are educational programs available?

Safety and Cleanliness.

- Does the facility have a medical adviser for any special medical needs you have?
- Are the instructors certified in cardiopulmonary resuscitation (CPR) and first aid?
- Is the exercise area uncluttered and well monitored for safety?
- Is it clean and well maintained?

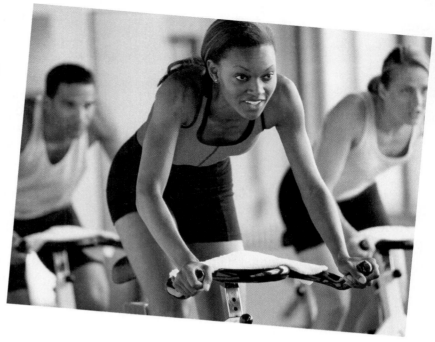

▲ If you join a health and fitness center or club, find one that meets your specific needs. *What are some strategies for achieving this goal?*

Lesson 4 Review

Using complete sentences, answer the following questions on a sheet of paper.

Reviewing Facts and Vocabulary

1. **Vocabulary** What is a *commercial fitness center?*
2. **Recall** What is the reason why corporate fitness centers have begun to appear?

Thinking Critically

3. **Explain** In what way do hospital-based wellness centers and corporate fitness centers share a similar outlook?

4. **Evaluate** Which of the questions used in choosing a fitness facility would be the most important to you? The least important? Why?

Personal Fitness Planning

Investigating Facilities Prepare a list of questions that may be used to survey the fitness facilities in your community. Use the questions suggested in this lesson to help you prepare your survey. Contact the fitness facilities in your community and see how they compare. Which one best meets your needs at present?

TRUE/FALSE

On a sheet of paper, write the numbers 1–10. Write True or False for each statement.

1. You can have a positive impact on your risk for chronic diseases.
2. Your resting metabolic rate does not decrease with age.
3. Developing positive attitudes and behaviors while you age may speed up the aging process.
4. Leisure-time activities will not help you reduce your stress levels.
5. Rock climbing requires high levels of muscular strength and endurance.
6. Volleyball is a leisure-time activity that helps develop coordination.
7. Podiatrists are physicians who specialize in disorders of the heart and lungs.
8. Physicians do not require a state license to practice medicine.
9. Testimonials that a product yielded great results are usually proof that a fitness product claim is valid.
10. Not all health and fitness facilities are alike.

MULTIPLE CHOICE

On a sheet of paper, write the letter of the word or phrase that best completes each statement.

11. From ages 30 to 90, a person's lung capacity is likely to decrease by approximately
    a. 10 percent.   c. 40 percent.
    b. 25 percent.   d. 60 percent.
12. Of the following changes associated with aging, the one that can be controlled by being physically active and eating healthfully is
    a. increased body fat.   c. inherited diseases.
    b. graying of hair.   d. balding.
13. The statement that does NOT usually occur in people who remain sedentary as they age is:
    a. They get depressed.
    b. They maintain functional health.
    c. They lose self-esteem.
    d. They lose bone mass.

14. The top of the Physical Activity Pyramid consists of activities that you should
    a. cut down on.
    b. do 2 to 3 times a week.
    c. do every day.
    d. none of the above.
15. Leisure-time activities do all of the following EXCEPT
    a. provide an opportunity for social interaction.
    b. guarantee improvements in health-related or skill-related fitness.
    c. provide a source of recreation.
    d. burn calories.
16. Mountain biking should be done with all of the following EXCEPT
    a. a bike with a heavy frame.
    b. a bike with wide tires that provide better traction.
    c. a light-framed bike.
    d. a safety helmet.
17. Physical therapists primarily work with
    a. athletes.
    b. people who need to control their weight.
    c. people recovering from injuries.
    d. none of the above.
18. Podiatrists work with
    a. people who need to control their weight.
    b. people recovering from injuries.
    c. people with foot problems.
    d. none of the above.
19. When evaluating claims for fitness products you should be suspicious of all of the following EXCEPT
    a. claims of quick and simple results.
    b. miracle breakthroughs that have not been reported by reputable sources.
    c. mail-order sales or infomercials.
    d. writers of articles who have credentials.
20. All of the following are true of hospital-based wellness centers EXCEPT that they
    a. cater to patients recovering from serious injuries.
    b. are designed for people who require medical screening before beginning a fitness program.
    c. can be used by people who require medical supervision during physical activity.
    d. offer a variety of exercise and educational programs focusing on personal fitness.

DISCUSSION

Using complete sentences, answer the following questions on a sheet of paper.

21. **Identify** List the mental and physical functions that change with the aging process. Describe how you can control to some degree the rate at which these functions change.
22. **Describe** Explain how you can be a wiser health and fitness consumer.

VOCABULARY

On a sheet of paper, write the letter of the term in Column B that best fits the definition in Column A.

Column A

23. Professionals who specialize in providing nutritional advice and helping people control their weight.
24. Professionals specially trained to understand the body's physical reactions to exercise.
25. Sports and other action-oriented pursuits done for recreation.
26. Activities that combine exercise and relaxation techniques.
27. On-site health and fitness facilities available to employees and their families.
28. A branch of medicine that deals with bone and joint injuries and disorders.

Column B

a. registered dietitian
b. leisure-time activities
c. martial arts
d. orthopedics
e. exercise physiologists
f. corporate fitness centers

CRITICAL THINKING

Using complete sentences, answer the following questions on a sheet of paper.

29. **Identify** Develop a list of lifetime activities that you do now or would like to do now or in the future. Then explain why you enjoy these activities and how they can help you develop and maintain your personal fitness levels.

30. **Synthesize** React to this statement: Education can make you a better health and fitness consumer and can prevent you from being the victim of rip-offs.

CASE STUDY

MOLLY'S PROBLEM

Molly has just returned from a visit with her aunt, who is recovering from knee surgery. During their conversations, Molly's aunt talked about her concerns with getting older. She explained to Molly how she had begun to notice being out of breath while going up stairs and that she wanted to lose some weight. She further shared her concerns about fully recovering from her surgery.

HERE IS YOUR ASSIGNMENT:

Assume that you are Molly and you want to share with your aunt what you have learned about exercise and the aging process. Organize a list of benefits associated with exercise and nutrition and their relationship to the aging process. You should specifically address your aunt's concerns about her surgery and her desire to lose weight. Suggest specific professionals she should see.

KEYS TO HELP YOU

- Consider your aunt's current medical status.
- Consider your aunt's current fitness status and knowledge of fitness.
- Consider your aunt's needs and desires.
- Consider which fitness experts would be best for your aunt's fitness needs.
- Consider the types of fitness facilities that would be best for your aunt's fitness needs.

Contents

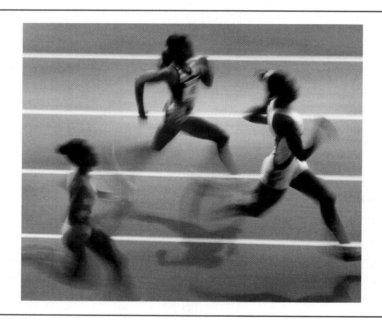

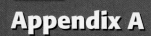

National Association for Sport and Physical Education (NASPE)
PHYSICAL EDUCATION STANDARDS

NASPE Content Standards for Grades K-12	A physically educated student:
Content Standard 1	Demonstrates competency in motor skills and movement patterns needed to perform a variety of physical activities.
Content Standard 2	Demonstrates understanding of movement concepts, principles, strategies, and tactics as they apply to the learning and performance of physical activities.
Content Standard 3	Participates regularly in physical activity.
Content Standard 4	Achieves and maintains a health-enhancing level of physical fitness.
Content Standard 5	Exhibits responsible personal and social behavior that respects self and others in physical activity settings.
Content Standard 6	Values physical activity for health, enjoyment, challenge, self-expression and/or social interaction.

Source: National Association for Sport and Physical Education Outcomes Committee Task Force, 2004.

Healthy People 2010

Healthy People 2010 is a set of 28 health objectives established for the nation to achieve over the first decade of the new century. The objectives, listed on these pages, were created after the Surgeon General's Report in 2000 identified specific National Health Promotion and Disease Prevention goals. The chapters in *Foundations of Personal Fitness* provide strategies for addressing many of these objectives.

1 Access to Quality Health Services Improve access to comprehensive, high-quality health care services.

2 Arthritis, Osteoporosis, and Chronic Back Conditions Prevent illness and disability related to arthritis and other rheumatic conditions, osteoporosis, and chronic back conditions.

3 Cancer Reduce the number of new cancer cases as well as the illness, disability, and death caused by cancer.

4 Chronic Kidney Disease Reduce new cases of chronic kidney disease and its complications, disability, death, and economic costs.

5 Diabetes Through prevention programs, reduce the disease and economic burden of diabetes, and improve the quality of life for all persons who have or are at risk for diabetes.

6 Disability and Secondary Conditions Promote the health of people with disabilities, prevent secondary conditions, and eliminate disparities between people with and without disabilities in the U.S. population.

7 Educational and Community-Based Programs Increase the quality, availability, and effectiveness of educational and community-based programs designed to prevent disease and improve health and quality of life.

8 Environmental Health Promote health for all through a healthy environment.

9 Family Planning Includes preventing unintended pregnancy.

10 Food Safety Reduce foodborne illnesses.

11 Health Communication Use communication strategically to improve health.

12 Heart Disease and Stroke Improve cardiovascular health and quality of life through the prevention, detection, and treatment of risk factors; early identification and treatment of heart attacks and strokes; and prevention of recurrent cardiovascular events.

13 HIV Prevent human immunodeficiency virus (HIV) infection and its related illness and death.

14 **Immunization and Infectious Diseases** Prevent disease, disability, and death from infectious diseases, including vaccine-preventable diseases.

15 **Injury and Violence Prevention** Reduce injuries, disabilities, and deaths due to unintentional injuries and violence.

16 **Maternal, Infant, and Child Health** Improve the health and well-being of women, infants, children, and families.

17 **Medical Product Safety** Ensure the safe and effective use of medical products.

18 **Mental Health and Mental Disorders** Improve mental health and ensure access to appropriate, quality mental health services.

19 **Nutrition and Overweight** Promote health and reduce chronic disease associated with diet and weight.

20 **Occupational Safety and Health** Promote the health and safety of people at work through prevention and early intervention.

21 **Oral Health** Prevent and control oral and craniofacial diseases, conditions, and injuries and improve access to related services.

22 **Physical Activity and Fitness** Improve health, fitness, and quality of life through daily physical activity.

23 **Public Health Infrastructure** Ensure that Federal, Tribal, State, and local health agencies have the infrastructure to provide essential public health services effectively.

24 **Respiratory Diseases** Promote respiratory health through better prevention, detection, treatment, and education efforts.

25 **Sexually Transmitted Diseases** Promote responsible sexual behaviors, strengthen community capacity, and increase access to quality services to prevent sexually transmitted diseases (STDs) and their complications.

26 **Substance Abuse** Reduce substance abuse to protect the health, safety, and quality of life for all, especially children.

27 **Tobacco** Reduce illness, disability, and death related to tobacco use and exposure to secondhand smoke.

28 **Vision and Hearing** Improve the visual and hearing health of the Nation through prevention, early detection, treatment, and rehabilitation.

The President's Challenge

Regular physical activity substantially reduces the risk of poor health. Physical activity need not be strenuous or very time-consuming to be beneficial, and all ages can benefit from modest physical activity. Every little bit of effort counts.

- **Adults, get at least 30 minutes of physical activity each day.** If it is too hard to set aside 30 minutes at one time, break it up into 10 or 15 minute segments. Developed by a panel of scientists under the leadership of the Department of Agriculture (USDA) and the Department of Health and Human Services (HHS) as a part of the *2000 Dietary Guidelines for Americans*, these recommendations for daily activity are based on the results of studies that examined the relationship between physical activity and health. If only 10 percent of American adults began regularly walking, $5.6 billion in health care costs associated with heart disease could be saved.

- **Children and teenagers, get at least 60 minutes of physical activity each day.** For children, setting aside time for physical activity should be easy. Unfortunately, even children have busy schedules today. According to the *Dietary Guidelines for Americans*, they can break activity up into segments. Regular activity for children is important. Normal childhood play or outdoor activity helps control blood pressure and manages weight while building and maintaining healthy bones, muscles, and joints.

- **Parents, commit to family activities that involve physical activity.** It can be easier to work physical activity into your daily routine if you combine it with family time.

PHYSICAL ACTIVITY AND FITNESS GUIDELINES

The Surgeon General's Report on Physical Activity and Health, along with the President's Council on Physical Fitness and Sports, identified fitness as a major public health concern. The Physical Fitness Objectives from *Healthy People 2010* for children and adolescents appear below.

Physical Activity in Children and Adolescents

- Increase the proportion of adolescents who engage in moderate physical activity for at least 30 minutes on 5 or more of the previous 7 days.

- Increase the proportion of adolescents who engage in vigorous physical activity that promotes cardiorespiratory fitness 3 or more

days per week for 20 or more minutes per occasion.
- Increase the proportion of the Nation's public and private schools that require daily physical education for all students.
- Increase the proportion of adolescents who participate in daily school physical education.

- Increase the proportion of adolescents who spend at least 50 percent of school physical education class time being physically active.
- Increase the proportion of adolescents who view television 2 or fewer hours on a school day.

PHYSICAL FITNESS GUIDELINES

Regular physical activity performed on a daily basis reduces the risk of developing illness or disease. Moderate physical activity can be achieved in a variety of ways, and the Centers for Disease Control and Prevention (CDC) have developed this list of examples showing moderate amounts of activity that can contribute to an individual's health.

Physical Activities Arranged by Energy Level and Time

- Washing and waxing a car for 45–60 minutes
- Washing windows or floors for 45–60 minutes
- Playing volleyball for 45 minutes
- Playing touch football for 30–45 minutes
- Gardening for 30–45 minutes
- Wheeling self in wheelchair for 30–40 minutes
- Walking $1\frac{3}{4}$ miles in 35 minutes (20 min/mile)
- Basketball (shooting baskets) for 30 minutes
- Bicycling 5 miles in 30 minutes
- Dancing fast (social) for 30 minutes

- Pushing a stroller $1\frac{1}{2}$ miles in 30 minutes
- Raking leaves for 30 minutes
- Walking 2 miles in 30 minutes (15 min/mile)
- Water aerobics for 30 minutes
- Swimming laps for 20 minutes
- Wheelchair basketball for 20 minutes
- Basketball (playing a game) for 15–20 minutes
- Bicycling 4 miles in 15 minutes
- Jumping rope for 15 minutes
- Running $1\frac{1}{2}$ miles in 15 minutes (10 min/mile)
- Shoveling snow for 15 minutes
- Stair walking for 15 minutes

Source: CDC, Physical Activity and Health, A Report of the Surgeon General, 1999.

Obesity and Diabetes in the United States

More than one-third of students in grades 9–12 do not regularly engage in vigorous physical activity. Daily participation in high school physical education classes dropped from 42 percent in 1991 to 29 percent in 1999. The prevalence of obesity and diabetes among adults in the U.S. has increased significantly in the past decade, as shown in the maps below. The CDC reports that regular physical activity, healthy eating, and creating an environment that supports these behaviors are essential to reducing this epidemic of obesity and diabetes. A commitment to lifelong physical activity and fitness can help reduce these trends.

Percentage of Obese Adults: 1995 and 2001

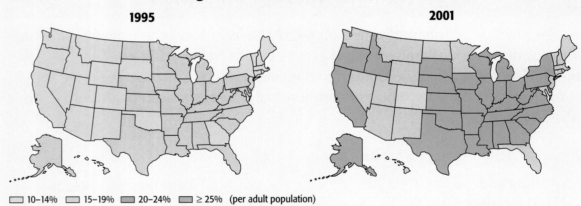

1995   2001

10–14%   15–19%   20–24%   ≥ 25%   (per adult population)

Percentage of Diabetes Among Adults: 1994 and 2001

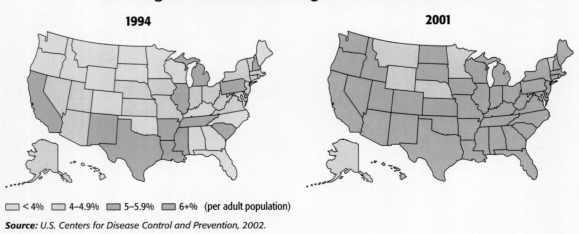

1994   2001

< 4%   4–4.9%   5–5.9%   6+%   (per adult population)

Source: U.S. Centers for Disease Control and Prevention, 2002.

Endnotes

Chapter 1

1. Centers for Disease Control and Prevention, Division of Nutrition and Physical Activity. "A Report of the Surgeon General, At-A-Glance, 1996." 14 Aug. 2003 < http://www.cdc.gov >
2. Adapted from U.S. Department of Health and Human Services; Centers for Disease Control and Prevention, National Center for Chronic Disease Prevention and Health Promotion, Division of Nutrition and Physical Activity. *Promoting Physical Activity: A Guide for Community Action.* Champaign, IL: Human Kinetics, 1999.
3. Reprinted with permission from Sizer, F.S., Whitney, E.N., Debuyne, L.K. *Health: Making Life Choices.* Lincolnwood: National Textbook Company, 2000. 236. Activity adapted from Russell Pate (University of South Carolina, Department of Exercise Science).

Chapter 2

1. U.S. Department of Health and Human Services. "The Surgeon General's Call to Action to Prevent and Decrease Overweight and Obesity." Rockville, MD, 2001.
2. Health Canada Online. "Canada's Physical Activity Guide to Healthy Active Living, Health Canada, 2002"©. Reproduced with permission of the Minister of Public Works and Government Services Canada, 2003. 14 Aug. 2003 < http://www.hc-sc.gc.ca >
3. Healthlink. Medical College of Wisconsin, 2001. 14 Aug. 2003 < http://healthlink.mcw.edu >
4. U.S. Consumer Product Safety Commission, 1999. 14 Aug. 2003 < http://www.cpsc.gov >
5. Modified from the *National Healthy People 2010 Objectives* as measured by the *National Youth Risk Behavior Survey,* 2001.

Chapter 3

1. Borg, Gunnar. *Borg's Perceived Exertion and Pain Scales.* Champaign, IL: Human Kinetics, 1998. 47.

Chapter 4

1. U.S. Department of Agriculture. "Dietary Guidelines for Americans, 2002." 14 Aug. 2003 < http://www.nal.usda.gov >
2. Jennings, D.S. and Steen, S.N. *Play Hard, Eat Right: A Parent's Guide to Sports Nutrition for Children.* New Jersey: John Wiley & Sons, ©1998. Reprinted by permission of John Wiley & Sons, Inc.
3. Jennings, D.S. and Steen, S.N. *Play Hard, Eat Right: A Parent's Guide to Sports Nutrition for Children.* New Jersey: John Wiley & Sons, ©1998. Reprinted by permission of John Wiley & Sons, Inc.
4. Jennings, D.S. and Steen, S.N. *Play Hard, Eat Right: A Parent's Guide to Sports Nutrition for Children.* New Jersey: John Wiley & Sons, ©1998. Reprinted by permission of John Wiley & Sons, Inc.

Chapter 5

1. Adapted from Jackson, A.S. and Ross, R.M. *Understanding Exercise for Health and Disease, 3rd Edition.* Dubuque, Iowa: Kendall Hunt Publishers, 1997.
2. McArdle, William D., Katch, Frank I., Katch, Victor L. *Exercise Physiology: Energy, Nutrition, and Human Performance, 5th Edition.* Philadelphia, PA: Lippincott Williams & Wilkins Publishers, 2001.
3. Town, G.P. and Wheeler, K.B. "Nutrition Concerns for the Endurance Athlete." *Dietetic Currents* 13 (1986): 7–12.

4. McArdle, William D., Katch, Frank I., Katch, Victor L. *Exercise Physiology: Energy, Nutrition, and Human Performance, 5th Edition.* Philadelphia, PA: Lippincott Williams & Wilkins Publishers, 2001.

Chapter 6

1. Centers for Disease Control and Prevention, National Center for Health Statistics. "Prevalence of Overweight and Obesity Among Children and Adolescents: United States, 1999-2000." 16 Jul. 2003 < http://www.cdc.gov >
2. U.S. Department of Health and Human Services. "The Surgeon General's Call to Action to Prevent and Decrease Overweight and Obesity." Rockville, MD, 2001.

Chapter 7

1. American Heart Association, *Heart Disease and Stroke Statistics – 2003 Update.* Dallas, TX: American Heart Association, 2002.
2. Centers for Disease Control and Prevention, Tobacco Information and Prevention Source (TIPS), "Comparative Causes of Annual Deaths in the United States, 2003." 14 Aug. 2003 < http://www.cdc.gov >
3. Borg, Gunnar. *Borg's Perceived Exertion and Pain Scales.* Champaign, IL: Human Kinetics, 1998. 47.

Chapter 8

1. Walker, J.L., Murray, T.D., Jackson, A.S., Morrow, J.R., Michaud, T.D., Rainey, D.L. "The Energy Cost of Horizontal Walking and Running in Adolescents." *Medicine and Science in Sports and Exercise,* 31:2 (1999): 311–322.
2. Blair, S.N. and Brodney, S. "Effects of Physical Inactivity and Obesity on Morbidity and Mortality: Current Evidence and Research Issues." *Medicine and Science in Sports and Exercise,* 33:11 (1999): 646–662.
3. Cooper, Kenneth H. *The Aerobics Program for Total Well-Being.* ©1982 by Kenneth H. Cooper. Used by permission of Bantam Books, a division of Random House Inc.
4. Blair, S.N. and Brodney, S. "Effects of Physical Inactivity and Obesity on Morbidity and Mortality: Current Evidence and Research Issues." *Medicine and Science in Sports and Exercise,* 33:11 (1999): 646–662.
5. Blair, S.N. and Brodney, S. "Effects of Physical Inactivity and Obesity on Morbidity and Mortality: Current Evidence and Research Issues." *Medicine and Science in Sports and Exercise,* 33:11 (1999): 646–662.

Chapter 9

1. National Osteoporosis Foundation. "Disease Statistics: 'Fast Facts'." Updated 2003. 14 Aug. 2003 < http://www.nof.org >

Chapter 11

1. President's Council on Physical Fitness and Sports, "Questionable Exercises." *President's Council on Physical Fitness and Sports, Research Digest,* 3: 8 (1999). 14 Aug. 2003 < http://www.fitness.gov >

Chapter 12

1. Reprinted with permission from Sizer, F.S., Whitney, E.N., Debuyne, L.K. *Health: Making Life Choices.* Lincolnwood: National Textbook Company, 2000. 630.
2. Adapted with permission from Kemper and Niemeyer. "The Importance of a Physically Active Lifestyle during Youth for Peak Bone Mass." *New Horizons in Pediatric Exercise Science,* ed. C. Blimkie and B. Oded. Champaign, IL: Human Kinetics, 1995.

Glossary

A

Absolute muscular strength The maximum force an individual is able to exert regardless of size, age, or weight (Ch. 9, p. 247)

Acclimatization The process of allowing the body to adapt slowly to weather conditions (Ch. 2, p. 42)

Active warm-up Exercises that raise body temperature by actively working the body systems centering on the muscles, skeleton, heart, and lungs (Ch. 3, p. 103)

Addiction Physical and mental dependence on a substance or activity (Ch. 2, p. 63)

Adductor muscles The muscles on the inside of the leg that pull the legs together (Ch. 11, p. 348)

Adherence The ability to stick to a plan of action (Ch. 1, p. 21)

Adipose tissue Body fat (Ch. 4, p. 117)

Aerobic activity Continuous activity that requires large amounts of oxygen (Ch. 7, p. 193)

Agility The ability to change and control the direction and position of the body while maintaining a constant, rapid motion (Ch. 3, p. 75)

Aging process The manner in which the body changes as a natural result of growing older (Ch. 12, p. 357)

Alternated grip A position in which a barbell is grasped with one palm facing downward and the other palm facing upward (Ch. 10, p. 277)

Amino acids The building blocks of proteins (Ch. 4, p. 118)

Anabolic steroids Chemicals similar in structure to the male hormone testosterone (Ch. 2, p. 66)

Anaerobic fitness High levels of muscular strength, muscular endurance, and flexibility (Ch. 7, p. 212)

Anaerobic activity Activity that requires high levels of energy and is done for only a few seconds or minutes at a high level of intensity (Ch. 7, p. 212)

Androstenedione A chemical agent that aids the body in its production of testosterone (Ch. 4, p. 143)

Anorexia nervosa An eating disorder in which a person abnormally restricts his or her calorie intake (Ch. 6, p. 177)

Antioxidants Substances that protect body cells, including those of the immune system, from damage (Ch. 4, p. 124)

Arteries Blood vessels that carry blood from the heart to the major extremities of the body (Ch. 7, p. 194)

Asthma A disease in which the small airways of the lungs become narrowed, making it difficult to breathe (Ch. 2, p. 36)

Atherosclerosis A condition in which a fatty deposit called plaque builds up inside arteries, restricting or cutting off blood flow (Ch. 7, p. 36)

Athletic trainers Professionals who work with athletes undergoing rehabilitation (Ch. 12, p. 371)

Attitude An individual's mindset or outlook toward a given topic or subject (Ch. 1, p. 18)

B

Balance The ability to control or stabilize the body while standing or moving (Ch. 3, p. 75)

Ballistic stretching Quick up-and-down movements in which stretches are held very briefly (Ch. 11, p. 342)

Behavioral-change stairway A step-by-step approach to setting and achieving fitness goals (Ch. 1, p. 26)

Bigorexia A disorder in which an individual falsely believes he or she is underweight or undersized (Ch. 6, p. 178)

Binge eating disorder An eating disorder where individuals eat more rapidly than normal until they cannot eat any more (Ch. 6, p. 178)

Biomechanics The study and application of the principles of physics to human motion (Ch. 2, p. 54)

Blood pooling A condition in which blood collects in the large veins of the legs and lower body (Ch. 3, p. 108)

Blood pressure The force of the blood in the main arteries (Ch. 7, p. 206)

Body composition The ratio of body fat to lean body tissue, including muscle, bone, water, and connective tissue (Ch. 5, p. 150)

Body image The way an individual sees his or her body (Ch. 6, p. 176)

Body mass index (BMI) A way to assess body size in relation to height and weight (Ch. 5, p. 149)

Bulimia nervosa An eating disorder in which people overeat and then force themselves to purge the food afterward (Ch. 6, p. 177)

C

Calipers A tweezer-like device used to pinch a fold of skin surrounding adipose tissue (Ch. 5, p. 161)

Calisthenic exercises Exercises that create resistance by using one's own body weight (Ch. 9, p. 266)

Calorie The amount of energy needed to raise the temperature of 1 kilogram (about a quart) of water 1 degree Celsius (Ch. 4, p. 115)

Calorie expenditure The total number of calories an individual burns or expends (Ch. 5, p. 154)

Calorie intake The total number of calories an individual takes in from food (Ch. 5, p. 154)

Capillaries Small blood vessels that deliver oxygen and other nutrients to individual cells (Ch. 7, p. 194)

Carbohydrates The starches and sugars found in food (Ch. 4, p. 115)

Cardiac muscle A special type of striated tissue that forms the walls of the heart (Ch. 9, p. 250)

Cardiorespiratory endurance The ability of the body to work continuously for extended periods of time (Ch. 7, p. 198)

Cardiovascular conditioning Exercises or activities that improve the efficiency of the heart, lungs, blood, and blood vessels (Ch. 3, p. 84)

Cardiovascular cooldown Moving about slowly and continuously for three to five minutes following physical activity or exercise (Ch. 3, p. 109)

Cardiovascular disease (CVD) A medical disorder that affects the heart or blood vessels (Ch. 7, p. 200)

Cartilage Tissue that surrounds the ends of bones at a joint to prevent the bones from rubbing against each other (Ch. 2, p. 57)

Cholesterol A fatlike substance that is produced in the liver and circulates in the blood (Ch. 4, p. 120)

Chronic disease A disease that is ongoing (Ch. 2, p. 36)

Circuit training An approach to resistance training that involves rotating from one exercise to the next in a particular sequence (Ch. 10, p. 298)

Circulatory system Consists of the heart, blood, and blood vessels (Ch. 7, p. 194)

Clips Clamp-like devices on a barbell that secure the weights in place (Ch. 10, p. 275)

Commercial fitness centers Health and fitness facilities that offer access to a wide variety of resistance- and aerobic-training equipment for a fee (Ch. 12, p. 376)

Commitment A pledge or promise (Ch. 1, p. 20)

Compound sets Alternate sets of exercises without rest between sets (Ch. 10, p. 320)

Conflicts Struggles or disagreements (Ch. 1, p. 7)

Contraction The shortening of a muscle (Ch. 9, p. 252)

Cooper's 1.5-mile run test A test that requires jogging or running 1.5 miles in as little time as possible (Ch. 8, p. 219)

Coordination The ability to use the senses to determine and direct the movement of your limbs and head (Ch. 3, p. 75)

Core stability The stretching and strengthening of muscles around the spine and pelvic muscles (Ch. 11, p. 338)

Corporate fitness centers On-site health and fitness facilities available to employees and their families (Ch. 12, p. 378)

Creatine A supplement that increases muscle size while enhancing the body's ability to use protein (Ch. 4, p. 143)

Credentials A summary of the person's professional training and experience in a given field (Ch. 12, p. 370)

Cross-contamination The spreading of bacteria or other pathogens from one food to another (Ch. 4, p. 136)

Cross-training Varying exercise or activity routine or type (Ch. 3, p. 98)

Culture The shared customs, traditions, and beliefs of a particular group (Ch. 4, p. 114)

D

Deconditioned Having been out of training for a significant period after achieving at least a moderate level of fitness (Ch. 8, p. 234)

Dehydration Body fluid loss (Ch. 2, p. 41)

Detraining The loss of functional fitness that occurs when one stops fitness conditioning (Ch. 3, p. 98)

Diaphragm A muscle found between the chest cavity and abdomen (Ch. 7, p. 194)

Dietary fiber A special subclass of complex carbohydrates that has several functions, including aiding the body in digestion (Ch. 4, p. 117)

Dietary Reference Intakes (DRI) Daily nutrient recommendations for healthy people of both genders and different age groups (Ch. 4, p. 130)

Dietary supplement A nonfood form of one or more nutrients (Ch. 4, p. 128)

Dynamic contraction A type of muscle contraction that occurs when the resistance force is movable (Ch. 9, p. 252)

Dynamic posture The posture of the body while in motion or preparing to move (Ch. 11, p. 331)

E

Eating disorders Psychological illnesses that cause people to undereat, overeat, or practice other dangerous nutrition-related behaviors (Ch. 6, p. 176)

Ectomorph A body type characterized by a low percentage of body fat, small bone size, and a small amount of muscle mass and size (Ch. 5, p. 147)

Elasticity The ability of the muscles and connective tissues to stretch and give (Ch. 11, p. 326)

Elliptical motion trainer An exercise machine that simulates the natural motions of running but without placing stress on the joints (Ch. 8, p. 227)

Emphysema A disease in which the small airways of the lungs lose their normal elasticity, making them less efficient in helping to move air in and out of the lungs (Ch. 7, p. 204)

Endomorph A body type characterized by a high percentage of body fat, large bone size, and a small amount of muscle mass and size (Ch. 5, p. 147)

Energy cost The amount of energy needed to perform physical activities or exercises (Ch. 3, p. 73)

Ephedrine A compound that increases the rate at which the body converts calories to energy (Ch. 4, p. 143)

Essential fat The minimum amount of body fat necessary for good health (Ch. 5, p. 151)

Excessive leanness Having a percentage of body fat that is below the acceptable range for an individual's age and gender (Ch. 5, p. 151)

Excessive weight disabilities Health problems and diseases linked to or resulting directly from long-term overweight or obesity (Ch. 6, p. 173)

Exercise Physical activity that is planned, structured, and repetitive, and that results in improvements in fitness (Ch. 1, p. 4)

Exercise bands Elastic bands or tubing made of latex that are used to develop muscular strength and endurance (Ch. 9, p. 265)

Exercise bulimia An eating disorder in which people purge calories by exercising excessively (Ch. 6, p. 177)

Exercise physiologists Specially trained professionals who understand the body's physical reactions to exercise and evaluate a person's fitness (Ch. 12, p. 372)

Exercise prescription A breakdown of a fitness program, based on the frequency, intensity, time, and type of physical activity or exercise (Ch. 3, p. 83)

Exercise stress test An evaluation of cardiovascular fitness that involves walking on a treadmill or riding a stationary bicycle under medical supervision (Ch. 8, p. 220)

Extension The stretching of a muscle (Ch. 9, p. 252)

F

Fad diets Weight-loss plans that are popular for only a short time (Ch. 6, p. 182)

Fast-twitch muscle fiber Muscle fiber that contracts rapidly, thus allowing for greater muscle strength (Ch. 7, p. 208)

Fatigue The feeling of being tired all the time (Ch. 3, p. 99)

Fats Substances that supply a concentrated form of energy and help transport other nutrients to locations in the body where they are needed (Ch. 4, p. 115)

Flexibility A joint's ability to move through its full range of motion (Ch. 11, p. 325)

Fluid balance The body's ability to balance the amounts of fluid taken in with the amounts lost through perspiration or excretion (Ch. 2, p. 41)

Food Guide Pyramid A visual guide to help make healthful food choices (Ch. 4, p. 130)

Foodborne illnesses Illnesses that result from consuming food contaminated with disease-causing organisms, the poisons they produce, or chemical contaminants (Ch. 4, p. 136)

Free weights A term applied collectively to dumbbells, barbells, plates, and clips (Ch. 9, p. 262)

Frequency The number of times per week an individual engages in physical activity or exercise (Ch. 3, p. 84)

Frostbite Damage to body tissue that results from freezing (Ch. 2, p .44)

Functional fitness A person's physical ability to function independently in life, without assistance (Ch. 1, p. 7)

Functional health The ability to maintain high levels of health and wellness by reducing the risks of developing health problems (Ch. 1, p. 7)

G

Girth The distance around a body part (Ch. 5, p. 159)

H

Health A combination of physical, mental/emotional, and social well-being (Ch. 1, p. 6)

Health-related fitness The ability to become and stay physically healthy (Ch. 1, p. 11)

Heart rate monitor A device that records the heart beat by means of a chest transmitter and wrist monitor (Ch. 8, p. 229)

Heart rate The number of times a person's heart beats per minute (Ch. 3, p. 85)

Heat cramps Muscle spasms resulting from the loss of large amounts of salt and water through perspiration (Ch. 2, p. 41)

Heat exhaustion An overheating of the body resulting in cold, clammy skin and symptoms of shock (Ch. 2, p. 41)

Heat stress index A scientific measure of the combined effects of heat and humidity on the body (Ch. 2, p. 43)

Heatstroke A condition in which the body can no longer rid itself of excessive heat through perspiration (Ch. 2, p. 41)

Hemoglobin An iron-rich compound in the blood that helps to carry oxygen from lungs to cells and tissues (Ch. 7, p. 194)

Heredity The sum of the physical and mental traits that are inherited from one's parents (Ch. 1, p. 13)

Hernia A condition that occurs when muscle fibers from the intestine protrude through the wall of the abdomen (Ch. 2, p. 37)

High-density lipoprotein (HDL) A type of compound that picks up excess cholesterol and returns it to the liver (Ch. 4, p. 121)

Hyperflexibility Excessive amount of flexibility (Ch. 11, p. 334)

Hypertension High blood pressure (Ch. 7, p. 203)

Hypertrophy A thickening of existing muscle fibers (Ch. 9, p. 253)

Hypothermia A condition in which the body temperature drops below normal (Ch. 2, p. 44)

I

Impaired glucose tolerance (IGT) A disorder in which blood glucose levels become elevated (Ch. 6, p. 173)

Insomnia Sleeplessness (Ch. 3, p. 99)

Insulin A hormone produced by the pancreas (Ch. 6, p. 173)

Intensity The difficulty or exertion level of a physical activity or exercise (Ch. 3, p. 85)

Interval training A program in which high-intensity physical activities alternate with low intensity recovery bouts for several minutes at a time (Ch. 7, p. 215)

L

Large muscle group Any group of muscles of large size or any large number of muscles being used at one time (Ch. 10, p. 302)

Lean body weight The combined weight of bone, muscle, and connective tissue (Ch. 5, p. 148)

Leisure-time activities Sports and other action-oriented pursuits done for recreation (Ch. 12, p. 362)

Lifestyle diseases Diseases that are the result of certain lifestyle choices, such as smoking, eating plan, and inactivity (Ch. 7, p. 199)

Ligament Bands of tissue that connect bone to bone and limit the movement of joints (Ch. 2, p. 57)

Long-term goal A goal that you plan to reach over an extended length of time (Ch. 3, p. 91)

Low-density lipoprotein (LDL) A type of compound that carries cholesterol from the liver to areas of the body where it is needed (Ch. 4, p. 120)

M

Martial arts Activities that combine exercise and relaxation techniques (Ch. 12, p. 367)

Maximal oxygen consumption (VO$_{2max}$) The largest amount of oxygen the body is able to process during strenuous aerobic exercise (Ch. 7, p. 207)

Media The collective forms of mass communication found within society at any given time (Ch. 1, p. 20)

Medical history A record of past health problems and illnesses (Ch. 2, p. 39)

Medical screening A basic assessment of a person's overall health and personal fitness (Ch. 2, p. 35)

Mesomorph A body type characterized by a low-to-medium percentage of body fat, medium-to-large bone size, and a large amount of muscle mass and size (Ch. 5, p. 147)

Metabolism The process by which the body converts calories from food to energy (Ch. 5, p. 155)

Microtear Microscopic rips in the muscle fiber and/or surrounding tissues (Ch. 9, p. 255)

Minerals Elements the body cannot manufacture but that help regulate the body's processes, such as the conversion of glucose to energy (Ch. 4, p. 125)

Moderate physical activity or exercise Any activity or exercise that ranges in intensity from light-to-borderline-heavy exertion (Ch. 1, p. 28)

Multiple hypertrophy sets Lifting the same amount of weight to the point of fatigue (Ch. 10, p. 321)

Multiple sets The lifter uses the same amount of weight for three to five sets at a training load of 80 to 95 percent of his or her 1RM (Ch. 10, p. 318)

Muscle fiber The specific structure in the muscle that receives signals from the nerves (Ch. 9, p. 253)

Muscle hyperplasia An increase in the number of muscle fibers (Ch. 9, p. 253)

Muscle imbalance A condition in which one muscle group becomes too strong in relation to a complementary group (Ch. 11, p. 334)

Muscle tone A muscle's firmness and definition (Ch. 9, p. 259)

Muscular endurance The ability of the same muscle or muscle group to contract for an extended period of time without undue fatigue (Ch. 9, p. 248)

Muscular strength The maximum amount of force a muscle or muscle group can exert against an opposing force (Ch. 9, p. 247)

N

Negative reps Performing the eccentric, or negative, phase of an exercise only, using a weight 10 to 15 percent greater than one's 1RM (Ch. 10, p. 318)

Nerves Pathways that deliver messages from the brain to other body parts (Ch. 9, p. 253)

Nutrient-dense foods Foods that are high in nutrients as compared with their calorie content (Ch. 5, p. 165)

Nutrients Substances in food that the body needs for energy, proper growth, body maintenance, and functioning (Ch. 4, p. 113)

Nutrition The study of food and how the body uses the substances in food (Ch. 4, p. 113)

Nutrition Facts panel A thumbnail analysis of a food's calories and nutrient content for one serving (Ch. 4, p. 132)

O

Obesity A medical condition in which a person's ratio of body fat to lean muscle mass is excessively high (Ch. 2, p. 36)

One-rep maximum (1RM) A measure of a lifter's absolute maximum strength for any given exercise (Ch. 10, p. 307)

Orthopedics A branch of medicine that deals with bone and joint injuries and disorders (Ch. 12, p. 371)

Osteoporosis A bone disease that causes decreased bone mass and density, especially in older women (Ch. 9, p. 258)

Overfat Carrying too much body fat for one's age and gender (Ch. 5, p. 151)

Overhand grip A position in which a barbell is grasped with the palms facing downward and the knuckles facing upward (Ch. 10, p. 277)

Overload principle A rule of exercise that states that in order to improve the level of fitness, one must increase the amount of regular activity or exercise he or she normally does (Ch. 3, p. 83)

Overtraining Exercising or being active to a point where it begins to have negative effects (Ch. 3, p. 99)

Overuse injury A muscular injury that results from overloading a muscle beyond a healthful point (Ch. 3, p. 95)

Overweight A condition in which a person is heavier than the standard weight range for his or her height (Ch. 5, p. 150)

P

Passive stretching A type of stretching against a counter force and in which there is little or no movement (Ch. 11, p. 342)

Passive warm-up Using outside heat sources to raise body temperature (Ch. 3, p. 103)

Pedometer A device that measures the number of steps a person takes and records the distance traveled (Ch. 8, p. 228)

Peers People the same age who share a common range of interests and beliefs (Ch. 1, p. 19)

Perceived exertion A measure of how intensely an individual feels he or she is working during physical activity or exercise (Ch. 3, p. 86)

Peripheral vascular disease A CVD that occurs mainly in the legs and, less frequently, in the arms (Ch. 7, p. 202)

Personal fitness Total, overall fitness achieved by maintaining acceptable levels of physical activity, a healthy eating plan, and avoiding harmful substances (Ch. 1, p. 4)

Physical activity Any movement that works the larger muscles of the body, such as arm, leg, and back muscles (Ch. 1, p. 4)

Physical fitness The body's ability to carry out daily tasks and still have enough reserve energy to respond to unexpected demands (Ch. 1, p. 4)

Physical therapists Health professionals specially trained to work with people recovering from injuries (Ch. 12, p. 371)

Phytonutrients Health-promoting substances found in plant foods (Ch. 4, p. 127)

Plyometric exercises Quick, powerful muscular movements that require the muscle to be pre-stretched just before a quick contraction (Ch. 9, p. 266)

Podiatrist Physician trained specifically to treat disorders of the feet (Ch. 12, p. 371)

Posture The alignment of the body's muscles and skeleton as they provide support for the total body (Ch. 11, p. 329)

Power The ability to move the body parts swiftly while simultaneously applying the maximum force of the muscles (Ch. 3, p. 76)

Pre-event meal The last full meal consumed prior to a practice session or the competitive event itself (Ch. 4, p. 139)

Progression principle A rule of exercise that states as fitness levels increase, so do the factors in FITT (Ch. 3, p. 95)

Progressive resistance Continued systematic increase of muscle workload by the addition of more weight or resistance (Ch. 9, p. 248)

Pronation The normal motion of the foot as one walks or runs, from the outside of the heel striking the ground through the normal inward roll of the foot (Ch. 2, p. 49)

Proteins Nutrients that help build, maintain, and repair body tissues (Ch. 4, p. 115)

Pyramid training An approach to training that uses progressively heavier weights and fewer reps through successive sets of an exercise (Ch. 10, p. 317)

R

Range of motion (ROM) The degrees of motion allowed around a joint (Ch. 11, p. 325)

Reaction time The ability to react or respond quickly to what you hear, see, or feel (Ch. 3, p. 76)

Recovery time The duration of the rest periods taken between workout components (Ch. 10, p. 311)

Recumbent cycles Reclining exercise cycles (Ch. 8, p. 239)

Reflex-assisted stretching Stretching movements that challenge the reflexes to adapt (Ch. 11, p. 342)

Reflexes The automatic responses that the nerves and muscles provide to various movements (Ch. 11, p. 342)

Registered dietitians (RDs) Professionals who specialize in providing nutritional advice and helping people control their weight (Ch. 12, p. 372)

Regular physical activity or exercise Any activity or exercise performed most days of the week, preferably daily (Ch. 1, p. 28)

Rehydrate To restore lost water (Ch. 2, p. 42)

Relative muscular endurance The maximum number of times an individual can repeatedly perform a resistance activity in relation to his or her body weight (Ch. 9, p. 248)

Relative muscular strength The maximum force an individual is able to exert in relation to his or her body weight (Ch. 9, p. 247)

Repetition (rep) One completion of an activity or exercise (Ch. 10, p. 296)

Resistance training A systematic program of exercises designed to increase an individual's ability to resist or exert force (Ch. 9, p. 245)

Resistance-training cycle Modified programs, designed to meet the needs of off-season, pre-season, and in-season (Ch. 10, p. 312)

Respiratory system The body system that exchanges gases between the body and the environment (Ch. 7, p. 194)

Resting metabolic rate (RMR) The amount of calories expended for body processes while at rest (Ch. 5, p. 155)

Restoration Ways in which an individual can optimize recovery from physical activity or exercise (Ch. 3, p. 100)

RICE (Rest, Ice, Compress, and Elevate) A first-aid procedure indicating proper treatment for strains and sprains that become swollen (Ch. 2, p. 58)

Risk factors Conditions and behaviors that represent a potential threat to an individual's well-being (Ch. 1, p. 12)

S

Saturated fatty acids Fats that come mainly from animal fats and are often solid at room temperature (Ch. 4, p. 119)

Sedentary Physically inactive (Ch. 1, p. 7)

Self-concept The view an individual has of his- or herself (Ch. 1, p. 22)

Self-esteem Feelings of self-confidence and personal worth (Ch. 1, p. 7)

Set A group of consecutive reps for any exercise (Ch. 10, p. 296)

Shinsplint Inflammation of a tendon or muscle in the leg (Ch. 2, p. 59)

Skeletal muscles Muscles attached to bones that cause body movement (Ch. 9, p. 250)

Skill-related fitness The ability to perform successfully in various games and sports (Ch. 1, p. 11)

Sleep apnea A condition in which a person stops breathing during sleep, due to obstructed or reduced air passages (Ch. 6, p. 173)

Slow-twitch muscle fiber Muscle fiber that contracts at a slow rate, allowing for greater muscle endurance (Ch. 7, p. 208)

Small muscle group Any group of muscles of small size or any small number of muscles being used at one time (Ch. 10, p. 302)

Smokeless tobacco Tobacco that is sniffed through the nose or chewed (Ch. 2, p. 64)

Smooth muscles Muscles responsible for the movements of the internal organs (Ch. 9, p. 250)

Specificity principle A rule of exercise that states overloading a particular component will lead to fitness improvements in that component alone (Ch. 3, p. 90)

Speed The ability to move the body or body parts swiftly (Ch. 3, p. 76)

Split workout A fitness program that exercises three or four body areas at each session, at a high intensity (Ch. 10, p. 306)

Sports medicine clinic Centers that focus on research promoting health and fitness, as well as on the development and operation of health, fitness, recreation, and educational programs (Ch. 12, p. 378)

Spotter A partner who can assist with the safe handling of weights and offer encouragement during a session (Ch. 9, p. 262)

Sprain A condition in which the ligaments that hold joints in position are stretched or torn (Ch. 2, p. 58)

Static contraction A type of muscle contraction that occurs absent of any significant movement (Ch. 9, p. 252)

Static posture The posture of the body while in a resting position (Ch. 11, p. 331)

Static stretching Exercises that stretch muscles slowly, smoothly, and in a sustained fashion for 20 to 30 seconds (Ch. 11, p. 341)

Steady-state cycle test A test that requires one to pedal for 20 minutes on a stationary cycle and try to achieve a specific goal distance (Ch. 8, p. 220)

Steady-state jog test A test that requires you to pace yourself steadily as you jog for 20 minutes and try to achieve a specific goal distance (Ch. 8, p. 219)

Steady-state swim test A test that requires one to swim for 20 minutes and try to achieve a specific goal distance (Ch. 8, p. 220)

Steady-state walk test A test that requires you to pace yourself steadily as you briskly walk for 30 minutes and try to achieve a specific goal distance (Ch. 8, p. 219)

Strain A pull in a muscle or tendon (Ch. 2, p. 58)

Stress fracture A break in the bone caused by overuse (Ch. 2, p. 59)

Stress The mind and body's response to the demands and threats of everyday life (Ch. 1, p. 16)

Stretching cooldown Three to five minutes of stretching following physical activity or exercise (Ch. 3, p. 109)

Stroke When blood flow to a person's brain is interrupted or cut off entirely by a blocked artery (Ch. 7, p. 202)

Stroke volume The amount of blood pumped per beat of the heart (Ch. 7, p. 194)

Substance abuse Any unnecessary or improper use of chemical substances for nonmedical purposes (Ch. 2, p. 63)

Supersets Alternately perform sets of exercises that train opposing muscles, without resting between sets (Ch. 10, p. 319)

Supination The normal outward roll of the foot as it hits the ground (Ch. 2, p. 49)

T

T'ai chi A martial art that involves fluid, graceful movements, demanding precise muscular control (Ch. 12, p. 367)

Talk test A measure of one's ability to carry on a conversation while engaged in physical activity or exercise (Ch. 3, p. 86)

Target heart rate range The range one's heart rate should be in during aerobic exercise or activity for maximum cardiorespiratory endurance (Ch. 8, p. 234)

Tendons Bands of tissue that connect muscles to bones (Ch. 2, p. 57)

Testosterone A chemical produced by the body that plays an important role in building muscles (Ch. 9, p. 257)

Time The duration of a single workout, measured in either minutes or hours (Ch. 3, p. 88)

Toe box The part of the shoe that surrounds the toes (Ch. 2, p. 50)

Total-body workout One in which all major muscle groups are worked three times a week, with at least one day off between workouts (Ch. 10, p. 306)

Trainability The rate at which an individual's fitness levels increase during fitness training (Ch. 3, p. 97)

Training load The amount of weight an individual should lift for a given exercise (Ch. 10, p. 307)

Training plateau A period of time during training when little, if any, fitness improvement occurs (Ch. 3, p. 98)

Trans fatty acids Fats that are formed when certain oils are processed into solids (Ch. 4, p. 119)

Type The particular type of physical activity or exercise you choose to do (Ch. 3, p. 89)

U

Underhand grip A position in which a barbell is grasped with the palms facing upward and the knuckles facing downward (Ch. 10, p. 277)

Underweight Having a Body Mass Index (BMI) that is below the 5th percentile for one's age (Ch. 6, p. 175)

Unsaturated fatty acids Fats that are usually liquid at room temperature and come mainly from plant sources (Ch. 4, p. 119)

V

Vegetarian A person who eats mostly or only foods that come from plant sources. (Ch. 4, p. 118)

Veins Blood vessels that deliver the blood back to the heart (Ch. 7, p. 194)

Vigorous physical activity or exercise Any activity or exercise that ranges in intensity from heavy-to-maximum exertion (Ch. 1, p. 29)

Vitamins Micronutrients that help control body processes and help the body release energy to do work (Ch. 4, p. 123)

W

Warm-up Portion of a complete workout that consists of a variety of low-intensity activities that prepare the body for physical work (Ch. 3, p. 102)

Warranty A guarantee on the part of the manufacturer or representative of the manufacturer to repair or replace parts for a predetermined time period (Ch. 8, p. 238)

Weight cycling The cycle of losing, regaining, losing and regaining weight (Ch. 6, p. 188)

Weight machines Mechanical devices that move weights up and down using a system of cables and pulleys (Ch. 9, p. 263)

Weight-training belts Belts that protect the lower back and stomach when lifting heavy weights (Ch. 9, p. 269)

Weight-training gloves Gloves that prevent blisters and calluses from forming on your palms (Ch. 9, p. 269)

Wellness Total health in the areas of physical well-being, mental/emotional well-being, and social well-being (Ch. 1, p. 6)

Wind-chill factor The combined influence of wind and temperature on the body (Ch. 2, p. 44)

Glosario

A

Absolute muscular strength/Fuerza muscular absoluta La fuerza máxima que puede alcanzar un individuo, más allá del tamaño, el peso o la edad.

Acclimatization/Aclimatación Proceso que permite al cuerpo adaptarse lentamente a las condiciones del clima.

Active warm-up/Precalentamiento activo Ejercicios que elevan la temperatura del cuerpo al trabajar activamente los sistemas corporales, centrándose en músculos, esqueleto, corazón y pulmones.

Addiction/Adicción Dependencia física y mental a una substancia o actividad.

Adductor muscles/Músculos abductores Músculos de la parte interna de la pierna que controlan el cierre de las piernas.

Adherence/Adherencia Capacidad para atenerse a un plan de acción.

Adipose tissue/Tejido adiposo Grasa corporal.

Aerobic activity/Actividad aeróbica Actividad continua que exige gran cantidad de oxígeno.

Agility/Agilidad Capacidad para cambiar y controlar la dirección y posición del cuerpo mientras se mantiene un movimiento constante y rápido.

Aging process/Proceso de envejecimiento Modo en que cambia el cuerpo como resultado natural del paso de los años.

Alternated grip/Toma alternada Una posición en la cual la barra de pesas se toma con la palma de una mano hacia abajo y la otra palma hacia arriba.

Amino acids/Aminoácidos Los componentes básicos de las proteínas.

Anabolic steroids/Esteroides anabólicos Substancias químicas similares en estructura a la hormona masculina testosterona.

Anaerobic fitness/Buen estado físico anaeróbico Niveles elevados de fuerza muscular, resistencia muscular, y flexibilidad.

Anaerobic activity/Actividad anaeróbica Actividad que exige altos niveles de energía y se realiza sólo por pocos segundos o minutos a un elevado grado de intensidad.

Androstenedione/Androstenediona Agente químico que ayuda al cuerpo en la producción de testosterona.

Anorexia nervosa/Anorexia nerviosa Trastorno alimenticio en el que el individuo restringe en forma anormal su ingestión calórica.

Antioxidants/Antioxidantes Substancias que previenen el deterioro de las células corporales, incluyendo aquellas que pertenecen al sistema inmunológico.

Arteries/Arterias Vasos sanguíneos que transportan la sangre desde el corazón hacia las principales extremidades del cuerpo.

Asthma/Asma Enfermedad en la que las vías respiratorias inferiores de los pulmones se estrechan, provocando dificultades para respirar.

Atherosclerosis/Aterosclerosis Afección por la que un depósito graso denominado placa se acumula en el interior de las arterias, restringiendo o cortando el flujo sanguíneo.

Athletic trainers/Entrenadores atléticos Profesionales que trabajan con atletas en proceso de rehabilitación.

Attitude/Actitud La mentalidad de un individuo fija en un tópico o tema definido, o con una visión definida hacia ese tópico o tema.

B

Balance/Equilibrio Habilidad para controlar o estabilizar el cuerpo de pie o en movimiento.

Ballistic stretching/Estiramiento balístico Movimientos rápidos hacia arriba y abajo en los que el estiramiento se mantiene en forma muy breve.

Behavioral-change stairway/Cambio de conducta escalonado Método paso a paso, para establecer y alcanzar un objetivo personal para el logro de un buen estado físico.

Bigorexia/Bigorexia Trastorno por el que un individuo cree erróneamente ser de bajo peso, o tener un cuerpo subdesarrollado.

Binge eating disorder/Trastorno alimenticio por ingestión inmoderada Trastorno en la alimentación por el que un individuo come más rápido de lo normal, hasta que no puede seguir comiendo.

Biomechanics/Biomecánica Estudio y aplicación de principios de la física a la motricidad humana.

Blood pooling/Flebitis Afección por la que la sangre se acumula en las principales venas de las piernas, y en la parte inferior del cuerpo.

Blood pressure/Presión sanguínea Fuerza de la sangre en las principales arterias.

Body composition/Composición corporal Proporción entre grasa corporal y tejido corporal magro incluyendo músculo, hueso, agua y tejido conectivo.

Body image/Imagen corporal Forma en que un individuo ve su cuerpo.

Body mass index (BMI)/Índice de masa corporal Método de evaluación de las dimensiones del cuerpo con relación a altura y peso.

Bulimia nervosa/Bulimia nerviosa Trastorno en la alimentación a raíz del cual los individuos comen en exceso, y luego fuerzan la eliminación de lo ingerido.

C

Calipers/Calibrador Aparato con forma de tenaza, que se usa para pinzar un pliegue de piel que rodea tejido adiposo.

Calisthenic exercises/Ejercicios calisténicos Ejercicios que generan resistencia al utilizar el propio peso del cuerpo.

Calorie/Caloría Cantidad de energía necesaria para elevar 1 grado Celsius la temperatura de 1 kilogramo (aproximadamente un cuarto) de agua.

Calorie expenditure/Consumo calórico Número total de calorías que un individuo quema o consume.

Calorie intake/Ingestión calórica Número total de calorías que un individuo ingiere a través de los alimentos.

Capillaries/Capilares Pequeños vasos sanguíneos que proveen oxígeno y otros nutrientes a las células.

Carbohydrates/Carbohidratos Almidones y azúcares que aportan los alimentos.

Cardiac muscle/Músculo cardiaco Clase especial de tejido estriado que forma las paredes del corazón.

Cardiorespiratory endurance/Resistencia cardiorrespiratoria Capacidad del cuerpo para trabajar en forma continua durante prolongados períodos de tiempo.

Cardiovascular conditioning/Acondicionamiento cardiovascular Ejercicios o actividades que mejoran el rendimiento del corazón, los pulmones, la sangre, y los vasos sanguíneos.

Cardiovascular cooldown/Recuperación cardiovascular Consiste en moverse lenta y constantemente durante tres a cinco minutos, a continuación de la actividad física o el ejercicio.

Cardiovascular disease (CVD)/Enfermedad cardiovascular Término aplicado a todo trastorno que afecte al corazón o a los vasos sanguíneos.

Cartilage/Cartílago Tejido que rodea los extremos de los huesos en las articulaciones, y evita que friccionen entre sí.

Cholesterol/Colesterol Substancia de tipo graso que se produce en el hígado y circula por la sangre.

Chronic disease/Enfermedades crónico Enfermedades habitual o continuo.

Circuit training/Entrenamiento en circuitos Método de entrenamiento de resistencia, en el que se pasa de un ejercicio a otro en una secuencia determinada.

Circulatory system/Sistema circulatorio Comprende el corazón, la sangre y los vasos sanguíneos.

Clips/Topes o sujetadores Aparatos con forma de pinza—que a veces cargan peso—para mantener la barra de pesas en su lugar.

Commercial fitness centers/Centros comerciales de preparación física Instalaciones dedicadas a la salud y a la preparación física, que mediante el pago de una cuota, permiten el acceso a una amplia variedad de aparatos de resistencia y entrenamiento aeróbico.

Commitment/Compromiso Voto o promesa.

Compound sets/Series compuestas Series alternadas de ejercicios que se efectúan sin descanso entre las series.

Conflicts/Conflictos Luchas o desacuerdos.

Contraction/Contracción Acortamiento de un músculo.

Cooper's 1.5-mile run test/Test de Cooper de 1.5 millas Prueba que exige trotar/correr 1.5 millas tan rápido como sea posible.

Coordination/Coordinación Capacidad para utilizar los sentidos a fin de determinar y orientar los movimientos de las extremidades y la cabeza.

Core stability/Estabilidad central Estiramiento y fortalecimiento de los músculos que rodean la columna y los músculos pélvicos.

Corporate fitness centers/Centros empresariales de preparación física Instalaciones dedicadas a la salud y a la preparación física dentro de la propia empresa, a disposición de los empleados y sus familias.

Creatine/Creatina Suplemento que aumenta el tamaño de los músculos, al tiempo que potencia la capacidad del cuerpo para utilizar proteínas.

Credentials/Credenciales Resumen de la experiencia y el entrenamiento profesional de un individuo en determinada área.

Cross-contamination/Contaminación cruzada Propagación de bacterias u otros patógenos de un alimento a otro.

Cross-training/Entrenamiento cruzado Variación en el ejercicio, o en la rutina de la actividad, o bien, en el estilo.

Culture/Cultura Usos y costumbres, tradiciones y creencias que comparte un grupo determinado.

D

Deconditioned/Fuera de estado Carencia de entrenamiento durante un período significativo, que se produce tras haber alcanzado, al menos, un nivel moderado de preparación física.

Dehydration/Deshidratación Pérdida de líquido corporal.

Detraining/Desentrenamiento Pérdida en el nivel de funcionamiento físico, como resultado de un cese en el acondicionamiento del estado físico.

Diaphragm/Diafragma Músculo que se halla entre la cavidad torácica y el abdomen.

Dietary fiber/Fibra dietética Subclase especial de carbohidratos complejos que posee varias funciones, entre otras la de asistir al cuerpo en la digestión.

Dietary Reference Intakes (DRI)/Referencia Dietética para la alimentación Recomendaciones de nutrientes diarios para individuos saludables de ambos sexos y diferentes grupos de edad.

Dietary supplement/Suplemento dietético Formula no alimenticia que consta de uno o más nutrientes.

Dynamic contraction/Contracción dinámica Tipo de contracción muscular que se produce cuando la fuerza de resistencia es móvil.

Dynamic posture/Postura dinámica Postura del cuerpo en movimiento o preparándose para moverse.

E

Eating disorders/Trastornos en la alimentación Enfermedades psicológicas que provocan que un individuo coma de menos o de más, o que ejerza una conducta peligrosa para su nutrición.

Ectomorph/Ectomorfo Tipo de cuerpo caracterizado por poseer un bajo porcentaje de grasa corporal, huesos pequeños, y reducida cantidad de masa y tamaño muscular.

Elasticity/Elasticidad Capacidad de los músculos y los tejidos conectivos para estirarse y dar de sí.

Elliptical motion trainer/Máquina de movimiento elíptico Aparato de ejercicios que simula el movimiento natural de correr, pero no genera tensión en las articulaciones.

Emphysema/Enfisema Enfermedad por la que las vías respiratorias inferiores de los pulmones pierden su elasticidad normal, haciéndolas menos eficientes en su función de facilitar la salida y entrada de aire a los pulmones.

Endomorph/Endomorfo Tipo de cuerpo caracterizado por poseer un alto porcentaje de grasa corporal, huesos grandes y cantidades reducidas de masa y tamaño muscular.

Energy cost/Consumo energético Cantidad de energía necesaria para realizar diferentes actividades físicas o ejercicios.

Ephedrine/Efedrina Compuesto que incrementa la proporción en que el cuerpo convierte calorías en energía.

Essential fat/Grasas esenciales Cantidad mínima de grasa corporal necesaria para gozar de buena salud.

Excessive leanness/Delgadez excesiva Poseer un nivel de grasa corporal por debajo de los valores aceptables según el sexo y la edad del individuo.

Excessive weight disabilities/Incapacidad por peso excesivo Problemas de salud y enfermedades relacionadas con o provocadas directamente por exceso de peso u obesidad prolongados.

Exercise/Ejercicio Una actividad física planeada, estructurada y repetitiva, que resulta en mejoras del estado físico.

Exercise bands/Bandas elásticas Bandas elásticas o tubulares de látex que se usan para desarrollar fuerza y resistencia muscular.

Exercise bulimia/Bulimia por ejercicio Trastorno en la alimentación por el que el individuo elimina calorías ejercitándose en exceso.

Exercise physiologists/Fisiólogos del ejercicio Especialistas entrenados para comprender las reacciones físicas del cuerpo hacia el ejercicio, y evaluar el estado físico de un individuo.

Exercise prescription/Plan de entrenamiento Información detallada de un programa de preparación física, basado en frecuencia, intensidad, tiempo y tipo de actividad física o ejercicio.

Exercise stress test/Test de stress por ejercicio Evaluación del estado cardiovascular de un individuo, que implica caminata en la cinta o pedaleo en la bicicleta fija, bajo supervisión médica.

Extension/Extensión Estiramiento del músculo.

F

Fad diets/Dietas de moda Planes para perder peso que se ponen de moda sólo por un breve período de tiempo.

Fast-twitch muscle fiber/Contracción de fibra muscular por espasmo rápido Contracción veloz, que permite una mayor fuerza muscular.

Fatigue/Fatiga Sentirse cansado todo el tiempo.

Fats/Reserva Provisión de una forma concentrada de energía, y asistencia en el transporte de otros nutrientes a los lugares donde el cuerpo los necesita.

Flexibility/Flexibilidad Capacidad de la articulación para moverse en la totalidad de su margen de movimiento.

Fluid balance/Equilibrio de líquidos Capacidad corporal para equilibrar la cantidad de líquido que se incorpora y que se pierde, por transpiración o excreciones.

Food Guide Pyramid/Pirámide nutricional Guía visual que orienta una elección saludable en la alimentación.

Foodborne illnesses/Intoxicación Enfermedad provocada por el consumo de alimentos que poseen organismos causantes de afecciones, los intoxicantes derivados de su mal estado, o contaminantes químicos.

Free weights/Pesas libres Término que se aplica en forma colectiva a mancuernas, barras de pesas, discos y topes de seguridad con sus cargas respectivas.

Frequency/Frecuencia Cantidad de veces por semana en que un individuo realiza actividad física o ejercicio.

Frostbite/Congelación Daño en el tejido corporal producido por congelamiento.

Functional fitness/Buen estado físico funcional Capacidad física de un individuo para funcionar independientemente en la vida, sin asistencia.

Functional health/Salud funcional Capacidad para mantener altos niveles de salud y bienestar, al reducir riesgos para desarrollar problemas de salud.

G

Girth/Contorno Medida alrededor de una parte del cuerpo.

H

Health/Salud Combinación de bienestar físico, mental/emocional, y social.

Health-related fitness/Buen estado físico conectado a la salud Resistencia cardiorrespiratoria, composición corporal, fuerza muscular, resistencia muscular y flexibilidad.

Heart rate monitor/Monitor de frecuencia cardiaca Aparato que registra los latidos del corazón por medio de un transmisor de pecho y de un monitor de pulsera.

Heart rate/Frecuencia cardiaca Cantidad de veces por minuto que late el corazón de un individuo.

Heat cramps/Calambres por calor Espasmos musculares resultantes de la pérdida de grandes cantidades de sal y agua a través de la transpiración.

Heat exhaustion/Agotamiento por calor Sobrecalentamiento corporal que se manifiesta por piel fría y húmeda, a la vez que conlleva síntomas de shock.

Heat stress index/Tabla de estrés por calor Medida científica que registra los efectos combinados del calor y la humedad sobre el cuerpo.

Heatstroke/Golpe de calor Afección por la cual el cuerpo ya no logra librarse del calor excesivo a través de la transpiración.

Hemoglobin/Hemoglobina Compuesto sanguíneo rico en hierro que ayuda a transportar oxígeno desde los pulmones a células y tejidos.

Heredity/Hereditario Suma de rasgos físicos y mentales que se heredan de los padres.

Hernia/Hernia Lesión que se produce cuando las fibras musculares del intestino sobresalen a través de las paredes del abdomen.

High-density lipoprotein (HDL)/Lipoproteína de alta densidad Tipo de compuesto que recoge el excedente de colesterol y lo devuelve al hígado.

Hyperflexibility/Hiperflexibilidad Excesiva cantidad de flexibilidad.

Hypertension/Hipertensión Alta presión sanguínea.

Hypertrophy/Hipertrofia Engrosamiento de fibras musculares preexistentes.

Hypothermia/Hipotermia Estado por el que la temperatura corporal desciende por debajo de lo normal.

I

Impaired glucose tolerance (IGT)/Deficiencia en la tolerancia a la glucosa Trastorno por el que se elevan los niveles de glucosa en sangre.

Insomnia/Insomnio Incapacidad para conciliar el sueño.

Insulin/Insulina Hormona producida por el páncreas.

Intensity/Intensidad Nivel de dificultad o esfuerzo en la actividad física o en el ejercicio.

Interval training/Entrenamiento por intervalos Programa en el que las actividades. físicas de alta intensidad, se alternan con tandas de recuperación de baja intensidad durante varios minutos por vez.

L

Large muscle group/Grupo grande de músculos Todo grupo de músculos de grandes. dimensiones, como así también, una cantidad grande de músculos utilizados al mismo tiempo.

Lean body weight/Peso corporal magro Peso combinado de hueso, músculo y tejido conectivo.

Leisure-time activities/Actividades recreativas Deportes y demás actividades orientadas al movimiento, con fines recreativos.

Lifestyle diseases/Enfermedades por estilo de vida Enfermedades resultantes de ciertas elecciones relacionadas con el estilo de vida, por ejemplo, el fumar, la inactividad o ciertos planes alimenticios.

Ligament/Ligamento Franjas de tejido que se extienden de un hueso a otro y limitan el movimiento de las articulaciones.

Long-term goal/meta a largo plazo Un objetivo que una persona trata de alcanzar durante un largo período de tiempo.

Low-density lipoprotein (LDL)/Lipoproteína de baja densidad Tipo de compuesto que transporta el colesterol desde el hígado hacia áreas del cuerpo donde se lo necesita.

M

Martial arts/Artes Marciales Actividades que combinan ejercicios físicos y técnicas de relajación.

Maximal oxygen consumption (VO_{2max})/Máximo consumo de oxígeno (VO_{2max}) Cantidad máxima de oxígeno que el cuerpo puede procesar durante ejercicios aeróbicos enérgicos.

Media/Medios Sistema colectivo de comunicación masiva, instalados en la sociedad en un momento dado.

Medical history/Historia clínica Registro de los antecedentes de enfermedades y problemas de salud de un individuo.

Medical screening/Chequeo médico Evaluación básica del estado de salud general y condición física personal de un individuo.

Mesomorph/Mesomorfo Tipo de cuerpo caracterizado por un bajo a mediano porcentaje de grasa corporal, huesos medianos a grandes, y gran cantidad y tamaño de masa muscular.

Metabolism/Metabolismo Proceso por el que el cuerpo convierte en energía las calorías aportadas por la alimentación.

Microtear/Micro desgarro Desgarro microscópico de fibras musculares y/o tejidos circundantes.

Minerals/Minerales Elementos que el cuerpo no puede generar, pero que ayudan a regular los procesos corporales, tales como la conversión de glucosa en energía.

Moderate physical activity or exercise/Actividad física o ejercicio moderados Toda actividad o ejercicio que varía en intensidad de leve al límite del esfuerzo máximo.

Multiple hypertrophy sets/Series múltiples de hipertrofia Levantamiento de igual carga de peso hasta el punto de fatiga.

Multiple sets/Serie múltiple Levantamiento de pesas en el que el individuo usa la misma cantidad de peso durante tres a cinco series, a una carga de entrenamiento del 80 al 95 por ciento de su 1RM.

Muscle fiber/Fibra muscular Estructura específica en el músculo que recibe la señal nerviosa.

Muscle hyperplasia/Hiperplasia muscular Aumento en la cantidad de fibras musculares.

Muscle imbalance/Desequilibrio muscular Estado en que un grupo de músculos se torna más fuerte, con relación a un grupo complementario.

Muscle tone/Tono muscular Definición y firmeza de un músculo.

Muscular endurance/Resistencia muscular Capacidad del propio músculo o grupo muscular para contraerse durante un período prolongado de tiempo, sin presentar fatiga excesiva.

Muscular strength/Fuerza muscular Máxima cantidad de fuerza que un músculo o grupo muscular puede ejercer contra una fuerza de oposición.

N

Negative reps/Repetición negativa Ejercitación que comprende sólo la fase excéntrica o negativa de un ejercicio, al utilizar un peso de un 10 o 15 por ciento superior al propio 1RM.

Nerves/Nervios Conductores que descargan mensajes desde el cerebro a otras partes del cuerpo.

Nutrient-dense foods/Alimentos de alta densidad nutritiva Alimentos que proporcionan altos valores nutritivos, en comparación con su contenido calórico

Nutrients/Nutrientes Substancias en los alimentos que aseguran al cuerpo energía, crecimiento apropiado, mantenimiento corporal y funcionamiento.

Nutrition/Nutrición Estudio de los alimentos y de la forma en que el cuerpo utiliza las substancias que estos aportan.

Nutrition Facts panel/Información nutricional Análisis condensado del valor calórico y nutritivo por porción de alimento.

O

Obesity/Obesidad Problema de salud en el que, la diferencia entre la grasa corporal y la masa muscular magra de un individuo, es extremadamente elevada.

One-rep maximum (1RM)/Máximo por ejercicio (1RM) Medida de levantamiento de pesas para fuerza máxima absoluta en cualquier ejercicio dado.

Orthopedics/Ortopedia Rama de la medicina que trata sobre esqueleto, lesiones y trastornos articulares.

Osteoporosis/Osteoporosis Enfermedad de los huesos que provoca disminución en la densidad y en la masa ósea, especialmente en mujeres mayores.

Overfat/Sobrepeso Exceso de grasa corporal en proporción a edad y sexo.

Overhand grip/Toma en prono Una posición en la cual la barra de pesas se toma con las palmas de las manos hacia abajo y los nudillos hacia arriba.

Overload principle/Principio de sobrecarga Regla de ejercitación que establece que, a fin de mejorar el nivel de preparación física, debe incrementarse la cantidad de actividad o ejercicio regular que se efectúa habitualmente.

Overtraining/Sobreentrenamiento Ejercitarse o entrenarse hasta un punto en el que comienzan a aparecer efectos negativos.

Overuse injury/Lesión por sobrecarga Lesión muscular ocasionada al sobrecargar un músculo más allá de un punto saludable.

Overweight /Sobrepeso Estado en el que un individuo pesa más que los valores establecidos según su altura.

P

Passive stretching/Estiramiento pasivo Tipo de estiramiento contra una contra fuerza en el que hay escaso o ningún movimiento.

Passive warm-up/Precalentamiento pasivo Utilización de fuentes de calor externas para elevar la temperatura corporal.

Pedometer/Podómetro Aparato que mide el número de pasos que da un individuo, y registra la distancia recorrida a pie.

Peers/Pares Individuos de la misma edad que comparten un marco común de intereses y creencias.

Perceived exertion/Percepción de esfuerzo Medida que denota en qué grado un individuo siente el trabajo durante la actividad o el ejercicio físico.

Peripheral vascular disease/Enfermedad vascular periférica Enfermedad cardiovascular que ocurre principalmente en las piernas y, con menor frecuencia, en los brazos.

Personal fitness/Buen estado físico personal Preparación física total y general, que se logra manteniendo niveles aceptables de actividad física, buena alimentación y evitando el consumo de sustancias perjudiciales.

Physical activity/Actividad física Todo movimiento que trabaja los músculos mayores del cuerpo, tales como los de brazos, piernas y músculos de la espalda.

Physical fitness/Buen estado físico Capacidad del cuerpo para llevar a cabo las tareas cotidianas, y aún conservar una suficiente reserva de energía para responder a exigencias inesperadas.

Physical therapists/Fisioterapeutas Profesionales de la salud especialmente entrenados para trabajar con individuos que se recuperan de lesiones.

Phytonutrients/Fitonutrientes Substancias aportadas por alimentos vegetales, que contribuyen a mantener la salud.

Plyometric exercises/Ejercicios pliométricos Movimientos musculares veloces y poderosos, que exigen un pre-estiramiento muscular exactamente antes de una rápida contracción.

Podiatrist/Podiatra Médico entrenado específicamente para tratar trastornos en los pies.

Posture/Postura Alineación de los músculos corporales y del esqueleto al sostener la totalidad del cuerpo.

Power/Fuerza Capacidad para mover las partes del cuerpo en forma veloz, mientras se aplica al mismo tiempo la fuerza máxima de los músculos.

Pre-event meal/Comida pre-evento La última comida completa consumida en forma previa a la sesión de ejercicios, o al propio evento competitivo.

Progression principle/Principio de progresión Regla de ejercitación que establece que, a medida que los niveles de acondicionamiento físico aumentan, se incrementan los factores en el FITT.

Progressive resistance/Resistencia progresiva Aumento de la carga del músculo, continuado y sistemático, al agregarse mayor peso o resistencia.

Pronation/Pronación Movimiento normal del pie al caminar o al correr, desde el talón hacia fuera al pisar el suelo, hasta la propulsión hacia adentro, normal en un pie.

Proteins/Proteínas Nutrientes que contribuyen a la construcción, mantenimiento y reparación de los tejidos del cuerpo.

Pyramid training/Entrenamiento piramidal Sistema de entrenamiento que recurre al incremento de peso progresivo en las pesas, y a una menor cantidad de repeticiones, a través de sucesivas series de ejercicios.

R

Range of motion (ROM)/Alcance de movilidad
Grados de movimiento posibles alrededor de una
articulación.

Reaction time/Tiempo de reacción Capacidad
para reaccionar o responder velozmente a lo que
se oye, se ve o se siente.

Recovery time/Tiempo de recuperación
Duración del período de descanso que se toma
entre los componentes del entrenamiento.

Recumbent cycles/Ciclos de reposo Ciclos de
ejercicio en posición reclinada.

**Reflex-assisted stretching/Estiramiento asistido
por reflejos** Movimientos de estiramiento que
estimulan la adaptación de los reflejos.

Reflexes/Reflejos Respuesta automática que
ofrecen nervios y músculos a variados
movimientos.

**Registered dietitians (RDs)/Dietólogos
matriculados** Profesionales que se especializan
en proveer asesoraramiento nutricional a las
personas, a la vez que los ayudan a controlar su
peso.

**Regular physical activity or exercise/Ejercicio o
actividad física regular** Toda actividad o
ejercicio que se realiza la mayor parte de la
semana, preferentemente, a diario.

Rehydrate/Rehidratación Reposición del agua
perdida.

**Relative muscular endurance/Resistencia
muscular relativa** Número máximo de veces
que un individuo puede repetir una actividad de
resistencia, en relación al peso corporal.

**Relative muscular strength/Fuerza muscular
relativa** Máxima fuerza que un individuo es
capaz de ejercer, con relación a su peso corporal.

Repetition (rep)/Repetición La ejecución
completa de una actividad o ejercicio dado.

**Resistance training/Entrenamiento de
resistencia** Programa sistemático de ejercicios,
diseñado para incrementar la habilidad de un
individuo para resistir o ejercer fuerza.

**Resistance-training cycle/Ciclo de
entrenamiento para resistencia** Programas
modificados, diseñados para cubrir las
necesidades de pre temporada, temporada y
fuera de temporada.

Respiratory system/Sistema respiratorio Sistema
corporal de intercambio de gases entre el cuerpo
y el medio ambiente.

**Resting metabolic rate (RMR)/Tasa metabólica
en reposo** Cantidad de calorías que se gastan en
los procesos corporales mientras se está en
reposo.

Restoration/Recuperación Formas en que un
individuo puede optimizar la recuperación por
actividad física o ejercicios.

**RICE (Rest, Ice, Compress, and
Elevate)/Primeros auxilios deportivos
(Reposo, Hielo, Compresión y Elevación)**
Procedimiento de primeros auxilios que
establece el tratamiento indicado en caso de
tirones y espasmos que se inflaman.

Risk factors/Factores de riesgo Condiciones y
conductas que representan una amenaza
potencial para el bienestar de un individuo.

S

Saturated fatty acids/Ácidos grasos saturados
Grasas que provienen principalmente de grasas
animales, y que generalmente son sólidas a
temperatura ambiente.

Sedentary/Sedentario Físicamente inactivo.

Self-concept/Concepto personal La idea que se
tiene de uno mismo.

Self-esteem/Estima personal Sentimiento de auto
confianza y valor personal.

Set/Serie Grupo de repeticiones consecutivas de
cualquier ejercicio.

Shinsplint/Herida a la espinilla Inflamación de
un tendon o músculo de la canilla.

Skeletal muscles/Músculos del esqueleto
Músculos adheridos al hueso que causan
movimiento corporal.

**Skill-related fitness/Buen estado físico
relacionado con la habilidad** Agilidad,
equilibrio, fuerza, velocidad, coordinación y
tiempo de reacción.

Sleep apnea/Apnea del sueño Afección por la
que el individuo deja de respirar durante el
sueño, debido a la obstrucción o reducción de
los pasajes de aire.

**Slow-twitch muscle fiber/Contracción lenta de
fibra muscular** Fibra muscular que se contrae a

un ritmo bajo, permitiendo mayor resistencia muscular.

Small muscle group/Grupo de músculos pequeños Todo grupo de músculos de menor tamaño, o bien, una pequeña cantidad de músculos utilizados al mismo tiempo.

Smokeless tobacco/Tabaco sin humo Tabaco que se inhala por la nariz o se mastica.

Smooth muscles/Músculos lisos Músculos a cargo del movimiento de los órganos internos.

Specificity principle/Principio de especificidad Establece que, sobrecargar determinado componente derivará en mejoras del estado físico de dicho único componente.

Speed/Velocidad Capacidad para mover el cuerpo o partes del mismo rápidamente.

Split workout/Serie de ejercicios dividida Programa de preparación física en el que se ejercitan tres o cuatro áreas corporales por sesión, trabajando a una elevada intensidad.

Sports medicine clinic/Centros clínicos de medicina deportiva Centros que se concentran en la investigación, con el fin de promover la salud y el buen estado físico, como así también, el desarrollo y la operatividad de la salud, la preparación física, la recreación y los programas educativos.

Spotter/Compañero Compañero que puede, tanto asistir a un individuo en el manejo seguro de las pesas, como alentarlo durante la sesión.

Sprain/torcedura Una condición en que los ligamentos que mantienen las articulaciones en su lugar están distendidos o quebrados.

Static contraction/Contracción estática Tipo de contracción muscular que se produce en ausencia de cualquier movimiento considerable.

Static posture/Postura estática Postura del cuerpo en posición de reposo.

Static stretching/Estiramiento estático Ejercicios que estiran el músculo despacio, suavemente y en forma sostenida, entre 20 y 30 segundos.

Steady-state cycle test/Test de bicicleta a ritmo sostenido Prueba que exige pedalear durante 20 minutos en bicicleta fija, y tratar de alcanzar una distancia predeterminada.

Steady-state jog test/Test de trote a ritmo sostenido Prueba que exige mantener el ritmo del trote durante 20 minutos hasta alcanzar una distancia específicamente determinada.

Steady-state swim test/Test de natación a ritmo sostenido Prueba que exige nadar durante 20 minutos, y tratar de alcanzar una distancia predeterminada.

Steady-state walk test/Test de caminata a ritmo sostenido Prueba que exige sostener el ritmo a paso vivo durante 30 minutos, y tratar de alcanzar una distancia predeterminada.

Strain/Desgarro Desgarro de un músculo o tendón.

Stress fracture/Fractura por estrés Ruptura del hueso provocada por carga excesiva.

Stress/Estrés Respuesta del cuerpo y la mente a las exigencias y amenazas de la vida diaria.

Stretching cooldown/Estiramiento de enfriamiento Comprende entre tres y cinco minutos de estiramiento posterior a actividad física o ejercicio.

Stroke/Apoplejía Cuando el flujo sanguíneo al cerebro de un individuo se interrumpe, o cesa por completo, a causa de una arteria obstruida.

Stroke volume/Volumen por impulso La cantidad de sangre bombeada con cada latido del corazón.

Substance abuse/Consumo de drogas Todo uso inapropiado o innecesario de substancias químicas con fines no medicinales.

Supersets/Superseries La ejecución alternada de series de ejercicios para entrenar músculos opuestos, sin descanso entre series.

Supination/Supinación Giro normal del pie hacia afuera cuando toca el piso.

T

T'ai chi/T'ai chi Arte marcial que incluye movimientos fluidos y gráciles, que exigen un preciso control muscular.

Talk test/Test del habla Medida de la habilidad que se tiene para sostener una conversación, mientras se realizan ejercicios o actividad física.

Target heart rate range/Valores óptimos de frecuencia cardiaca Valores a los que el ritmo cardiaco debería instalarse durante el ejercicio aeróbico, o actividad física, para rendir una máxima resistencia cardiorrespiratoria.

Tendons/Tendones Bandas de tejidos que conectan músculo con hueso.

Testosterone/Testosterona Químico producido por el cuerpo, que juega un importante rol en la construcción del músculo.

Time/Tiempo Duración de una serie completa de ejercicios, generalmente medido en minutos u horas.

Toe box/Capellada Parte del zapato que recubre los dedos de los pies.

Total-body workout/Serie de ejercicios completa Aquélla en que los principales grupos musculares se trabajan tres veces por semana, dejando, al menos, un día libre entre cada preparación física.

Trainability/Entrenabilidad Valores a los que los niveles de estado físico se incrementan durante la preparación física.

Training load/Carga de entrenamiento Cantidad de peso que un individuo debe levantar en un ejercicio dado.

Training plateau/Entrenamiento mesetario Período de tiempo durante el entrenamiento, en el que se producen pocos o ningún avance en el estado físico.

Trans fatty acids/Ácidos trans grasos Grasas que se forman cuando ciertos aceites se convierten en sólidos.

Type/Tipo El tipo particular de actividad física o ejercitación que se elige realizar.

U

Underhand grip/Toma supino Una posición en la cual la barra de pesas se toma con las palmas de las manos hacia arriba y los nudillos hacia abajo.

Underweight/Bajo peso Tener un índice de masa corporal (IMC) que es menor a un quinto del percentil de la edad correspondiente.

Unsaturated fatty acids/Ácidos grasos no saturados Grasas que son generalmente líquidas a temperatura ambiente y provienen principalmente de fuentes vegetales.

V

Vegetarian/Vegetariano Una persona que come principalmente o solamente alimentos que provienen de las plantas.

Veins/Venas Vasos sanguíneos que devuelven la sangre al corazón.

Vigorous physical activity or exercise/ Ejercitación o actividad física vigorosa Toda actividad o ejercitación que varía en intensidad de fuerte a máximo esfuerzo.

Vitamins/Vitaminas Micronutrientes que ayudan a controlar los procesos corporales, y contribuyen a que el cuerpo libere energía para trabajar.

W

Warm-up/Precalentamiento Porción de un plan de ejercicios completo, que consiste en una variedad de actividades de baja intensidad para preparar el cuerpo para el trabajo físico.

Warranty/Garantía Aval por parte del fabricante o representante para reparar o proporcionar durante un período limitado de tiempo.

Weight cycling/Ciclo del peso Ciclo en el que se baja y se sube de peso, alternativamente.

Weight machines/Máquinas con pesas Aparatos mecánicos que mueven pesas de arriba hacia abajo, utilizando un sistema de cables y poleas.

Weight-training belts/Cinturón de levantamiento de pesas Faja para proteger la parte baja de la espalda y del estómago cuando se levantan pesas pesadas.

Weight-training gloves/Guantes de levantamiento de pesas Guantes que previenen la formación de ampollas y callos en las palmas de las manos.

Wellness/Bienestar Salud total en las áreas de bienestar físico, bienestar mental/emocional, y bienestar social.

Wind-chill factor/Factor de viento helado Influencia combinada de viento y temperatura en el cuerpo.

Index

AFLO FOTO AGENCY **v**(b), **75**, **76**, **109**, **321**; AFP/CORBIS **xi**(r), **205**, **339**; Peter Ardito/Index Stock Imagery **129**; Bettmann/CORBIS **373**; Rudi Von Briel/PhotoEdit **368**; Burke/Triolo/Brand X Pictures/PictureQuest **136**; Ron Chapple/Thinkstock **41**, **362**; Mike Chew/CORBIS **47**; Dick Clintsaman/Stone/Getty Images **329**; Color Day Productions/The Image Bank/Getty Images **138**; Gary Conner/PhotoEdit **18**; Steve Craft/Masterfile **374**; Jim Cummins/CORBIS **46**, **357**, **379**; Ron Dahlquist/SuperStock **356**; Luis Delgado **50**, **58**, **181**; Mary Kate Denny/PhotoEdit **59**; Kevin Dodge/CORBIS **214**(l); Steve Dunwell/Index Stock Imagery **113**; Duomo/CORBIS **90**; Duomo/CORBIS **93**; Jon Feingersh/CORBIS **v**(t), **71**, **186**, **233**; Curt Fischer **258**; Ken Fisher/Stone/Getty Images **207**; FIUBIOMED/Custom Medical Stock Photo Inc. **173**; Tracy Frankel/Imagebank/Getty Images **363**; Tony Freeman/PhotoEdit **73**, **176**; Jose Galvez/PhotoEdit **99**; Garry Gay/ImageState **131**; Raymond Gehman/ CORBIS **40**; Glencoe/McGraw-Hill **3**(r), **8**(b), **8**(tc), **8**(tl), **8**(tr), **9**(bl), **9**(br), **9**(tl), **9**(tr), **78**(l), **78**(r), **79**(b), **79**(t), **80**(b), **80**(t), **86**(b), **86**(t), **95**, **106**(bcl), **106**(bcr), **106**(bl), **106**(br), **106**(c), **106**(cl), **106**(cr), **106**(tcl), **106**(tcr), **106**(tl), **106**(tr), **159**(l), **159**(r), **162**(b), **162**(t), **174**(b), **174**(tc), **174**(tl), **174**(tr), **239**, **240**, **261**(b), **265**(b), **265**(t), **266**, **267**(l), **267**(r), **268**, **273**, **275**, **277**(c), **277**(l), **277**(r), **278**(c), **278**(l), **278**(r), **279**(bc), **279**(bl), **279**(tl), **279**(tr), **280**(bl), **280**(br), **280**(tl), **280**(tr), **281**(b), **281**(t), **282**(bl), **282**(br), **282**(cl), **282**(cr), **282**(tl), **282**(tr), **283**(c), **283**(l), **283**(r), **284**(bc), **284**(bl), **284**(br), **284**(tc), **284**(tl), **284**(tr), **285**(bl), **285**(br), **285**(tc), **285**(tl), **285**(tr), **286**(c), **286**(l), **286**(r), **287**(bl), **287**(br), **287**(tc), **287**(tl), **287**(tr), **288**(c), **288**(l), **288**(r), **289**(bl), **289**(br), **289**(tc), **289**(tl), **289**(tr), **290**(bl), **290**(br), **290**(tc), **290**(tl), **290**(tr), **291**(bl), **291**(br), **291**(tl), **291**(tr), **292**(bl), **292**(br), **292**(tc), **292**(tl), **292**(tr), **293**(bl), **293**(br), **293**(tl), **293**(tr), **294**(tl), **294**(tr), **295**(l), **295**(r), **319**(l), **319**(r), **336**(l), **336**(r), **337**(b), **337**(t), **343**(l), **343**(r), **344**(l), **344**(r), **346**(br), **346**(cl), **346**(cr), **346**(tl), **346**(tr), **347**(b), **347**(bc), **347**(t), **347**(tc), **348**(b), **348**(c), **348**(t), **349**(b), **349**(t); Spencer Grant/PhotoEdit **375**; Jeff Greenberg/PhotoEdit **147**; Charles Gupton/CORBIS **153**; Brian Hagiwara/Foodpix/ Getty Images **184**; Michal Heron/CORBIS **101**; ICI Phamaceuticals Division, Cheshire, England **201**(br), **201**(tr); A.Inden/Masterfile **367**; Jiang Jin/SuperStock **171**; Tracy Kahn/CORBIS **214**(r); Chuck Keeler, Jr./ CORBIS **256**; Michael Keller/CORBIS **137**; Brooks Kraft/CORBIS **16**; Brian Leatart/FoodPix/Getty Images **117**; Roger Allyn Lee/SuperStock **272**; Lenz/Masterfile **vi**(t), **126**; Randy Lincks/CORBIS **364**; Robert Llewellyn/ SuperStock **338**; Dennis MacDonald/PhotoEdit **208**(t); David Madison/Stone/Getty Images **xi**(bcl), **xi**(tcl), **197**, **213**(bl), **325**, **382**; Felicia Martinez/PhotoEdit **70**; Scott Markewitz/FPG International/Getty Images **34**; Tom & Dee Ann McCarthy/CORBIS **212**; Ed McDonald Photography **6**(b), **6**(l), **6**(r); Wally McNamee/CORBIS **257**; Matt Meadows Photography **61**; men David Mendelsohn/Masterfile **vi**(b), **114**; Raoul Minsart/Masterfile **370**; Michael Newman/PhotoEdit **35**, **82**, **142**, **276**; Johnathan Nourok/PhotoEdit **72**, **180**, **236**; Dennis O'Clair/Stone/Getty Images **164**; Roy Ooms/Masterfile **56**; Laurie Adamski-Peek/Stone/Getty Images **193**(r); Jose Luis Pelaez,Inc./CORBIS **208**(b); Petit Format/Nestle/Photo Researchers **13**; Kevin Radford/SuperStock **366**(b); Ken Reid/Taxi/Getty Images **179**; Reuters NewMedia Inc./CORBIS **3**(l), **341**; Joel W.Rogers/CORBIS **193**(l); Bob Rowan; Progressive Image/CORBIS **15**; Royalty-Free/CORBIS **viii**(t), **12**, **248**; Royalty-free/ Photodisc/Getty Images **204**, **231**; Royalty-free/Thinkstock/PictureQuest **229**; Pete Saloutos/CORBIS **52**; John Schnack/SuperStock **200**; Mark Scott/Getty Images **7**; Steve Skjold/PhotoEdit **25**; Richard Hamilton Smith/ CORBIS **219**; Joseph Sohm; ChromoSohm Inc./CORBIS **103**; spi H.Spichtinger/Masterfile **vii**, **332**; Tom Stewart/CORBIS **196**(b), **296**; David Stoecklein/CORBIS **91**; Stock Image/SuperStock **27**; SuperStock **2**, **107**, **192**, **215**, **230**, **237**, **245**, **261**(t), **305**; Thinkstock **63**; Allen ThorntonStone/Getty Images **74**; V.C.L./Taxi/Getty Images **viii**(b); **366**(t); Joel W. Rogers/CORBIS **x**(l); Laurie Adamski-Peek/Stone/Getty Images **x**(r); E.H.Wallop/Corbis **324**; Ulf Wallin/Getty Images **45**; Karl Weatherly/CORBIS **218**; wel LWA-Stephen Welstead/ CORBIS **112**, **167**; Rosemary Weller/Stone/Getty Images **122**; Dana White/PhotoEdit **371**; H.Winkler/ Masterfile **39**; David Young-Wolff/Getty Images **250**; David Young-Wolff/PhotoEdit **37**, **53**, **170**, **199**, **227**, **244**, **313**, **345**, **372**; Kwame Zikomo/SuperStock **146**.